Advance Praise for *The Essential Oils Apothecary*

"Beginner-level essential oil information abounds, but when one begins to seek out based protocols for more complicated ailments, finding information you can trust is in difficult. *The Essential Oils Apothecary* is the volume I wish I had years ago. Solid, science- information combined with simple, proven recipes—I can't recommend this resource enough."

—Jill Winger, bestselling author of *The Prairie Homestead Cookbook* and host of the Old Fashioned on Purpose podcast

"The Zielinskis are on a mission to make essential oils the missing link in twenty-first-century medicine. Their *Essential Oils Apothecary* offers clear-cut, evidence-based strategies for treating the twenty-five most prevalent and urgent health conditions of the day with practical recipes, internal remedies and diffusions. This book does a masterful job of aligning ancient wisdom with modern-day science to soothe body, mind, and spirit with super natural plant power!!"

—Ann Louise Gittleman, award-winning multiple *New York Times* bestselling author of *Radical Longevity*

"Essential oils are powerful medicine, and nobody knows more about them than Dr. Eric and Sabrina Ann Zielinski. If you're looking for both state-of-the-art science and practical, hands-on information, this is the book you need."

—Dr. Kellyann Petrucci, *New York Times* bestselling author of *Dr. Kellyann's Bone Broth Diet*

"Essential oils are part of many traditional healing approaches. *The Essential Oils Apothecary* merges these traditional uses with available science to provide helpful techniques and recipes to harness their benefits, with a focus on holistic healing for a range of chronic illnesses. It's exciting to see all the creative ways essential oils and lifestyle changes can be applied for overall healthier living. This book is a must-have for the modern-day 'health library'!"

—Deanna Minich, PhD, nutritionist, educator, and author of *Whole Detox*

"Dr. Eric Zielinski has established himself as *the* go-to authority on the science and everyday use of essential oils. His work is always practical, easy to understand, and beautifully heartfelt. With *The Essential Oils Apothecary*, Dr. Z has taken the field to a whole new level by writing the first book ever on the prevention and treatment of chronic disease using these amazing God-given medicines. This book is a treasure chest of detailed information and insights. Dr. Z's deep understanding of natural health and living a vibrant life will no doubt inspire you to use essential oils to care for yourself and your loved ones. *The Essential Oils Apothecary* is truly breathtaking in its scope. I consider this is a must-have, one-of-a-kind reference book that you'll use for a lifetime."

—Marc David, founder of the Institute for the Psychology of Eating and bestselling author of *Nourishing Wisdom* and *The Slow Down Diet*

"This book is a great reference to powerful, plant-based medicine. Dr. Zielinski is the leading mind in essential oil education, and I will rely on this book to help me improve brain health, mood, and sleep, and to support a healthy immune response."

—Dr. David Jockers, bestselling author of *Keto Metabolic Breakthrough* and *The Fasting Transformation*

"Medicine tends to put pharmaceuticals first instead of honoring our God-given design and putting nature first. *The Essential Oils Apothecary* will give you the solid foundation of knowledge you need to do so. It's a book everyone should have in their household."

—Anna Cabeca, DO, OBGYN, author of *The Hormone Fix* and *Keto-Green 16*

"Essential oils are one of nature's greatest gifts, and they can help many chronic conditions both mental and physical. A concise, evidence-based, safety-first guide to their use, *The Essential Oils Apothecary* will help you easily begin to use essential oils for all your chronic health needs."

—Sylla Sheppard-Hanger, founder of the Atlantic Institute of Aromatherapy

"If you're someone who has had it with the synthetic drug scheme foisted on Americans, then this book should be a staple in your home. It is your first step in the important task of thinking independently and taking care of yourself and your family."

—Joette Calabrese, international homeopathy practitioner and speaker

"You won't cure the world with essential oils, but you certainly will enhance your health with their use. Expanding your 'medicine cabinet' to a 'medicine and health' cabinet is easy with this essential, go-to manual to nature's 'first responders.' The recipes here are straightforward and easy to apply. It's a book you'll use time and time again."

—Tom O'Bryan, DC, CCN, DACBN, CIFM

"Eric has done it again! *The Essential Oils Apothecary* is extremely well-researched and well-written. A must-have for any essential oil library!"

—Jodi Cohen, bestselling author of *Essential Oils to Boost the Brain and Heal the Body*

"A must-have book that every home, health expert, and wellness clinic needs. A reminder of how to use powerful, innate, and ancient wisdom confidently in our fast-paced, quick-fix, drug-induced, modern world."

—Kim Morrison, clinical aromatherapist, author, speaker, and health and wellness educator

THE
ESSENTIAL
OILS
APOTHECARY

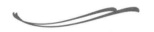

ALSO BY ERIC ZIELINSKI AND SABRINA ANN ZIELINSKI

The Essential Oils Diet

ALSO BY ERIC ZIELINSKI

The Healing Power of Essential Oils

THE
ESSENTIAL OILS APOTHECARY

Advanced Strategies and Protocols for
Chronic Disease and Conditions

Eric Zielinski, D.C., AND
Sabrina Ann Zielinski

RODALE.
NEW YORK

Published in the United States by Rodale Books, an imprint of Random House, a division of Penguin Random House LLC, New York.
rodalebooks.com

RODALE and the Plant colophon are registered trademarks of Penguin Random House LLC.

Library of Congress Cataloging-in-Publication Data
Names: Zielinski, Eric, author. | Zielinski, Sabrina Ann, author. Title: The essential oils apothecary / Eric Zielinski and Sabrina Ann Zielinski. Description: New York : Rodale, 2021. | Includes bibliographical references and index. Identifiers: LCCN 2020052332 (print) | LCCN 2020052333 (ebook) | ISBN 9780593139271 (trade paperback) | ISBN 9780593139288 (ebook) Subjects: LCSH: Essences and essential oils—Therapeutic use. Classification: LCC RM666.A68 Z536 2021 (print) | LCC RM666.A68 (ebook) | DDC 615.3/219—dc23 LC record available at https://lccn.loc.gov/2020052332 LC ebook record available at https://lccn.loc.gov/2020052333

ISBN 978-0-593-13927-1
Ebook ISBN 978-0-593-13928-8

Printed in the United States of America

Some of the recipes in this work were adapted or taken from *The Healing Power of Essential Oils* by Eric Zielinski and *The Essential Oils Diet* by Eric Zielinski and Sabrina Ann Zielinski.

Book design by Andrea Lau
Cover photograph by Science Photo Library/Getty Images

1st Printing

First Edition

Esther, Isaiah, Elijah, Isabella, and Ezekiel—we love you with all our hearts. Our challenge to you and the next generation is to pick up the baton and carry the message of biblical health and natural healing to new heights. May this book be a tool to help you accomplish this!

Love,
Daddy and Mommy

Natural Living Family—thank you. COVID-19 challenged our online community in more ways than we could have ever imagined, yet it brought us closer together. We are so grateful and thankful for each and every one of you. As always, our hope and prayer are that you and your family experience the abundant life!

Love,
Dr. Z and Mama Z

Contents

Preface

"If you're not a part of the solution, you're a part of the problem."

—*AFRICAN PROVERB*

Unless someone is a medical professional, there are surprisingly few health books devoted to chronic disease management, and even fewer discussing how to use natural therapies. This remains a paradox to us because more than 60 percent of the American population (nearly 200 million people) are affected by at least one chronic illness, and more than 40 percent have two or more, according to the Centers for Disease Control and Prevention.

Even more shocking, there were zero books devoted to the topic of using essential oils to prevent and/or treat chronic disease at the time we wrote this book. That's right, you read it correctly. Zero.

There is obviously a gap here, and the book you now hold in your hands is our attempt at filling it.

OUR PRAYERS ARE WITH YOU

Hi, my name is Dr. Eric Zielinski, and people online know me as "Dr. Z." With my wife, Sabrina (aka "Mama Z"), at my side, we are thrilled to present to you our latest installment of books devoted to learning how to use essential oils to experience the abundant life.

Before we begin, I'd like to offer my sincere and humble recognition that cancer, depression, obesity, and the other chronic conditions mentioned in this book can be absolutely devastating. I am personally acquainted with several of them, having suffered not only from depression, panic attacks, anxiety, and suicidal thoughts in my late teens and early twenties but alcohol and substance abuse as well.

First and foremost, know that Mama Z and I are praying for you. In addition, there are thousands of people across the globe who have joined us through our private groups and fan pages in an effort to support those battling chronic disease.

Second, there's hope. I am living proof that someone can overcome debilitating chronic disease, including mental health issues! I credit my healing experience to my faith in Christ, because it wasn't until I became a Christian that I was able to get sober and experience the fullness of joy and happiness. Today, eighteen years later, I can confidently boast in the Lord that I am still free! Sabrina has her own healing story of how God delivered her from an eating disorder and freed her from ten prescription drugs in her mid-twenties. So trust me when I say that we truly empathize with people who suffer from chronic health issues.

Third, Mama Z and I wholeheartedly believe that it is our God-given right to enjoy the abundant life that Christ refers to in John 10:10—the fullest expression of health in all areas of your life: spiritual, physical, emotional, financial, occupational, social, and, of course, mental. However, Christ's promise of the abundant life is like a winning lottery ticket, and many people neglect to cash it in. We invite you to join us to claim this right, and enjoy a glorious mental health in all of its joyful abundance!

Fourth, speaking of joy, the Bible tells us "The joy of the Lord is your strength" (Nehemiah 8:10).

At the core of our very existence is how we feel, and these feelings are intricately tied into our day-to-day existence and how well we adapt to the never-ending stressors of life. To be unhealthy or unwell emotionally, mentally, or physically is to be vulnerable at the deepest level of your humanity. This puts you at risk of developing further problems with your health, finances, and relationships, on your job, and in your spiritual life. Remember, you're only as strong as your weakest link, and all areas of your life are interconnected. To be "strong," on the other hand, is necessitated by joy, as described by Nehemiah, which is arguably the most powerful, invigorating feeling one can have. Joy will fuel and empower you through all obstacles, and it's vital to overcome chronic disease.

Last, but certainly not least, it's okay (and oftentimes necessary) to get help. If you suffer from chronic disease of any sort, we highly encourage you to seek support from a qualified professional if it's impacting your mental well-being. We have found that, as well intentioned as our loved ones may be, they are oftentimes unable to help us through those rough times, and having someone stable in your life to act as an anchor can make all the difference in the world.

We love you, are rooting for you, and hope this book provides the answers that you're looking for!

—Dr. Z

Introduction

On April 15, 2020, when most of America and the world were under shelter-in-place orders due to the COVID-19 pandemic, Roger Seheult, MD, posted his "Coronavirus Pandemic Update 56: What Is 'Forest Bathing' & Can It Boost Immunity Against Viruses?" on YouTube.

It was a fascinating presentation that introduced the concept of "forest bathing" (the ancient Japanese practice of simply "being in nature") to people in Western civilization. *Shinrin-yoku* (*shinrin* meaning "forest" and *yoku* meaning "bath" in Japanese) refers to immersing yourself in the forest atmosphere and enjoying nature.

Not to be confused with hiking or any sort of exercise, the key to *shinrin-yoku* is to connect with nature through your five senses. Considered a bridge between the human experience and the natural world, forest bathing exposes us to volatile organic compounds (VOCs) that are being released into the air by the surrounding trees and plants. VOCs, of course, are the active chemical components emitted by plants and flowers that give them their distinct aroma. They are also more commonly referred to as "essential oils."

As shown in multiple clinical trials, the naturally occurring VOCs in nature have a profound, measurable effect on enhancing immune function by increasing the quantity and activity of natural killer cells (NK cells), among other health benefits.

As white blood cells that support immune function, NK cells are a component of the first line of defense against tumors, inflammation, and viral infections. Essentially, being out in nature is synonymous to wearing a personal aromatherapy inhaler or diffuser necklace. This was Dr. Seheult's point: if people *really* wanted to boost their immune function, they'd get outdoors and forest bathe!

As you may have guessed, when they evaluated how study participants fared indoors with aromatherapy diffusers running, they found an effect similar to being out in nature!

We can then, quite literally, bring the outside in with essential oils and obtain the same beneficial constituents that trees and plants release during forest bathing. And in doing so, we reap their powerful benefits: uplifting our mood, calming the nervous system, treating illnesses, and strengthening the immune system.

ESSENTIAL OILS IN HEALTH AND HEALING

Essential oils have been used since ancient times as natural remedies to enhance health and well-being. In recent years, an increased emphasis on holistic healing has led to a resurgence in the traditional use of essential oils for restoring health, treating diseases and their symptoms, and protecting us against illness.

The practice of using essential oils has now established itself as a viable health-care alternative (and complement) to conventional medicine. In fact, a recent study of integrative medicine practitioners uncovered that 96.8 percent of clinicians surveyed recommend using essential oils to their patients.

Since the mid-1990s, thousands of research studies have been conducted, and science has finally caught up with what our ancestors knew all along: the plant-based volatile organic compounds that compose our favorite essential oils contain wonderful medicinal properties and can help keep our families free of sickness and disease.

This resurgence has not come too soon! Consider that by 2050, 66 percent of the world's population is projected to be urban, and the recent coronavirus outbreak has given us a glimpse of the health concerns humanity must consider as it continues to separate itself from nature.

COVID-19 is a good example. The sharp rise in active cases during the summer of 2020 should be seen as a wake-up call to view this crisis as an opportunity to build a healthier and more disease-resilient society.

While infectious diseases like COVID-19 haunt us, this does not diminish the concern over *chronic diseases*, which are still the leading causes of death and disability worldwide. We're talking about heart disease, cancer, respiratory illnesses, stroke, diabetes, Alzheimer's and dementias, and mental health disorders, among many others. Disease rates from these conditions are accelerating globally, advancing across every region, and pervading all socioeconomic classes. By 2020, cases of chronic disease had already risen by 57 percent, according to the World Health Organization (WHO), and conditions like obesity were quickly discovered to be primary risk factors associated with mortality rate in COVID-19 patients!

What has been driving this surge? Medical experts cite the following reasons: accelerated urbanization, a more sedentary lifestyle, rising rates of weight gain and abdominal fat, unhealthy Westernized diets and poor nutrition, tobacco, excessive alcohol use, and drug abuse.

Look over that list again. Each one of the factors is *controllable*, meaning when you modify your lifestyle for the better, you knock out one or more factors that can lead to chronic disease, prevent it, and enhance your well-being.

The WHO concurs: "Chronic disease prevention and control helps people to live longer and healthier lives."

Who doesn't want to live a longer, healthier life! *The Essential Oils Apothecary* can help you do just that.

A MODERN APOTHECARY

In the nineteenth century, if you had a nasty cough, upset tummy, or other ailment, your mother would go to an apothecary, who would mix up an herbal concoction of some sort, maybe even some essential oils, and wait for it to work its magic.

An apothecary is (and was) a medical professional who prepares and sells medicines, usually of an herbal variety, as well as a healer who understands the power of nature to prevent and treat ailments. Benjamin Franklin was an apothecary, among his many other pursuits.

Apothecary, as a profession, goes back to around 2600 BC, when the ancient Babylonians were credited with the earliest records of the practice. Clay tablets from that period have been found with medical texts recording symptoms, the prescriptions, and the directions for mixing remedies.

Apothecaries were renowned for their investigations into herbal and chemical ingredients—a field of study that was a precursor to the modern sciences of chemistry and pharmacology. The modern equivalent of an apothecary is a pharmacist—a credentialed health-care professional who takes orders for medications and fills prescriptions.

At a time when the pharmaceutical industry has seemingly invented a drug for every ache and ailment, the idea of an apothecary seems almost quaint. But it is not! Nowhere is the craft of the apothecary more alive and relevant than in the practice of essential oils, especially the art of blending to create uplifting, pleasant, and therapeutic scents.

When you blend oils, all sorts of wonderful things can happen. Creating what's referred to as a "synergistic effect," various essential oils complement each other and bring out healing properties that you would not otherwise have experienced if you used only a single oil.

Essential oils generally work better when mixed with other essential oils. This quality is so unlike pharmaceutical drugs, which are made from isolated constituents that have a long list of adverse side effects.

There is also a system to blending—one that has its roots in the early work of apothecaries. Oils are blended either by fragrance families, such as floral oils, citrus oils, woody oils, or medicinal oils. Medicinal oils are usually combined according to their group—energizing, calming, detoxifying, or healing.

This book will introduce you to many essential oils and combinations of oils, help you gain confidence in blending, and discover scent combinations you like. Before long, you'll develop an instinct for creating your own essential oil solutions. Along the way, you will find it fun to channel your own inner apothecary!

BRING YOURSELF BACK TO BALANCE WITH
THE ESSENTIAL OILS APOTHECARY

If you or a loved one has had to deal with a physical chronic illness, you know the battle and the frustration. You have lived it. Chronic disease can also lead to emotional ailments, such as fear, sadness, depression, and stress. This makes life difficult for those who struggle daily. There are no vaccines that can prevent chronic illness, and there are no medications to cure them. Drugs can only alleviate the symptoms, and some don't even work that well. For this reason, many people turn to alternative therapies and treatments that can provide relief—including essential oils.

The purpose of *this* book is to push the boundaries of what essential oils can do, not only for your health but for society as a whole. In it, you will

- learn how to treat and prevent the leading forms of chronic disease with essential oils, based on scientific evidence from leading journals.
- adopt lifestyle actions that support the power of essential oils against chronic illness.
- acquire an accessible and comprehensive introduction to essential oils therapy.
- gain a truly holistic approach so that you can use essential oils to not only treat ailments but also boost your immunity against them.
- discover how to safely create your own remedies using essential oils you know and love and boost your energy, relieve stress and depression, enhance your focus, regain your well-being, and live a more natural lifestyle.
- experience the power of essential oils and aromatherapy to build a lifetime of wonderful health habits.

This book features profiles of hundreds of the most important essential oils, with information on their medicinal uses and recipes for common concerns. We have developed a huge array of healing recipes that will help you treat many complaints, from the mild to the serious. We use these essential oil remedies with ourselves and with our family, friends, clients, and colleagues. Obviously, we would not do this unless we had a high degree of confidence in the healing power of essential oils and their safety. Throughout this book, you'll find the essential oils and blends we know to be the most effective for leading diseases and health problems. Our information is based on our personal experience, as well as the ever-expanding database of scientific information about the VOCs found in plants.

This book comes not only from a lifetime of experience but from our hearts as we seek to do whatever we can to help people heal naturally.

So, if you're ready, let's have a look at *The Essential Oils Apothecary*.

→ To help you along the journey, we have created a series of free demo videos on preparing several of the essential oil remedies and recipes featured in *The Essential Oils Apothecary*. Each of the videos contains extra insights into the strategies and information covered in this book. You can access these videos at EOApothecary.com.

The Healing Power of Essential Oils

I f you're like us, you'll be pleasantly surprised to learn how far-reaching the healing power of essential oils can take you. Though, before you dive in, there are some basic principles that you must master.

Be sure to thoroughly review the following chapters not only to learn the context of using aromatherapy to prevent and manage chronic disease, but so you can master the fundamentals and ensure that you use them safely and effectively.

Trust us, as capable as they are of healing the body, they are equally as harmful if used incorrectly. This is not to scare you but to instill in you a deep respect for their potency to ensure that you use them with care. With that note, if you use them the right way, there are virtually no side effects, so you can add them to your natural health regimen without worry.

Once you get familiar with the nuances of aromatherapy and learn the basics, let your intuition be your guide. This is where the true healing power of essential oils happens!

Chapter 1

A Closer Look at Chronic Disease

"Behind every chronic illness is just a person trying to find their way in the world."
—*GLENN SCHWEITZER*

I f you think about it, up until COVID-19 turned our lives upside-down, twenty-first-century life was pretty nice for most of us. We live longer than our recent ancestors. We're fairly active, even in our golden years. Our kids have been surviving their childhood and teenage years at an unprecedented rate. Cigarette smoking has reached an all-time low among adults in the United States.

But are we healthier? Do we live better? What about you: do you enjoy great health and a fulfilled life?

Modern medicine has been able to keep people alive, sure, but what kind of life is it? Obesity is at an all-time high, and diabetes keeps climbing higher up the list. Heart disease is still the number one killer of men and women. The growing suicide rate points to a serious lack of mental health care.

While modern medicine has been able to greatly reduce infectious diseases (though new strains like COVID-19 have exposed some serious holes in that arena), it is very ineffective at preventing or reducing chronic diseases.

So when we say "chronic disease," exactly what are we talking about?

It may come as a surprise, but despite all of our medical advances and our focus on unifying governing health agencies across the globe, there is no consensus as to what defines a chronic illness.

For example, the Centers for Disease Control and Prevention (CDC) classifies seven health conditions as chronic disease: heart disease, cancer, chronic lung disease, stroke, Alzheimer's disease, diabetes, and chronic kidney disease.

In contrast, the Centers for Medicare and Medicaid Services have a more extensive list of twenty-one chronic conditions, adding alcohol abuse, depression, and HIV/AIDS, but leaving out obesity.

The World Health Organization (WHO) also has a more extensive list and includes various mental disorders, vision and hearing impairments, oral diseases, bone and joint disorders, and genetic disorders.

And Medline, the US National Library of Medicine premier bibliographic database, branches out to include neurological disorders such as multiple sclerosis, Parkinson's disease, and epilepsy.

Not only is the list of chronic illnesses debated, but so are the qualifying definitions. The CDC defines a chronic disease as "conditions that last one year or more and require ongoing medical attention or limit activities of daily living or both." Whereas Medline takes a more nebulous approach: "a long-term health condition that may not have a cure."

To make matters even more complicated, chronic diseases appear under different headings. Sometimes the term *noncommunicable diseases* distinguishes itself from "communicable," or infectious, diseases. Yet several chronic diseases have an infectious component, such as cervical cancer and liver cancer. *Lifestyle-related disease* is a term that emphasizes the contribution of diet, exercise, and other behaviors to the development of chronic diseases. Yet many chronic diseases are heavily triggered by environmental circumstances, which are not the result of our individual choices.

Why is all of this important?

For one thing, it is confusing to the public. Not having a clearly defined understanding of what chronic disease is and isn't has led to widespread misunderstandings.

In fact, according to the WHO, there are several half-truths and common misunderstandings people across the globe share about chronic disease. Here's a brief summary:

- *"My grandfather smoked and was overweight—and he lived to ninety-six."* (Yes, this happens, but it is rare and not worth the risk of doing things you know are unhealthy.)
- *Chronic disease affects rich people and wealthy countries.* (On the contrary, the less affluent someone is, the more likely they are to develop a life-threatening chronic condition.)
- *Mostly older people are affected.* (Actually, nearly 50 percent of chronic disease deaths occur in people under seventy years of age.)
- *Usually men are affected—think heart disease.* (Not true. Men and women are equally at risk.)
- *Being healthy and preventing chronic disease is "too expensive."* (Again, not true, and we'll outline many budget-friendly options in this book.)
- *We will all die one day, and getting a chronic disease is inevitable.*

This last point is key. Nothing could be further from the truth, and this underlying suspicion that nothing can be done to prevent and successfully treat chronic disease is completely false.

For the sake of this book, we lean toward a WHO broad-stroke approach to defining chronic disease, its symptoms, and its management. Chronic disease:

- has its origins at young ages;
- takes decades to become fully established as epidemics;
- requires a long-term and systematic approach to treatment;
- and, most important, has many opportunities for prevention—even reversal.

RISK FACTORS FOR CHRONIC DISEASES

All of the leading chronic diseases—arthritis, cardiovascular disease, cancer, chronic fatigue, COPD, fatty liver, obesity, osteoporosis, sleep disorders, and type 2 diabetes— are linked by common and preventable risk factors, according to the CDC and other global health authorities, including the following:

- Tobacco use and exposure to secondhand smoke
- Inadequate, unbalanced nutrition, including diets low in fruits and vegetables and high in sugar, sodium, and processed foods
- Sedentary lifestyle
- Alcohol abuse

There are other risk factors for most chronic diseases, as well, that have emerged from major landmark studies.

Chronic Inflammation

This occurs if the body's normal inflammatory healing process does not end when it should, leaving your body in an unhealthy state of alarm that can hurt your physical and mental well-being. Over time, chronic inflammation may impair the function of your tissues and organs—a destructive condition that leads to many chronic diseases.

Toxic Burden

Indoor air pollution, fluoridated water, contaminants, pesticides, chemical cleaners, drugs, and other environmental exposures can accumulate in your tissues and cause disease.

Genotoxins

These are chemicals or agents, usually found in the environment, that can cause damage to genetic material and are also involved in many chronic diseases, such as liver disease, brain illnesses, cardiovascular disorders, diabetes, arthritis, cancer, chronic inflammation, and aging.

Over-Sanitization

People who live in areas with high levels of sanitation do not obtain the normal exposure to microbes, pollen, and other microscopic elements in the environment. The lack of that exposure negatively affects the development of the immune system, making people more susceptible to emerging viruses and even Alzheimer's disease.

Stress

It's widely known that stress damages health in many ways. It interferes with sleep, leads to a weakened immune system, causes digestive problems and obesity, and increases your risk of depression.

EMF Exposure

Cell phones, microwaves, Wi-Fi routers, and other devices are all forms of electromagnetic frequency (EMF) exposure, which emits radiation that can damage the immune system. Overexposure to even low levels of radiation from these sources has been known to trigger sleep disorders, headaches, fatigue, memory problems, cognitive problems, and many other health problems.

Comorbidities

This refers to other chronic diseases that make you more susceptible to additional chronic diseases. Remember that kids' song explaining how the bones in the body connect? We can still hear it in our heads—"The foot bone connects to the ankle bone. . . ." Well, the same goes for chronic disease. For example, obesity and type 2 diabetes can also be linked to cancer, arthritis, and chronic pain and will put you at risk of developing every chronic disease known to man. And recent research has linked type 2 diabetes with Alzheimer's and other dementias.

Social Isolation

Based on a growing number of studies, it turns out that being socially isolated may prove even deadlier than a poor diet, obesity, or smoking.

Spanish and US researchers published a study on this issue in 2018, leading them to conclude that "social isolation increases the risk of being diagnosed with chronic illnesses. That is, people with greater social participation have lower risk of suffering from multiple chronic diseases."

The most common chronic diseases associated with social isolation are heart disease, brain illnesses, and dementia. Humans, like other social species, are wired for social connection. Without it, we experience stress, and our health can fail as a result. Suicide is also an outcome of the intense stress associated with social isolation and chronic illness. *In fact, during the early stages of the 2020 pandemic, the intense stress, coupled with unemployment, fear of contracting the virus, disturbed routines, social isolation, and increasing substance abuse, led experts to refer to COVID-19 as the "perfect storm" when it comes to suicide.*

Leaky Skin

Here's a risk factor for chronic disease that no one is talking about: leaky skin.

You may have heard the term *leaky gut*—a situation that describes an abnormal permeability in your intestinal lining. Under normal conditions, this lining forms an impermeable barrier that regulates what is absorbed into your bloodstream. However, a compromised—or permeable—gut lining lets toxins, undigested food particles, and bad bacteria "leak" out and then move through your body via your bloodstream.

In much the same way, you can have leaky skin. If your skin microbiome—the microorganisms that are normal residents on your skin—is off-balance, meaning that the healthy balance of good bacteria on your skin is not intact, your skin's natural barrier can be compromised. This leads to inflammation, which in turn results in chronic skin conditions like acne, eczema, rosacea, and psoriasis.

The main symptom is itchy skin. Skin is also often dry, because water leaks out.

Scratching makes the skin red, chafed, and thickened. Leaky skin is often caused by using antibacterial and conventional body-care products that dry and damage the skin. Using organic or DIY household cleaners and body-care products can go a long way to prevent leaky skin.

It is beyond a shadow of a doubt that eliminating these primary risk factors of chronic disease could prevent more than 40 percent of all cancers and at least 80 percent of heart disease, stroke, and type 2 diabetes.

So, yes, chronic disease can be reversed and prevented—with positive lifestyle changes that include diet; exercise; avoidance of drugs, tobacco, and excessive alcohol; stress relief; and reduced exposure to environmental toxins.

But here's a huge problem: Doctors and their patients tend not to address problems until the latter get very sick. At best, they usually prescribe only moderate weight loss and exercise programs—without any real specifics or follow-up. Also, physicians tend to prescribe drugs—diabetes drugs like metformin are a good example—that are far less effective with more side effects than healthful lifestyle changes. And so the cycle of chronic disease is perpetuated, even accelerated, by resigning ourselves to drugs and haphazard attempts at lifestyle changes.

Growing evidence points to the value of prevention, not only as a way to save and improve lives but also as a way to address out-of-control health-care costs and overhaul a health-care system traditionally focused on treating the sick rather than keeping people well.

Resigning yourself to debilitating, lingering ill-health does not have to be your portion in life, and the purpose of this book is to give you the tools you need to enjoy an abundant life through a ripe old age!

ENTER ESSENTIAL OILS TO TREAT CHRONIC DISEASE

"And the leaves of the tree are for the healing of the nations" (Revelations 22:2). We can think of no other substance on Earth that epitomizes this Bible verse better than essential oils.

Extracted directly from the bark, flowers, leaves, resins, and roots of plants, essential oils are highly concentrated plant-based chemical compounds recognized for thousands of years for their healing prowess.

Just one drop of essential oil contains up to three hundred powerfully life-changing chemicals found naturally in plants that serve to resist disease, attract bees and other pollinators, and protect plants from predators. They are plant-based medicine in their purest form.

In fact, the very chemicals that make up most pharmaceuticals on the market today are based on the chemical constituents that can be found in essential oils. However, unlike the drugs used to treat chronic disease, when you use essential oils properly, there are virtually no side effects!

When it comes to chronic disease, the health benefits of essential oils are extensive and well researched. They are also validated by countless testimonials from the millions of daily users across the globe.

Are you ready to harness the power of the world's most proven healing compounds to fight chronic disease? Are you ready to learn a whole new approach to healthy, natural living?

If so, open your mind to a whole new way of preventing and reversing health conditions that you've been battling for years.

We invite you to turn the page to see how to get started!

Chapter 2

All You Need to Know to Start Using Essential Oils

"The simplest solution is almost always the best."

—OCCAM'S RAZOR

A long time ago, before there was a CVS or Walgreens on every corner, you'd visit an apothecary shop to find something for an ailment. As you walked in, you'd be surrounded by herbs, teas, essential oils, soaps, and other handmade products. The earthy, rosy, palpable aromas wafting up from the distillates of flower blossoms, herbs, and plants would exert a magical feeling of calm and relaxation over your body.

The tools of the trade would be perched everywhere: essential oils and herbs with literally hundreds and hundreds of possibilities for formulas and remedies, mortars and pestles, handblown apothecary jars labeled in gold, recipe books filled with healing formulas, and more.

Over the years, we've had lots of people ask us where to begin when they want to start using essential oils and cultivate their own home apothecary for their health needs. This makes us super happy! It's so fun to create places in your home to use essential oils for good old-fashioned yet effective preventive and acute care.

Starting your own essential oils practice at home doesn't have to be done in one fell swoop—it's a process, one that depends on what you and your family need. In this chapter, we'll break down what to invest in—the "tools of the trade"—based on your experience with essential oils, so you can start trying them out to see which are most effective for you.

PURCHASE YOUR ESSENTIAL OILS

When you realize that it takes 50 lemon rinds, 3 pounds of lavender flowers, 189 pounds of lemon balm, or 726,000 rose petals to fill a single 15-milliliter bottle with essential oil, you appreciate how extraordinarily concentrated they are. As you can guess, it takes vastly different amounts of the various plant compounds to fill that itty-bitty container, which is one reason why the prices of various oils differ considerably.

You can buy essential oils from many different sources: online vendors and health-food stores top the list. Yes, you have probably seen essential oil sets on the shelves at national chain stores, but be careful. Often, these are labeled 100 percent pure yet sold at a dirt-cheap price. Don't buy into this! It has been shown that these products are often adulterated with synthetic versions of the natural and active ingredients in oils.

Read labels, for sure. You'll be looking for the plant taxonomy, plant sourcing, extraction method, and chemotype (a variation in the chemical components of an essential oil due to different conditions of growth and often distinguished by the letters "ct" after the name). Everything else will be marketing hype! An example is the term *therapeutic grade*, implying that the oils are of a superior quality, compared to nontherapeutic-grade oils. Reality check: This is marketing propaganda and means very little, because all essential oils are therapeutic if pure. But when companies put synthetic substances in the oils, they are not essential oils at all, just mostly chemicals that smell good.

There are several quality brands out there, and we use many of them. Here's what we do before we start before using new essential oils:

Ask the company for a report of their sourcing and quality standards. You can generally find a "batch report" on their website. This is technically a gas chromatography/mass spectrometry (GC/MS) report that breaks down the chemical components of individual oils. This can help you determine the chemotype and whether any adulterants or contaminants are in the oil.

Also, be aware that essential oils—even those certified as organic—can contain pesticide residues. Pesticides easily dissolve in fats and lipids, making the transition to essential oils possible. This is where trust comes in. Yes, trust. The essential oil and supplement industries are like the Wild West, and federal organizations do not regulate what's on the market. Essentially, anyone can sell anything, so it's important to do your homework and make sure the company that you're buying from is legit.

Check for quality. Before jumping in and buying a bunch of oils from a company, consider asking these questions to help ensure quality:

- Does the company have relationships with their distillers?
- Can the company readily provide material safety data sheets upon request?
- What are the common name and Latin name (exact genus and species)? Many companies will indicate the Latin designation of the plant it comes from, in addition to its common name. As an example, *Lavandula angustifolia* is the name that we find on the bottles of the popular lavender oil. Also known as English lavender, *Lavandula angustifolia* contains a slightly different chemical makeup and aroma than its cousin *Lavandula stoechas* (French or Spanish lavender).
- What is the country of origin, part of the plant processed, and type of extraction (distillation or expression), and how was it grown (organic, wildcrafted, traditional)?
- What's the cost? Price matters, as you may guess from the sheer amount of plant matter required to extract just a 15-milliliter bottle as described above. If you see a bottle of rose oil, for example, that costs $10, you can be sure it's fake. Shopping online to get an average cost can help you set the benchmark for the going rate of essential oils.

Note the container. Unadulterated essential oils can go bad if exposed to ultraviolet radiation. Therefore, real oils are stored in dark-colored bottles (these may be amber or cobalt blue).

Pure essential oils must be stored in glass containers. This is absolutely crucial in order to maintain the quality of the oils, as the strong chemical compounds in the oils break down and react when they come into contact with plastic.

EXTEND THE SHELF LIFE OF YOUR ESSENTIAL OILS

If you use them and expose them to oxygen regularly, the shelf life of most oils ranges from two to four years. If you rarely open the bottle, they can last decades.

Here are some tips to for maximizing that shelf life:

- Store them in cool, dark places.
- Tightly cap the bottles.
- Keep them out of the sun and away from extreme heat (which accelerates oxidation).
- Store your essential oils in the refrigerator to extend their life beyond two to four years.
- When possible, mix your oils with fractionated coconut oil, which doesn't go rancid like other carrier oils. See Kitchen Carrier Oils on page 23.

Seek referrals. Contact a friend or family member who uses essential oils that you trust to be conscientious and a thorough researcher—be careful not to let hate speech and multilevel marketing propaganda get in the way of truth. *Everyone's* brand is the best, right? Especially when they're selling something.

Sample a few oils. Try a couple for yourself. In technical aromatherapy terms, this is referred to as an "organoleptic evaluation"—how your body perceives the oil through the six senses: taste, touch, smell, sight, hearing, and intuition—and you should perform this test every time you get a new oil just in case the oil's constituents don't jibe with your body's chemistry. Lemon, lavender, and peppermint are common, are relatively inexpensive, and should provide a good gauge to see if a particular brand is for you.

Check your sourcing. In our opinion, the most important factor is whether or not the oils are indigenously sourced and "organic in nature," meaning they are harvested where God planted them, which is why they are referred to as "native" plants. One reason is because the word *organic* is not always a guarantee of purity. The other reason, even more important, is because non-native plants pale in comparison to native plants when it comes to nutrition and chemical constituents.

Once you have a few oils ready to go, start by diffusing them on their own (see page 21) and then in combinations of a couple of drops of two or three of them at a time. You can buy a diffuser, or you can simply simmer a pot of water on the stove and add your drops to it.

When you are familiar and comfortable with the scents, you will start to learn what blends you like. As you discover more about their effects, you can begin to create blends for specific reasons, like energizing your sluggish afternoon or clearing the air after a virus passed through the house. This book will help you in this regard.

From there, you can begin to experiment with diluted topical applications, like a soothing peppermint rub or a calming massage.

The important thing is to always be learning—never stop learning! The more we learn and grow, the better we can utilize these precious, truly essential oils.

STOCK UP ON KEY SUPPLIES

You'll want to purchase amber-colored glass containers for your blends—and several of each. We suggest the following:

- 5-, 10-, and 15-milliliter bottles with screw tops for your blends.
- 2-ounce bottles with eye-dropper screw tops for massage and body oils.
- 10-milliliter roll-on bottles are best for healing remedies using fractionated coconut oil, perfumes, and colognes.

- 1-, 2-, 4-, 16-, and 32-ounce bottles with spray tops; these are best for spritzes (e.g., air fresheners, spot removers, hair spray, hand sanitation, and household cleaners).
- Several aromatherapy inhaler tubes—lip-balm-size glass tubes with tight-fitting caps—gives you on-the-go healing benefits without any mess.
- An aromatherapy necklace; also known as a "diffuser necklace" or "aromatherapy locket," these jewelry pieces resemble a fashionable locket with an open-air design, which allows the essential oils to permeate and benefit the wearer. Several recipes in this book work well with aromatherapy necklaces.
- Stainless-steel mini funnels and glass eye droppers for blending and mixing.
- Buy an ultrasonic water diffuser or two. They are an easy, effective way to enjoy the benefits of inhaling essential oils.
- Size 00 vegan gel or enteric-coated (time-delayed) capsules are also a must for most of the recipes in this book that recommend using essential oils internally.

Note, your bottles and glass droppers can be sanitized in the dishwasher between uses, and you'll want to clean them between batches so you don't cross-contaminate used oils with new blends. And, it's a good idea to wipe your diffuser reservoir clean with a dry paper towel between each use. To give it a more thorough cleaning, simply fill the reservoir halfway to the fill line, add 10 drops of white vinegar, and let run for a few minutes. Drain the water and clean the reservoir with a clean rag or paper towel. Rinse with water and allow to air-dry before using again.

DIFFERENT TYPES OF ESSENTIAL OIL PRODUCTS

Essential oils are extracted from plant materials (see the chart on page 18) through removal methods that are suited to the specific plant part containing the oils. The various forms of extraction produce different types of products. Understanding these differences will help you become not only an avid label reader but a more informed consumer who spends his or her money wisely to meet health goals. Here is a rundown.

Absolutes. Used in the perfume industry and aromatherapy, absolutes are similar to essential oils. They are concentrated, highly aromatic, oily mixtures extracted from plants. Whereas essential oils are extracted by distillation and other methods, absolutes are usually produced through a laboratory-intense process called enfleurage, which involves using odorless fats at room temperature to trap the essence of the plant compounds.

CO_2 Extraction. This process uses supercritical carbon dioxide (sCO_2), which is a fluid state in which CO_2 is held at or above its critical temperature and critical pressure. In this state, it has an uncanny ability to perform as a commercial and industrial solvent. Unlike commonly used toxic solvents, like hexane, CO_2 is safe and environmentally friendly. The resulting essential-oil-based extract is currently all the rage in the aromatherapy community.

Cold-Pressed Citrus Oils. Most essential oils are distilled, but oils from citrus peels are *cold-pressed*. This process involves puncturing the skins of either the whole fruit or just the fruit peel and pressing out the essential oil.

Distillation. This method utilizes steam to vaporize the plant material's volatile compounds, which eventually go through a condensation and collection process.

Extracts. These contain volatile and nonvolatile principals, extracted from the plant using nonalcoholic solvents such as water, glycerin, or vinegar.

Hydrosols. These are collected from the distillation of the plant matter. They contain the water-soluble components of the plant material used as well as minute amounts of the more water-soluble essential oil constituents. Very little essential oil is actually present in the waters.

Infused Oils. An infusion of an essential oil is made by blending plant material into a carrier oil. The essential oil is then said to be "infused" into the carrier oil.

Tinctures. This is typically an extract of plant or animal material dissolved in ethanol (ethyl alcohol).

PLANT PARTS THAT PRODUCE ESSENTIAL OILS

PART	PLANT
Balsam, gum, and resin	Elemi, frankincense, galbanum, myrrh, Peru balsam
Bark	Cassia, cinnamon
Berries and fruit	Allspice, black pepper, juniper berry, may chang (also known as *Litsea cubeba*)
Flowers and leaves	Basil, catnip, clary sage, hyssop, lavender, marjoram, Melissa (lemon balm), oregano, orange blossom, peppermint, rosemary, sage, spearmint, thyme
Flowers, petals, and buds	Chamomile, clove, helichrysum, jasmine, neroli, rose, ylang ylang
Leaves	Bay, cajuput, cinnamon, eucalyptus, geranium, myrtle, niaouli, patchouli, petitgrain, tea tree
Needles	Cypress, fir, Scotch pine, spruce
Peel/rind	Bergamot, lemon, lime, mandarin, orange, tangerine, yuzu
Roots	Angelica, ginger, spikenard, valerian, vetiver
Seeds	Anise, cardamom, carrot, coriander, cumin, dill, fennel, nutmeg, parsley
Wood	Cedarwood, palo santo, rosewood, sandalwood

THE WIDESPREAD USE OF ESSENTIAL OILS

You may be surprised to learn that essential oils are used commercially in many industries—as agrochemicals, fragrances, flavors, industrial cleaners, and even pharmaceuticals.

Here's a breakdown of the industries that use essential oils and the approximate percentage of all the essential oils on the market that you will find in these products:

- Food and flavors: 50 percent
- Fragrance: 25 percent
- Pharmaceuticals: 20 percent (used to flavor medicine—menthol is a good example)
- Industrial: 3 percent
- Aromatherapy: 2 percent

THREE WAYS TO HARNESS THE THERAPEUTIC PROPERTIES OF ESSENTIAL OILS

There are three basic ways to use essential oils: inhale them, apply them on your skin, or consume them. All three come into play when dealing with chronic disease, and we'll share with you how to specifically use them in each chapter in Parts 2 and 3, but let's briefly look at each approach.

Inhalation

Not only is inhalation the oldest form of aromatherapeutic essential oil use, it is also arguably the safest. Oils diffused throughout a room are relatively risk-free, in most cases, for people of all ages and pets due to the low level of concentration when used correctly.

We recommend getting an ultrasonic water diffuser to start your essential oils practice. Alternatively, more direct effects can be obtained by using a nebulizer, breathing in a steam directly, or inhaling right from the bottle or from a few drops on a cloth.

You can also fill a glass spray bottle with water and a few drops of essential oil and spritz your clothes, pillow, or air as you do with an air freshener. Many people like to use a technique called cupping, in which you put a drop of oil in your hand, rub your hands together, and breathe into your hands. All of these techniques carry the volatile oil directly into your respiratory system and mucous membranes, diffused throughout either the steam or air molecules.

Safety Tips: Make sure the room in which you use a diffuser or nebulizer is well ventilated, especially if there are children or pets in your home. When you start to use one of these devices to diffuse essential oils, run the diffuser for only a few minutes to gauge your reaction. Likewise, when you use a new scent or new blend, take it slowly. Assuming you don't get a headache, experience sinus issues, or have another adverse reaction, slowly but surely increase the amount of time you run the diffuser, up to several hours.

Purchase a diffuser. Throw away those toxin-emitting plug-ins and air fresheners! Instead invest in diffusers. Similar to a humidifier, these small machines break down essential oils into minuscule components and disperse them through the air and ultimately into your respiratory system. We run them in every room of our home. They enhance sleep, mood, and the health of everyone in the family.

There are many different types of diffusers from which to choose. These are just a few:

- Ultrasonic or humidifying (our favorite because it is super easy to clean)
- Heat diffusers
- Nebulizers
- Reed diffusers
- USB car diffusers

BASIC DIFFUSER RECIPE

4 to 6 drops essential oil per 150 ml water

SUPPLIES

Diffuser

1. Fill your diffuser with purified water as directed in the manufacturer's instructions.

2. Add the essential oil.

3. Run the diffuser in a well-ventilated room until the water is used.

NOTE: *As a rule of thumb, it is okay to use purified water in your diffuser recipes because they are designed to be used up in a few hours, or a couple days at most. However, since spritzer recipes are designed to be used over a longer span of time, it is best to use distilled water because we're trying to reduce bacteria overgrowth.*

BASIC INHALER RECIPE

20 drops essential oil

SUPPLIES

Precut organic cotton pad

Aromatherapy inhaler

1. Place a cotton pad in the inhaler tube.

2. Drop the essential oil directly onto the cotton pad inside the tube. Alternatively, you can drop the oil into a glass bowl, roll the cotton pad in the oil to absorb it, and then insert it into the inhaler tube using tweezers.

3. Secure the cap and store the inhaler in a desk drawer, purse, or glove compartment so it's handy.

4. When desired, simply open the inhaler and take a few deep breaths of vapor from the tube.

Topical

Topical use is a step further than traditional inhalation-based aromatherapy, though it's still familiar in the context of massage therapy, which often utilizes aromatherapy for massage applications.

Instead of the broad diffusion through air droplets that inhalation provides, topical use of essential oils is much more direct. Research has found that once diluted essential oils are applied on the skin, the individual components can be detected in the bloodstream within five minutes.

With topical application, the oil is absorbed through the layers of your skin, while inhalation moves quickly through the thinner mucous membranes. Knowing your oil and the goal you have in mind can help you determine which application is more appropriate.

In theory and in some professional practices, certain essential oils can be used on the skin undiluted. However, the safest application is via dilution. These carrier oils usually have benefits of their own, and you can easily combine a couple of drops in a teaspoon to dilute the oils and help bypass potential irritation. (See more on carrier oils on page 23.)

Diluting essential oils in appropriate levels for applications is one of the basic standards of safe use, especially when applying them directly to the body. Depending on what you're trying to accomplish, it is generally advised that you dilute as follows:

- 0.5 to 1 percent: For children, the face, and sensitive skin like genitals and underarms
- 2 percent: Standard adult dilution for most DIY applications
- 3 to 5 percent: For chronic conditions like aches and pains
- 5 to 25 percent: For acute conditions like burns and cuts and for specifically treating a disease up to one week at a time
- 25 percent plus: To be used with great care and only for a very short period of time
- 50 percent plus: To be used only under the supervision of a trained health-care provider

Two quick dilution guides to knowing how many drops of essential oil to add to your topical preparations can be found on pages 26–28.

UNDERSTAND THE IMPORTANCE OF CARRIER OILS

The main purpose of a carrier oil (also known as vegetable oil or base oil) is to dilute the essential oil before it is used, especially on the skin. They are usually derived from kernels or seeds and hence are a plant's fatty portions. You can use different carrier oils to dilute multiple essential oils together.

Another term for carrier oils is *fixed oils*. You know these best as fatty oils derived from both animals and plants. Common examples include cooking oils, such as coconut, olive, and other vegetable oils you see in your grocery stores. In contrast to essential oils, fixed oils do not evaporate. In fact, they will leave a stain on absorbent surfaces. These oils vary in consistency and can be solid, semisolid, or liquid.

If you do not use carrier oils for essential oils, your skin may experience burns, irritation, sensitivity, redness, and inflammation.

Because they are volatile, essential oils quickly evaporate off your skin. The fats in the carrier oil prevent this from happening and ensure that the essential oils easily penetrate into your pores.

There are many different carrier oils from which to choose. We like to group them into beginner, intermediate, and advanced—based on where you are in your knowledge and experience of using essential oils.

Kitchen Carrier Oils: Olive and Coconut

Produced from pressed olives, olive oil is best known as a healthy edible oil with a fruity aroma. But it's also used in aromatherapy as a carrier oil. It's packed with fatty acids and plant sterols, which make it very effective at cleansing and moisturizing dry skin.

Organic virgin coconut oil is an edible oil, too, produced from the meat of mature coconuts. It contains skin-nourishing fatty acids and plant compounds, which make it a great carrier oil for massage oils and skin-care preparations.

Excellent for dry or sensitive skin, "fractionated" coconut oil contains literally only a fraction of the oil; all of the long-chain fatty acids have been removed so the oil stays liquid at room temperature. Sold as a medium-chain triglyceride (MCT) oil in the low-carb/high-fat diet industry, this oil will never turn rancid and helps preserve the shelf life of essential oils when blended.

Traditional Carrier Oils: Sweet Almond and Jojoba

Sweet almond oil is an edible oil made from the kernels of almonds. Used widely in aromatherapy, it is a great moisturizer for dry skin.

Jojoba oil comes from the seeds of the jojoba plant. Technically, jojoba isn't an oil but a wax with powerful moisturizing properties. Jojoba oil absorbs easily into the skin.

Herbal-infused oils like calendula and other extracts provide healing benefits in their own right and work wonderfully as carrier oils. We explain how to make these on page 209 in chapter 11.

Additional Carrier Oils

Apricot kernel oil is made from apricot kernels. It's a luxurious oil high in fatty acids and vitamin E. It absorbs easily into the skin. Use it as a carrier oil to make massage oils, bath oil, and hair-care preparations.

Avocado oil is a heavy, thick edible oil made from the avocado fruit. This can be a good carrier oil for dry skin remedies and body creams—unless you're dealing with acne. Avocado oil may increase sebum production, so if you are acne-prone, check with your dermatologist prior to using it.

Grapeseed oil is extracted from *Vitis vinifera*, which is usually grown to produce wine or grape juice. Usually, the seeds and oil are discarded, even though the seeds have a lot of nutritional value. Grapeseed oil is good for skin and hair essential-oil blends.

Borage oil comes from an herb notable for its vibrant purple flowers and medicinal properties. It is especially rich in gamma linoleic acid (GLA), which is an omega-6 fatty acid that has been shown to decrease inflammation.

Evening primrose oil comes from the evening primrose plant. It is a good carrier-oil option for people with dry or mature skin. It also contains a large amount of GLA and can be combined with other carrier oils for a good massage oil.

Cannabidiol (CBD) has taken the natural health world by storm, and we have found it to be an extremely useful and healing carrier. Similar to essential oils, most of the CBD on the market is adulterated, and it's critical to buy a product that's pure and uncontaminated and with little to no THC, which is the chief intoxicant in marijuana.

In fact, according to the Food and Drug Administration's newest report in 2020, most products on the market are mislabeled. Of those products that indicate the amount of CBD on the label, only 45 percent contain CBD within 20 percent of the labeled amount, with the remaining 55 percent containing either more or less CBD than listed, or none at all.

Safety Tip: Dimethyl sulfoxide (DMSO) is a popular carrier-oil option available online, but it's important to note that it is a by-product of the paper-making industry. It comes from a substance found in wood and has been used as an industrial solvent since the mid-1800s. We see this as a major red flag, because it is highly manufactured and not regulated. Is the wood organic? Fair trade? Wild crafted? It's the Wild West when it comes to DMSO, and we simply don't trust it. No matter the fantastic claims we see online, we recommend avoiding it and sticking with the oils listed above.

MAMA Z'S OIL BASE

This is our favorite carrier oil. It's extremely healing in its own right, let alone when you add essential oils to it! Making the recipe below will set you up for dozens of remedies and uses that we'll outline in subsequent chapters. Also, this recipe makes a lot. Divide all ingredients in half or quarters to make a smaller batch.

54 ounces organic virgin coconut oil, melted

16 ounces sweet almond oil

8 ounces jojoba oil

4 ounces vitamin E oil

continues

SUPPLIES

Quart- or pint-size wide-mouthed mason jars or other glass containers with lids

1. In a large glass bowl or stock pot, combine the coconut oil with the sweet almond, jojoba, and vitamin E oils. Using a wooden spoon, mix until thoroughly combined.

2. Pour the mixture into mason jars and tightly close the lids. Store in a cool (see Notes), dark place for up to two years. The saturated fats in the coconut oil won't spoil, but the sweet almond oil may get stale if not properly stored.

NOTES: *If your coconut oil has hardened, the easiest way to melt it is to fill the kitchen sink with hot tap water and set the jar of coconut oil in it until it liquifies.*

Coconut oil has a melting point of 76°F. Depending on the temperature in your house, this base may revert to a solid or semisolid state. To reliquefy it, rub some in your hands or place the container close to a heating vent or in warm water.

DIY DILUTION GUIDE:
MEASURED IN OUNCES AND TABLESPOONS

When making topical essential oil (EO) preparations, the following dilution guidelines are the recommended aromatherapy standard.

Note: There are 2 tablespoons in 1 fluid ounce. So, if working with tablespoons is more comfortable for you, please use that chart.

OUNCES		TABLESPOONS	
INFANTS AND CHILDREN		*INFANTS AND CHILDREN*	
0.5%	3 drops of EOs per ounce of carrier	0.5%	1.5 drops of EOs per tablespoon of carrier
1%	6 drops of EOs per ounce of carrier	1%	3 drops of EOs per tablespoon of carrier

OUNCES		TABLESPOONS	
ADULTS		*ADULTS*	
2%	12 drops of EOs per ounce of carrier	2%	6 drops of EOs per tablespoon of carrier
3%	18 drops of EOs per ounce of carrier	3%	9 drops of EOs per tablespoon of carrier
5%	30 drops of EOs per ounce of carrier	5%	15 drops of EO per tablespoon of carrier
10%	60 drops of EOs per ounce of carrier	10%	30 drops of EOs per tablespoon of carrier

ROLLER BOTTLE GUIDE—BASED ON PERCENTAGE

We love roller bottles for topical application of essential oils. Simply dilute your oils as suggested below and roll them directly on your body. Use your roller bottle on your wrists, the bottoms of your feet, the back of your neck, on your face, belly, spine—virtually anywhere on your body.

ROLLER BOTTLE DILUTION GUIDE

	5 ML BOTTLE (1 TEASPOON CARRIER OIL)	10 ML BOTTLE (2 TEASPOONS CARRIER OIL)
0.5%	Less than a drop	1 drop
1%	1.5 drops	3 drops
2%	3 drops	6 drops
3%	4.5 drops	9 drops
4%	6 drops	12 drops
5%	7.5 drops	15 drops
10%	15 drops	30 drops

- Good carrier oils for roller bottles include fractionated coconut, almond, and jojoba.
- Always do a "skin patch" test prior to applying new essential oils on your skin.
- Start by using the lowest concentration and add more essential oils as needed.
- 0.5 to 1 percent is for sensitive skin and for application on sensitive areas like the face and underarm.
- 0.5 percent is for children under three years old.
- 1 percent is for children three to ten years old.
- 2 to 3 percent is the standard adult dilution and for children over ten years old.
- 5 percent plus is for acute, short-term application such as treatment for migraines and muscle soreness. Do not exceed 25 percent.
- A little goes a long way. The more carrier oil you use, the less risk of irritation and sensitization.

Where to Apply Essential Oils. You may have heard that applying essential oils to the bottom of your feet is the most effective way to get the healing compounds into your bloodstream. This is not actually true. Research has determined that this is the order of areas of the body where the skin is most permeable, from highest to lowest:

1. Genital region
2. Head and neck region
3. Trunk (chest, stomach, back)
4. Arms (including the hands and fingers)
5. Legs (including the bottom of the feet)

This doesn't mean you should apply essential oils to your genitals however! Due to general safety and skin permeability, if you want essential oils to reach your bloodstream and have a total body (systemic) effect, we recommend applying them on your abdomen, chest, and neck.

Skin Patch Test. Before putting a new oil or blend on your skin, do a skin patch test by applying a 1 percent dilution on the back of your hand or the bottom of your foot—this is the same concept as testing carpet cleaner on an inconspicuous spot first before potentially staining a large area. Let the mixture settle for a few minutes and observe. If you experience no adverse reactions (bumps, burns, rashes, etc.) within ten minutes, this is a good sign that you can gradually scale up to more concentrated dilutions.

Safety Tip: Certain essential oils, especially citrus oils, are potential photosensitizers. (See the charts below.) This means that if you apply them to your skin and go out in the sun, you may experience serious skin damage, such as redness, itching, burns, blisters, and permanent skin discoloration. Diluting these oils to a 2 percent concentration can help minimize this risk, but be careful if you have light skin. The best precaution is to avoid direct sun contact for at least an hour after applying these oils.

PHOTOSENSITIZERS

ESSENTIAL OIL	LATIN NAME
Angelica root	*Angelica archangelica*
Bergamot	*Citrus bergamia*
Bitter orange, expressed	*Citrus aurantium*
Cumin	*Cuminum cyminum*
Grapefruit	*Citrus paradisi*
Lemon	*Citrus limon*
Lime	*Citrus aurantifolia*
Rue	*Ruta graveolens*

NONPHOTOTOXIC CITRUS OILS

ESSENTIAL OIL	LATIN NAME
Bergamot: *Bergaptenless* (FCF: Furanocoumarin Free)* *A specially formulated bergamot essential oil with the bergapten removed so it is safe to use in the sun.*	*Citrus bergamia*
Blood, Sweet, and Wild orange	*Citrus sinensis*
Lemon, distilled	*Citrus limon*
Lime, distilled	*Citrus aurantifolia*
Mandarin	*Citrus reticulata*

Tangelo	Citrus tangelo
Tangerine, expressed	Citrus reticulata
Yuzu	Citrus junos

BASIC BODY OIL RECIPE

1 ounce Mama Z's Oil Base (page 25) or carrier oil of your choice

12 drops essential oils

SUPPLIES

Small glass bowl

Lidded glass jar or lotion dispenser

1. In a glass bowl, mix the oil base and essential oils thoroughly.

2. Use as a moisturizer or body or massage oil.

3. Store any leftover oil in a glass jar or lotion container.

MAMA Z'S HEALING SKIN SERUM

1 tablespoon aloe vera gel

1 tablespoon organic virgin coconut oil, softened or melted

5 drops lavender essential oil

2 drops frankincense essential oil

SUPPLIES

High-speed blender or food processor

Lidded glass jar, lotion dispenser, or salve container

1. In a high-speed blender or food processor, blend the aloe, coconut oil, and essential oils until smooth.

2. Once well mixed, store in a glass jar, lotion dispenser, or salve container in the fridge or a cool place so the coconut oil remains hardened.

3. Use and enjoy the serum at least once per day. Make a fresh batch each month.

BASIC BATH SALTS RECIPE

1 cup Epsom salts

¼ cup unfiltered, raw apple cider vinegar

1 ounce carrier oil (do not use coconut oil, which can harden and clog pipes)

5 to 10 drops essential oils

SUPPLIES

Medium glass bowl

1. In a glass bowl, mix the Epsom salts, vinegar, and carrier and essential oils thoroughly.

2. Pour all of the contents into the tub while drawing a bath, using the warmest water you can tolerate to fully dissolve the ingredients.

Internal

Finally, and most controversially, many essential oils are safe for ingestion. Let us mention that many aromatherapists believe essential oils should never be ingested, and most will suggest only trained professionals utilize internal methods. We wholeheartedly disagree with this, because research and traditional aromatherapy use suggest otherwise.

What do you think flavors your favorite cola or flavored ice cream? Essential oils! It's all a matter of dosage.

The most basic form of ingestion is in culinary doses. Take cinnamon, for example. You could use cinnamon-bark essential oil in a cake batter, but you'd only need one drop for the whole batch versus a teaspoon or more of the bark powder.

Another common internal preparation is to combine it into a drink. Do remember that oil and water *do not mix*, so simply adding a drop to water will leave that drop undiluted. Some oils are irritants, and all oils are very strong, so it's best to be safe and dilute it first into some coconut milk, honey, or liquid stevia extract.

Medicinal doses, the ones discussed in this book, are always taken in capsule form and within maximum oral dosing limits. (See the sidebar on page 32.)

Safety Tip: Never put undiluted essential oils in your mouth. Doing so could burn your mucous membranes. Instead, dilute two or three drops with an edible carrier oil (such as olive, coconut, or avocado oil) and place the mixture in a vegan gelatin capsule.

SAFETY TIP: MAXIMUM DAILY ORAL DOSE

Depending on the oil, the maximum daily oral dose for adults ranges from six to twenty drops per day, up to three doses in one day, or two to six drops per application.

As a general rule, unless your doctor recommends otherwise, use only one essential oil remedy at a time when you're treating a health condition—meaning, don't take three or four of the remedies every day. By consuming only one, you can more easily determine if it's working. If you're taking multiple remedies, you won't know which one is effective.

Additionally, taking multiple remedies puts you at risk of phytochemical accumulation ("overdosing") and developing liver damage—the very thing we're trying to prevent with chronic disease prevention and management!

We have also found that it's wise to switch up protocols every month or so. This prevents the possibility that your body will develop some resistance. Otherwise, you may find yourself in a position where you need to increase the dose to get the same results, which we see with people using painkillers, antibiotics, and other pharmaceuticals, and that's never a good idea.

With ingestion comes greater risk of drug interactions and adverse effects, so discontinue use immediately if you experience any negative reaction to the oils. See Appendix B for an exhaustive list of known drug reactions that may occur if you ingest essential oils. As always, be sure to consult with your physician before starting a new protocol, especially if you're currently taking any medications.

BASIC CAPSULE RECIPE

Makes 1 dose

2 to 6 drops essential oils
Organic virgin coconut oil or extra-virgin olive oil

SUPPLIES
Pipette
Size 00 vegan gel capsule

1. Using a pipette, drop the essential oils into the bottom half (the longer, narrower one) of the capsule. Fill this half to the brim with coconut or extra-virgin olive oil.

2. Fit the wider top half of the capsule over the bottom half and secure it snugly.

3. Immediately swallow the capsule with water after breakfast and/or dinner. Take once or twice daily and monitor your symptoms.

4. Start with 2 drops and work your way up to increasing doses under the guidance of your physician.

As you begin your healing journey with essential oils, we know you're eager to learn many things: What essential oil should I use with my diabetes? Which oils can relieve my depression or anxiety? Is there an oil I can use to improve my memory?

The last thing we want to do is treat essential oils as we do pharmaceutical drugs, like a quick fix rather than lasting change. Essential oils enhance your body's innate, natural ability to heal itself and can improve your experience of treating chronic disease, as well as help you prevent it. Oils will not help you, however, if you are unwilling to change your lifestyle. They are a powerful adjunct to living a healthy, abundant life.

Chapter 3

Preventing Chronic Disease by Creating a Healthier Home

"Anything that's human is mentionable, and anything that is mentionable can be more manageable."

—MR. ROGERS

Using essential oils while living a "fast food" lifestyle is like taking one step forward but two steps back. In other words, for essential oils to help you enjoy abundant health and wellness—free from chronic disease—it is vital to use them within the context of a healthy lifestyle by creating a toxin-free home, right down to your emotional and spiritual well-being.

Whether we like to admit it, or even whether we're aware, we live in a toxic world, and toxins are one of the major risk factors for chronic disease. A toxin is anything foreign to your body that your built-in detoxification system is called upon to eliminate. Examples are commercial pesticides, mercury, lead, chemicals in self-care products, commercial household-cleaning solutions, and harmful substances that leach from plastics, among many other offenders. Even toxic thoughts and feelings brought on by stress can harm your health. Toxins, whether physical substances or emotions, increase your risk of developing chronic disease.

As we come into contact with microdoses of toxins over a long period of time, the damage accumulates, and our immune system weakens, leading to chronic inflammation and illness. This is why chronic stress is so dangerous, because it wears us down emotionally and makes us more susceptible to a plethora of other conditions that affect the mind as well as the body.

We have found that incorporating essential oils as a lifestyle practice is the most efficient strategy to mitigate these risks. In a very direct yet passive approach to our health care, we don't actually use essential oils every day as a way to prevent disease per se but to promote a healthy lifestyle free of toxins and stressful, inflammation-causing chemicals.

Thus, in this chapter we share some of our favorite healthy lifestyle tips and recipes, but before we do, let's unwrap what essential oils are so we understand them better.

ESSENTIAL OILS DEFINED

It may surprise you to learn two things about essential oils. First, essential oils are not essential. And, second, they are not oils.

The scientific term for essential oils is *volatile organic compound*, which paints a much better picture of what we're referring to. The volatile components of a plant are the parts that are released quickly into the air. The essential oil is why you smell lavender when you lean down and sniff the blooms.

The *Encyclopedia Britannica* describes the naming rationale this way, describing essential oil as a "highly volatile substance isolated by a physical process from an odoriferous plant of a single botanical species. . . . Such oils were called essential because they were thought to represent the very essence of odour and flavour." However, they are not essential to life.

Because they are airborne (volatile), essential oils interact with your olfactory system (sense of smell), which is responsible for immediately sending signals to the brain upon stimulation. Specifically, upon inhalation, a cascade of events occurs unique to the olfactory system that directly impacts your limbic system, that part of the brain responsible for your mood, emotions, memory, and also autonomic functions that control blood pressure, breathing, heart rate, hormone levels, and stress levels. Thus, we see the basis for much of the research discussed in this book explaining how essential oils can help prevent and treat chronic conditions. Additionally, the healing components that make up essential oils are also circulated through your respiratory system when you inhale them.

In biological terms, essential oils are referred to as "secondary metabolites," chemicals produced by plants that don't play a role in vital functions that are essential to human life such as growth, development, or reproduction. Meaning, unlike "primary metabolites" that are vital for us to consume in order to live (e.g., carbohydrates, proteins, vitamins, minerals, etc.), we don't need essential oils to survive. Still, we can think of no better remedy to have on hand to enjoy abundant health and wellness!

Essential oils also are not oils, which are the liquid form of fats (i.e., lipids) at room temperature. Like lipids, essential oils are insoluble in water; hence the misnomer *essential oil*. However, because the components of essential oils are terpenoids (a large class of organic compounds including terpenes, diterpenes, and sesquiterpenes), they differ from fatty oils because they do not contain the glycerides of fatty acids.

Rather, they are the lipophilic (i.e., fat-loving) and hydrophobic (i.e., water-hating) volatile organic compounds found in plants. In practical terms, this means essential oils dissolve readily in fat but don't mix easily with water. It's also the reason why they penetrate through the skin after topical application, enter into the bloodstream, and can cross the blood-brain barrier.

ESSENTIAL OILS AS ADAPTOGENS AND HARMONIZERS

While exposure to emotional and environmental toxins is not pleasant to think about, we have some very good news: essential oils work powerfully, along with other solutions, to support your body, mind, and spirit.

And, no, it's not "magic." It's all based on real science, and it's important to first understand that the real *healing* power of essential oils can be found in their ability to facilitate peace and harmony in the body. Using the right essential oils can help your mind and body reach a state of balance and homeostasis. Known as "harmonization," this is a well-known phenomenon in the medical literature and has been confirmed in studies evaluating ylang ylang and sandalwood.

The "outside-in" medical approach prescribes a drug or intervention to treat a disease or symptom in an attempt to overpower the body's natural physiological response (i.e., prescribing a mood-boosting drug that forces the brain to produce more dopamine for depression patients). Contrary to this, the proper use of essential oils should be to support the body to heal itself. This "inside-out" approach is more in line with a vitalistic philosophy where an intervention (i.e., aromatherapy) is used to stimulate the innate, inborn intelligence of the body to reach a state of homeostasis.

This is why essential oils can be referred to as "adaptogens." Defined as "a non-toxic substance and especially a plant extract that is held to increase the body's ability to resist the damaging effects of stress," adaptogens are well known to "promote or restore normal physiological functioning."

This is why inhaling ylang ylang today, for example, can help support your body to *elevate* blood pressure if needed, whereas tomorrow, if your blood pressure is a bit too high, ylang ylang will support your body in *reducing* it. Hence, we see studies debunking the myth that ylang ylang is always a sedative, calming agent. Yes, it can be, but it can also increase attentiveness and alertness.

Contrary to what we see online, this means that there is no "Oil for That," referring to the common marketing slogan that there is an essential oil for virtually every disease known to man.

This is also one of the reasons why aromatherapists like Gabriel Mojay define aromatherapy as "the controlled use of essential oils to maintain and promote physical, psychological, and spiritual well-being."

SIX MAJOR SOURCES OF TOXINS IN YOUR HOME AND HOW ESSENTIAL OILS HELP

1. Indoor Air

Here is a startling statistic: according to the US Environmental Protection Agency (EPA), indoor air is two to five times more polluted than outdoor air, regardless of where you live. And research shows that, on average, we spend approximately 90 percent of our time indoors, breathing in air filled with odors, potentially harmful gases and chemicals, pollen, dust, and viruses.

What is this doing to us? According to the American Heart Association, poor indoor air quality can cause heart problems and certain types of cancer, especially lung cancer. We see similar reports linking indoor air pollution to autoimmunity, Alzheimer's, and general cognitive impairment.

In that context, it's certain that indoor air quality should be a high priority.

Our Solutions

- Diffuse essential oils throughout your home to help kill airborne pathogens and provide a natural, healing scent to your rooms. We recommend starting with our Immune-Boosting Diffuser Blend (page 53).
- Stop using commercial air fresheners. They may contain solvents, stabilizers, UV absorbers, preservatives, and dyes as well as harmful chemicals. Many of these chemicals are carcinogens, respiratory irritants, hormone disruptors, neurotoxins (which cause damage to the brain), and allergens. Try making the Sweet Earth Spritzer (page 39) instead!
- To further clean the air, there are a number of natural alternatives: Himalayan salt lamps, charcoal bags, houseplants, or essential oils diffused into the air.
- Get rid of candles. They contain mostly synthetic chemicals for the fragrance. There are some natural versions that can be purchased if you cannot live without candles. Or try using a diffuser with essential oils to scent rooms, while obtaining all the therapeutic benefits they offer.
- Purchase a portable filtration system. It helps minimize all the main sources of air pollution in your home. An efficient one can even filter out virus-sized particles!

➡ Our favorite air purifier is AirDoctor Pro. We've been using them for years and have five units running throughout our home at all times. Visit NaturalLivingFamily.com/AirDr to learn more.

SWEET EARTH SPRITZER

We just stumbled upon this sweet, earthy blend and it makes for a wonderful spritzer to promote health and vitality.

10 drops organic 190-proof grain alcohol

5 drops cardamom essential oil

5 drops palo santo essential oil

5 drops pink pepper essential oil

5 drops vetiver essential oil

10 drops witch hazel

Distilled water, as needed

SUPPLIES

1-ounce spray bottle

1. Mix the grain alcohol, essential oils, and witch hazel in the bottle.

2. Fill with distilled water and shake gently to mix well.

3. Use as you normally would an aerosol spray for an invigorating aromatic escape and to promote overall health and vitality.

4. These oils also work great in a diffuser. Use just 1 drop of each oil.

NOTE: *These types of formulas will only be effective for a couple of weeks. We've had them last for as long as two months without noticing any bacterial overgrowth, which can happen with any water-based products. This may not be obvious at first, but the smell will become rancid and you will notice a change in color if it is contaminated. If so, discard and make another batch.*

2. Water

Is tap water safe? The answer is complicated.

No, drinking tap water won't kill you, but it will expose you to chemical contamination that may, in the long run, post harmful effects to your body. Some nasty contaminants may be flowing out of your faucets, to name just a few:

Fluoride—a neurotoxin and hormone disruptor

Chlorine—a trigger for respiratory problems and memory loss

Lead—highly damaging to children, as well as to the heart, brain, and reproductive organs

Mercury—related to brain damage, blindness, cognitive disability, impairment of motor functions, headaches, tremors, mood swings, memory loss, and skin rashes

PCBs—may cause cancer and immune damage

Our Solutions

- Detox your water supply with an excellent water filter. We recommend reverse-osmosis filters. They remove virtually all of the toxic chemicals from your tap water.
- Hydrate yourself. Drink several glasses of filtered water daily, as well as herbal teas. Doing so will also help you flush toxins from your body.
- Make Dr. Z's Citrus Soda Pop recipe on page 267 in chapter 15, or try Mama Z's Essential Oil Detox Water recipe below.

ESSENTIAL OIL DETOX WATER

Makes 1 gallon of concentrate; 2 gallons of drinking water

1 dropperful plain or flavored liquid stevia

10 drops lemon essential oil

10 drops grapefruit essential oil

1 teaspoon freshly squeezed lime or lemon juice

1 tablespoon unfiltered, raw apple cider vinegar

1 gallon purified water

SUPPLIES

1-gallon jug

1. Combine the stevia, essential oils, lime juice, and cider vinegar in the jug.
2. Top it all off with filtered water.
3. Use concentrate as the base for your drinking water each day. Dilute it further by mixing equal parts of concentrate and filtered water.
4. Drink 2 to 3 glasses per day.

➔ To watch us make this recipe and learn more about how to detox your home with essential oils, go to EOApothecary.com.

3. EMFs

Most of us love the conveniences of modern life. But few of us are aware of the possible health risks presented by the gadgets that make our world work.

It turns out that our cell phones, microwaves, Wi-Fi routers, computers, and other appliances send out a stream of invisible energy through electromagnetic fields (EMFs) that concerns some experts.

EMFs are known to trigger oxidative stress on various tissues throughout the body and they can cause free radical damage to your cells. So please remain aware of these negative effects of EMFs. Although the impact of the waves varies at different frequencies, it is better to stay as far as possible from their source because of the health risks.

Our Solutions

- Use essential oils as a way of life in your body care and cleaning products, and diffuse them throughout the day in your home. Essential oils are rich in free radical–fighting antioxidants and can help reduce the effects of these waves.
- Use the speaker function or headphones so your phone is not right by your ear when talking. Avoid wireless earbuds and Bluetooth technology.
- Turn off your phone or put it on "airplane mode" when you sleep.
- Turn off your Wi-Fi router at night.

- Live without a microwave. We do it, and it's not as hard as you might expect. You can reheat foods quickly on the stovetop or in your oven. Toaster ovens come in handy for the same reason. Water boils quickly in an electric kettle, and you can defrost foods overnight in your refrigerator.
- Use EMF-protection devices to help create a protected environment in your home, office, and car.

➜ Our favorite protection against EMF stress is the Harmoni Pendant. Our entire family wears it, and we noticed a difference the day we put it on! Go to NaturalLivingFamily.com/HarmoniPendant to learn more.

4. Household Cleaning Products

When you do laundry or housework, be aware that many household products are loaded with toxins that can contribute to autoimmunity and other chronic health issues.

Some of the most toxic chemicals are parabens, which are hormone disruptors and may lead to breast cancer; chlorine, associated with sneezing and skin, eye, nasal, and throat irritations; triclosan, another hormone disruptor; ammonia, which is corrosive to the lungs; and phthalates, which are carcinogens. Also, be wary of antibacterial cleaners. When you use them, good bacteria are also killed. This could be harmful to your skin microbiome if the ratio of good to bad bacteria is disturbed, and bad bacteria get the upper hand.

Our Solutions: Your Laundry Room

- Look for better modern detergents, such as green detergents that are formulated with natural, plant-based ingredients.
- Use baking soda. There's not much that baking soda cannot do. It's the jack-of-all-trades when it comes to cleaning. Baking soda washes clothing, is a natural stain remover, and can even dry-clean your clothes.

- Try washing soda. This natural cleaner is also a powerful water softener. The watchdog organization the Environmental Working Group ranks it as an "A," so it passes with flying colors, making it safe and nontoxic.
- Clean with distilled white vinegar. Simply put ½ cup in your washing machine's detergent compartment. You don't need to add any other detergents.

→ Making your own laundry soap can be very messy and a bit tricky, which is why we recommend using MyGreenFills, the best nontoxic, truly chemical-free laundry solution that actually works! Visit NaturalLivingFamily.com/MyGreenFills to learn more.

Our Solutions: Household Cleaners

- Distilled white and apple cider vinegars are all-natural disinfectants. You can even clean glass and other surfaces with them.
- Baking soda is extremely helpful for scrubbing down surfaces (including ovens), cleaning smelly drains, cleaning grout, mopping floors, and refreshing furniture.
- Definitely use essential oils in your cleaning products. They impart two big benefits: they are disinfectants, and they bring a pleasant scent to the job you're doing.
- MyGreenFills also has household cleaners that work great. If you don't have time to DIY (we don't), check out the cleaning products from this company. Everything is *truly* clean—no fragrances, dyes, fillers, formaldehyde, triclosan, ammonia, chlorine, or other harmful chemicals.

TEA TREE–CITRUS BATHROOM CLEANER

Adapted from *The Healing Power of Essential Oils*

2 tablespoons Dr. Bronner's Pure-Castile liquid soap

2 tablespoons baking soda

25 drops tea tree essential oil

30 drops orange or lemon essential oil

2 cups distilled water

SUPPLIES

16-ounce glass spray bottle

1. Combine the liquid soap, baking soda, and essential oils in the spray bottle and mix well.

2. Pour in the water and shake thoroughly.

3. Use as you would any other bathroom cleaner. Shake before each use.

4. Store in a cool, dark place.

CITRUS-POWERED GLASS CLEANER SPRAY

½ teaspoon Dr. Bronner's Pure-Castile liquid soap

¼ cup distilled white vinegar

25 drops essential oils (see Note)

1½ cups distilled water

SUPPLIES

16-ounce glass spray bottle

1. Add liquid soap, vinegar, and essential oils to the spray bottle and mix well.

2. Pour in the distilled water and shake thoroughly.

3. Spray the mixture directly on glass windows and mirrors for cleaning. Shake before each use.

4. Store in a cool, dark place.

NOTE: *Essential oils for cleaning glass include lemon, lime, bergamot, and grapefruit.*

5. Cosmetics and Personal Care Products

This is a biggie. Our skin is an organ—the largest organ, actually. And because our skin is porous, it absorbs anything and everything we put on it. That means all the body creams, perfumes, deodorants, hair-care products, shampoos, and even our nail polishes and all the chemicals in these products eventually wind up inside our body.

These are some of the chemicals we're concerned about:

Diethanolamine (DEA), found in moisturizers, shampoos, sunscreens, and cleansers, is a possible carcinogen.

Petroleum, found in hair products, lip balm, lipsticks, and many skin-care products such as petroleum jelly and baby oils, is often contaminated with cancer-causing substances.

Talc is commonly found in baby powders, face powders, and body powders. It is a mineral shown to be a major cause of ovarian cancer.

Lead is present in many cosmetics, including lipsticks. It is a neurotoxin that can damage the brain.

Parabens are chemicals commonly found in cosmetics and skin- and hair-care products. As noted earlier, they are hormone disruptors.

Methanol, or wood alcohol, is a poisonous chemical found in a number of hand sanitizers. It is an anti-germ product that has been in high demand due to COVID-19. In June 2020, the US Food and Drug Administration (FDA) warned consumers not to use nine brands of hand sanitizers.

Phthalates are typically found in moisturizers, perfumes, nail polishes, soaps, and hair sprays. They are a carcinogen.

Aluminum is most commonly found in deodorants and antiperspirants. Studies link aluminum to Alzheimer's disease and brain disorders.

Most store-bought hand sanitizers are the worst. Filled with cancer-causing registered pesticides like triclosan and artificial fragrances, they do nothing but dry your skin and hurt your skin's microbiome, leading to "leaky skin." (See page 8 for more information.)

Our Solutions

- Castile soap: Available in bars or liquid, castile soap replaces almost any commercial soap or cleanser alone or in recipes.
- Unfiltered, raw apple cider vinegar: Use this exceptional natural product as a clarifying hair rinse. It gets rid of residue buildup from hair products.
- Aloe gel: Fresh from the leaves or bottled, this gel is both healing and soothing to skin of all types and ages. It can replace many lotions and creams, alone or in recipes. See Mama Z's recipe for Quick and Easy Hand Sanitizer below.
- Witch hazel: From shrinking pores to fighting aging, witch hazel is a natural astringent with many skin-boosting benefits.
- Avocado: Mashed and used alone as a mask, an avocado is loaded with many minerals, vitamins, and antioxidants, all of which contribute to skin health in no uncertain terms. Avocado also contains fats that keep the skin moisturized as well as combat inflammation.
- Fatty oils: These include coconut, jojoba, olive, and sweet almond oils. They can be used alone as healing cleansing oils or as carrier oils in recipes to very convincingly replace commercial lotions and creams.
- Diluted essential oils: Oils such as lavender, frankincense, Roman chamomile, neroli, helichrysum, sandalwood, and rose are all popular choices for cosmetic or skin care in conjunction with many natural healing recipes.
- Flaxseeds: So often the skin needs exfoliation to get rid of dead skin cells and dry flaky areas. One of the best ways to exfoliate naturally is with ground flaxseeds, used in skin scrub recipes.
- Bentonite/French clay: Historically, clay is a top clarifying and detox mask ingredient that will give you glowing skin.
- Honey: Because honey is antibacterial, it is very healing for the skin and

helps promote probiotic activity (which may fight "leaky skin") and reduce acne.

- Fruit acids: Mashed, blended, or freshly juiced fruits are natural sources of alpha and beta hydroxy acids—both of which provide antiaging benefits to the skin. Try lemon, apple, cream of tartar (from grapes), or strawberries.

QUICK AND EASY HAND SANITIZER

10 drops essential oils (see Notes)

Organic 190-proof grain alcohol (or the highest proof alcohol you can get; see Notes)

SUPPLIES

1-ounce glass spray bottle or polyethylene terephthalate (PET) plastic flip-top bottle (PET is recognized as a safe material for food storage).

1. Drop the essential oils into the bottle, then add alcohol to fill the bottle.
2. Cover and shake vigorously to mix thoroughly.
3. Be sure to give your hands a thorough soak with the mixture, rub them vigorously, and let them air-dry, keeping them wet for as long as possible.

NOTES: *Since all essential oils are antimicrobial, you can pretty much choose whatever you want. Want to calm down? Use lavender. Want to boost your mood? Use citrus oils. Want to boost immune function? Use our Immune-Boosting Blend (page 49). The sky's the limit!*

At least 70 percent alcohol is necessary to sanitize the hands, but this concentration is not adequate for solubilizing essential oils.

HEALTHY LIQUID HAND SOAP

From *The Healing Power of Essential Oils*

¼ cup distilled water

¼ cup Dr. Bronner's Pure-Castile liquid soap

1½ teaspoons vitamin E oil

1½ teaspoons sweet almond or jojoba oil

20 drops of the essential oil or blend of your choice

SUPPLIES

8-ounce glass bottle with pump or glass foaming soap dispenser

1. In the glass bottle combine the water and liquid soap.
2. Add your vitamin E, sweet almond or jojoba oil, and essential oils.
3. Screw on the lid and shake well.

NOTE: *If you make this soap in a larger amount, store the leftovers in a glass jar until your containers need a refill; just remember to always shake well before using.*

6. Processed Junk Food

We talked about nutrition and diet extensively in our last book, *The Essential Oils Diet*, and we showed you how to use essential oils to help burn fat and boost your energy. We encourage you to read it from cover to cover. You'll gain wonderful insight into the toxins in many of our foods, including added sugar, saturated fats, additives, colorings, preservatives, artificial sweeteners, and more. Found mostly in processed foods, fast foods, and junk foods of every type, these bad ingredients are among the leading reasons chronic disease is on the rise.

Our Solutions

- Adding foods rich in *bioactive compounds* to your diet along with essential oils (which are also bioactive) to your routine can help ensure that you are getting the nourishment your body needs. Bioactive compounds are antioxidants and phytochemicals (plant-based chemicals) that help boost metabolism, prevent disease, and make you feel great. They are found mostly in plant foods—vegetables, fruits, healthy oils, nuts, and seeds.

- Avoid unsafe items like bleached sugars and white flour—and products made with them. Also on the list are vegetable oils like canola, which have been linked to numerous chronic diseases; commercial fruit juices (most store-bought versions are pasteurized, which renders them useless because they are void of nutrition); and artificial sweeteners.

- As for nonorganic, GMO meat products, these are absolute death foods. So eat organically grown or raised foods whenever possible. They are free of pesticides, insecticides, hormones, antibiotics, and other toxins known to cause harm to humans.

➜ To learn more about eating healthy, bioactive-rich foods and to discover how essential oils can enhance your diet, read our book *The Essential Oils Diet*. Go to EssentialOilsDiet.com to learn more.

ESSENTIAL OILS FOR IMMUNITY

With all of this being said, toxic exposure can harm the all-important immune system that keeps us well when it's strong. Fortunately, there are some very practical things we can do under the scope of aromatherapy to help mitigate these risks.

In addition to the lifestyle hacks we suggest in Appendix A, the aromatherapy approach we suggest you start to promote optimal immune function is our Immune-Boosting Blend and other recipes below. When mixed together, these oils have a synergistic effect, which research has shown can literally kill the flu virus!

IMMUNE-BOOSTING BLEND

10 drops cinnamon bark essential oil

10 drops clove bud essential oil

10 drops eucalyptus essential oil (*Eucalyptus globulus* or *E. radiata*)

continues

10 drops lemon essential oil

10 drops orange essential oil

10 drops rosemary essential oil

SUPPLIES

5 ml essential oils bottle with cap

1. Mix the essential oils in a 5 ml bottle.

2. Use as directed in the following recipes.

IMMUNE-BOOSTING CAPSULE

Makes 1 dose

2 to 4 drops Immune-Boosting Blend (page 49)

Organic virgin coconut oil or extra-virgin olive oil

SUPPLIES

Pipette

Size 00 vegan gel capsule

1. Using a pipette, drop the essential oil blend into the bottom half (the longer, narrower one) of the capsule. Fill this half to the brim with coconut or extra-virgin olive oil.

2. Fit the wider top half of the capsule over the bottom half and secure it snugly.

3. Immediately swallow the capsule with water after breakfast and/or dinner (see Note). Take once or twice daily during cold and flu season and monitor your symptoms.

NOTE: *Do not make and store these capsules for future use. This is not a long-term solution, and using it for more than three or four weeks at a time is not advisable. Be sure to consult with your health-care provider if you're taking immune-suppressing medications, blood thinners, or other medications that can interact with these essential oils. Discontinue use immediately if adverse reactions occur.*

DR. Z'S IMMUNE-BOOSTING SNACK

1 tablespoon unsweetened creamy almond or sunflower butter

1 serving liposomal vitamin C (this is a form of the vitamin that makes it highly absorbable by the body)

1 teaspoon raw honey (manuka is best)

1 teaspoon organic virgin coconut oil

1 to 2 drops Immune-Boosting Blend (page 49)

¼ teaspoon organic pumpkin pie spice

Tiny pinch of Himalayan pink sea salt

SUPPLIES

Small glass bowl

1. Mix all the ingredients together in a glass bowl.

2. Whenever you want a healthy immune-boosting snack, eat it solo or with some freshly cut veggie sticks or apple slices.

3. During cold and flu season, this recipe can replace the Immune-Boosting Capsule (page 50) remedy. Simply enjoy it twice daily at the onset of a cold, or once per day for prevention during cold and flu season.

NOTE: *Be sure to consult with your health-care provider if you're taking immune-suppressing medications, blood thinners, or other medications that can interact with these essential oils. Discontinue use immediately if adverse reactions occur.*

To watch us make this recipe and learn more about how to naturally boost your immune system with essential oils, go to EOApothecary.com.

IMMUNE-BOOSTING ROLL-ON

12 drops Immune-Boosting Blend (page 49)

Carrier oil of choice—jojoba and fractionated coconut oil absorb quickly and work best—as needed

SUPPLIES

10 ml glass roller bottle

1. Drop the essential oil blend into your roll-on bottle.

2. Fill the remaining space in the bottle with carrier oil.

3. Massage the mixture over your abdomen, chest, and back of the neck for immune support.

IMMUNE-BOOSTING BODY OIL

16 drops Immune-Boosting Blend (page 49)

2 ounces carrier oil or Mama Z's Oil Base (page 25)

SUPPLIES

Medium glass bowl

Lidded glass jar or lotion dispenser

1. Drop the essential oil blend into the glass bowl.

2. Add the carrier oil and mix until combined.

3. Apply after you shower to enhance your immune system or as a moisturizer or body oil throughout the day.

4. Store in a glass jar or lotion dispenser.

IMMUNE-BOOSTING DIFFUSER BLEND

6 drops Immune-Boosting Blend (page 49)

SUPPLIES

Diffuser

1. Fill your diffuser with purified water as directed in the manufacturer's instructions.

2. Add the essential oil blend.

3. Turn on the diffuser throughout the day to kill airborne pathogens and help boost your immune function.

IMMUNE-BOOSTING INHALER

20 drops Immune-Boosting Blend (page 49)

SUPPLIES

Precut organic cotton pad

Aromatherapy inhaler

1. Place a cotton pad in the inhaler tube.

2. Drop the essential oil blend directly onto the cotton pad in the tube. Alternatively, you can drop the blend into a glass bowl, roll the cotton pad in the oils to absorb them, and then insert it into the inhaler tube using tweezers.

3. When you're in public places, like the office, the local shopping mall, on an airplane, or wherever you want an aromatic escape and healthy immune boost, open the inhaler and take 10 deep breaths of the vapor from the tube. This recipe works well in an aromatherapy necklace.

IMPORTANT NOTE ON TELOMERE LENGTH, IMMUNITY, AND AGING

Regrettably, one of the enormous opponents of the immune system is also unalterable: length of life. As the body ages, immune functions dwindle. Lymphocytes are not as widespread, and their response to invaders is sluggish. But while we can't stop time, we can actively strive to turn back its influence.

One well-researched way to do this might be to lengthen our telomeres. Structurally, telomeres are the protective caps at the end of our chromosomes. They have been compared to the plastic caps at the end of shoelaces, and they help prevent our DNA from degrading. The length of our telomeres predicts the length of healthy life.

Studies over twenty years have shown that telomeres shorten with age, and shortened telomeres have been associated with several chronic diseases, including cancer and cardiovascular disease. That's where an enzyme called telomerase comes in. It's found in certain cells and helps prevent too much wear and tear, including shortening of your telomeres. Telomerase does this by adding additional telomere sequences to the ends of your chromosomes.

Given the links between telomere shortening and disease, some people are now interested in finding ways to lengthen their telomeres. But is this even possible?

Research surrounding telomere lengthening is still very new. But so far, the results do show some promise. We might be able to lengthen our telomeres and preserve telomerase through simple lifestyle changes, including the following:

- Following a healthy diet
- Getting regular exercise
- Managing stress through activities such as yoga and support groups
- Using essential oils. Preliminary research has shown that basil, clove, and rosemary essential oils contain telomere-protective effects and can help prevent and treat damage caused by environmental toxins. These oils seem to exert their benefits by reducing oxidative stress (a threat to telomere length and to immunity) and directly absorbing cell-damaging free radicals.

So, if you are looking for a way to live a more youthful life, using natural remedies like essential oils and using healthy lifestyle strategies are musts!

Using Essential Oils for Chronic Conditions

I n this section, we cover some of the most prevalent chronic health conditions today. Not always referred to as "chronic diseases" by global health agencies, these issues often precipitate or exacerbate the main causes of death worldwide.

For all of the essential oils listed in this section, and in Part 3 for that matter, we have decided to use common English names instead of Latin botanical names for ease and consistency.

We acknowledge that there are different chemotypes and species of plants. We are also fully aware that there are unique indigenous sources and harvest locations, which alter the plant chemistry. Take orange essential oil, for instance. It's probably the most complicated of all oils on the market today.

The botanical name for orange is *Citrus sinensis*, and common origins include California, Belize, Florida, Greece, and Italy. Manufacturers commonly label their orange essential oil as orange, blood orange, sweet orange, or wild orange—all the while referring to the botanical name of *Citrus sinensis*!

It is also very rare to see scientists reveal any detail other than the fact that they are evaluating "orange oil" or *Citrus sinensis* in their research studies. Meaning, when the medical literature reports that researchers are investigating *Citrus sinensis* or "orange oil," we don't know if they are referring to blood, sweet, or wild orange. Thus, we are left to assume that all varieties of *Citrus sinensis* referred to are interchangeable for the purposes found in this book.

With that said, we offer suggestions as to which orange you should use throughout the book based on our own experience. However, if you only have "wild" orange on hand, for instance, and the remedy calls for "sweet" orange, you'll be fine if you use wild orange.

Same with *Eucalyptus globulus* and *E. radiata* when eucalyptus is indicated. Or, one of the many different types of frankincense: *Boswellia carterii, B. sacra, B. frereana, B. rivae, B. neglecta, B. papyrifera, B. serrata.*

Of course, there are significant differences in the chemical makeup of cinnamon bark versus cinnamon leaf, because the oil is extracted from different plant parts, so we're sure to indicate whether cinnamon leaf or bark is indicated.

For the most part, researchers aren't concerned with studying various chemotypes and species. The bottom line is that we let the research do the talking, and we're simply reporting what the scientists are evaluating.

Chapter 4

Sleep Disorders and Insomnia

// I can't sleep. I toss and turn all night. Doctor, can you give me a pill or something to help me sleep?"

That's a question physicians hear often, and there are reasons for it.

Due to stress, shift work, illnesses, or sleep disorders, many people of all ages, income levels, and occupations get only a fraction of the sleep their weary bodies need.

In America, an estimated fifty to seventy million people (15 to 20 percent) suffer from sleep disorders. But don't think that this is an American problem. A recent study in the Netherlands uncovered that 27.3 percent of all people age twelve and above had some type of sleeping disorder.

We literally have a global epidemic on our hands, and this is something we all need to take seriously because the ramifications of sleep deprivation are sobering.

As you'll see over and over again in this book, one chronic health condition can increase your risk of developing another. Chronic insufficient and perpetual short sleep (less than seven hours per twenty-four-hour period) is:

- Associated with a range of negative health and social outcomes, including poor performance at school and at work.

- The known reason of several leading causes of death in the United States: cardiovascular disease, COPD, cancer, cerebrovascular disease, accidents, diabetes, kidney disease, arthritis, sepsis, Alzheimer's disease, and hypertension.
- Responsible for causing roughly 5 percent of all obesity cases in adults.
- Known to cause a tenfold increased risk of premature death.

AT LEAST SEVEN HOURS? EVERY SINGLE NIGHT?

Believe it not, the research is clear: adults need at least seven or more hours of sleep per night to experience optimal health and well-being. It's just how we're wired, and you cannot escape it. Eventually, it'll catch up with you. You can thank your circadian rhythm for that.

CIRCADIAN RHYTHM

Also known as your sleep/wake cycle, your circadian rhythm is basically a twenty-four-hour internal clock that runs in the background of your brain and cycles between alertness and sleepiness at regular intervals. Brainwave activity, hormone production, cell regeneration, and other important biological processes are determined by this cycle.

Working best when you have regular sleep habits, your circadian rhythm is disrupted when things get in the way, like jet lag, daylight savings time, or pulling an all-nighter. This makes you feel out of sorts, groggy, and irritable; can make it harder to pay attention; and will affect your eating habits and bowel regularity.

As you age, your sleep/wake cycle will most likely change. This is why it's critical that you pay close attention to your body and notice if abnormal feelings of alertness and drowsiness come up again and again, which may suggest that your cycle is adapting.

One of the best ways to support your circadian rhythm is to get proper sleep, and that can vary with age. The National Sleep Foundation compiled recommendations for sleep durations for people of all ages, and here is what they recommend:

- **Newborns (0 to 3 months):** 14 to 17 hours each day
- **Infants (4 to 11 months):** 12 to 15 hours
- **Toddlers (1 to 2 years):** 11 to 14 hours
- **Preschoolers (3 to 5):** 10 to 13 hours
- **School-age children (6 to 13):** 9 to 11 hours
- **Teenagers (14 to 17):** 8 to 10 hours
- **Younger adults (18 to 25):** 7 to 9 hours
- **Adults (26 to 64):** 7 to 9 hours
- **Older adults (65-plus):** 7 to 8 hours

Not getting seven hours of sleep every night? You're in good company.

According to the CDC, more than one-third of Americans don't get enough sleep. Princess Cruises, however, reports a much higher number: 53 percent.

In fact, according to Princess Cruises' tenth annual Relaxation Report published in 2019, America's numbers are on par with the rest of the world. More than half (52 percent) of adults worldwide reported they get less sleep than they need on an average night, and 80 percent of adults say they use weekend days to make up for sleep lost during the week.

A single night without sleep isn't usually a big deal, but too many sleepless nights can lead to more serious conditions. Longer term, too little sleep contributes to increased mortality and has been linked to most of the chronic diseases listed in this book. The big takeaway here is to practice good sleep habits, so that insomnia doesn't hijack your health or life.

Unfortunately, many people with sleep disorders are prescribed sedative drugs like benzodiazepines, which were originally designed to reduce anxiety. There are problems with these drugs.

An article published in the *British Medical Journal* states, "An estimated 6% to 10% of US adults took a hypnotic drug for poor sleep." That is a ton of people, especially considering the side effects! Benzodiazepine use has been associated with a 35 percent increase in developing cancer. In addition to the increased cancer risk, the big problem with prescribing benzodiazepines is that they are highly addictive.

Regarding over-the-counter drugs, most of those sleeping pills are anti-histamines. There's no proof that they work for insomnia, and they can cause some drowsiness the next day. Essential oils work much better and without side effects!

ARE YOU GETTING YOUR DAY OF REST?

Remember the Sabbath day and keep it holy. Six days you shall labor and do all your work, but the seventh day is a Sabbath to the Lord your God. On it you shall not do any work. . . . For in six days the Lord made heaven and earth, the sea, and all that is in them, and rested on the seventh day. Therefore, the Lord blessed the Sabbath day and made it holy.

—Exodus 20:8–11

Rest and proper sleep are part of God's design. Always was and always will be. We're made in His image, right? And, if He rested on the seventh day, then that means that we should, too. Don't you agree?

Obviously, He didn't *need* to rest. He was leading by example. And, when He included not working on the Sabbath as one of the Ten Commandments, He meant it.

Sure, pulling an all-nighter once in a while to get a project done or binge-watch a new show you found on Netflix is one thing (#guilty), but perpetually depriving yourself of sleep day after day, year after year, is a disaster waiting to happen.

And don't believe that because you "feel" fine after only getting five hours of sleep, that's it's still okay. That's not how God designed you. He intended for us to rest, but our tendency is to the contrary.

Like the Bible says, "Do not be deceived, God is not mocked; for whatever a man sows, that he will also reap" (Galatians 6:7).

We have been pushed by society to work all the time (school work, house work, yard work, business work—work, work, work) that we literally forget to rest. But we should not forget about the fourth commandment: remember the Sabbath day and keep it holy.

Taking a day off is a great way to unwind, let go, and give your body (and mind) time to recoup from the stressors of life.

EASY LIFESTYLE HABITS FOR OVERCOMING INSOMNIA

Can't sleep? Start with these easy tips:

Stick to a regular sleep/wake schedule. Make an effort to go to bed and wake up at roughly the same time every day. This reinforces your body's natural sleep/wake cycle.

Start your day off right. Might seem counterintuitive, but the manner in which you begin your day oftentimes mirrors how you will end it. Start off hurried, stressed, overwhelmed, groggy, and tired and you'll most likely crash into bed the same way. Set the tone with a short prayer, meditation, or positive affirmation. Having an uplifting essential oils routine can do wonders for you as well. Here's a list of some of the oils that have traditionally been used to increase alertness and get you ready to move.

Bay laurel	May chang (*Litsea cubeba*)
Bergamot	Mountain savory
Camphor	Orange
Eucalyptus	Peppermint
Grapefruit	Pine
Key lime	Ravensara
Lemon	Ravintsara
Lemon eucalyptus	Rosemary
Lemon myrtle	Spearmint
Lemon tea tree	Tea tree
Lemongrass	Wintergreen
Lime	

Take a midday nap. Research has shown that, for healthy younger people, taking a short nap can reduce sleepiness, enhance memory consolidation, prepare your mind for subsequent learning, and boost executive functioning and is linked to emotional well-being. Be careful not to overdo it, however, as napping too long (more than thirty minutes) or too often may prove to be counterproductive.

Limit your fluid intake at night. Try to avoid liquids an hour before bedtime so that you don't wake up to use the toilet. But stay well hydrated for the rest of the day. And don't forget not to drink coffee or caffeinated beverages after 2 p.m.

End the day with herbal tea. Make your last drink of the evening a nice cup of soothing caffeine-free Roman chamomile, valerian, or passionflower tea. For an extra dose of calm, add a drop of Roman chamomile or lavender essential oil and 1 teaspoon raw honey, which contains tryptophan (an amino acid precursor to the sleep-inducing serotonin and melatonin). For an added boost of sleepy time, add some CBD for a potent natural sleep remedy. We call this our Bee-Powered Sleepy Tea—check out the recipe on page 70.

Avoid late-night eating. Having a heavy or large meal within a couple of hours of bedtime can cause discomfort that might keep you awake. A little snack is okay, however. A small helping of nuts, bananas, dates, or tuna can help with a decent night's sleep. These foods are high in nutrients that promote sleep. The rule of thumb is don't eat after 7 p.m.

Avoid nighttime technology. This means no computer games, using your phone, or watching TV for at least thirty minutes prior to bedtime. Technology emits blue light, which interferes with brain signals that help you sleep. Plus, your body thinks you're not ready for sleep when you're engaged in these activities.

Create a tranquil sleep environment. Declutter your bedroom. Remove computers and TVs, if possible (or at least turn them off prior to bedtime.) Turn off your Wi-Fi router and put your phone on "airplane mode." These electromagnetic frequencies can disturb your sleep cycle. Keep your bedroom at a cool temperature; it's conducive to a good night's sleep. And make sure your bedroom is as dark as possible.

Be comfortable in bed. Hard mattresses aren't always the best. Comfort also extends to what you wear. Don't sleep in tight-fitting clothes. They can cause irritation and sweating and otherwise disturb your sleep.

Don't lose your temper at bedtime. Your nerves will be firing and stress hormones like cortisol will be surging when they're supposed to be dialing down. Designate the bedroom as a no-argument zone and decide with your partner that no one goes to bed angry. Issues can be resolved in the morning.

Take a warm bath. It always relaxes the body, especially when you add essential oils to your bathwater. See page 66 for our favorite aromatherapy bath recipe—give it a try!

Practice your faith or spirituality. There's no better way to settle down for bed than with prayer, spiritual reflection, and/or meditation. Act intentionally to always end the day on a positive note by starting a gratitude journal. Each night before you go to bed, write down two or three things that you are grateful for. It will put the challenges of the day into perspective, and you'll be surprised at how many good things happen to you each and every day as you look back at months' and years' worth of entries!

Diffusing essential oils during your faith practice will enhance the experience. Here's a list of some of the oils that have traditionally been used for mental clarity, meditation, and mindfulness. Chances are you have a couple of these on hand!

Amyris	Lime
Angelica root	Myrrh
Bergamot	Neroli
Buddha wood	Opoponax
Cedarwood	Orange
Chamomile, Roman or German	Palmarosa
Elemi	Palo santo
Frankincense	Patchouli
Helichrysum	Peru balsam
Key lime	Petitgrain
Lavender	Rose
Lemon	Rosemary

| Sandalwood | Valerian |
| Vitex | Ylang ylang |

If you decide to adjust your lifestyle for better sleep, don't try to change everything in one night. Cementing new habits can take time, and you don't want to overwhelm yourself with too many changes at once. In fact, research suggests it takes on average sixty-six days to form a new habit, so give yourself some grace and commit to long-term success, not fleeting victories.

THE ESSENTIAL OILS APPROACH FOR RESTFUL SLEEP

People across the globe have traditionally used natural remedies like essential oils for sleep. We certainly need to get back to those roots before sleep disorders ruin everyone's health!

Unlike common sleep aids and benzodiazepines, there are virtually no side effects when you use essential oils for sleeping. In the words of a 2014 systematic review of the literature, "A majority of the study findings suggested a positive effect of essential oils for sleep. Lavender was the most frequently studied essential oil. No adverse events were reported."

In fact, oils can possibly help get people off of drugs! Just be sure to consult with your physician, as going cold turkey can cause serious harm and withdrawal symptoms.

Here are some of the most popular essential oils that have been proven to aid sleep.

STOP Before you start implementing these essential oils for sleep, be sure to review the known drug interaction chart in Appendix B and consult with your physician if you're currently taking any medications. Also, don't forget that using essential oils while living a "fast food" lifestyle is like taking one step forward but two steps back! In other words, for essential oils to help you enjoy abundant health and wellness—free from chronic disease—it is vital to use them within the context of a healthy lifestyle. Go to Appendix A for our favorite "Disease-Busting Healthy Lifestyle Hacks" to learn more!

1. Lavender

In addition to its stress-reducing benefits, lavender is a powerful natural sleep aid. The chemical components of lavender have been shown to enter the bloodstream within five minutes of massaging the oil on the skin, so you can count on it working quickly as it relaxes your mind and body.

You can also diffuse lavender oil in your bedroom (it's safe for kids, too!). Research has shown that diffusion or inhalation of lavender oil has helped heart patients and women in midlife combat insomnia and improve sleep quality.

One interesting study from Korea explored the effects of lavender oil on female college students struggling with insomnia and depression. The students fell asleep more quickly, experienced less insomnia, and were more satisfied with their sleep when using the oil. The use of lavender oil also lessened the severity of their depression.

Since a clinical trial was conducted in the early 1990s, we have known that sleep duration significantly decreases in older patients who are dependent on benzodiazepines. However, once lavender aromatherapy was introduced into their lives, their sleep quality and duration could be restored to previous levels, despite not being on the drugs. According to the researchers who conducted this research, "This study suggested that ambient lavender oil might be used as a temporary relief from continued medication for insomnia and reduces the side-effects of these drugs." Note of caution: Be sure never to take yourself off benzodiazepines without medical guidance, because the side effects can be quite severe.

And if you're worried about lavender being a long-lasting sedative that will make you groggy upon waking, know that most of the lavender will leave your bloodstream within ninety minutes. By that time, you should be sound asleep!

Application: Make our Deep Sleep Blend and accompanying recipes for a total spirit, soul, and body approach to sound, rejuvenating sleep.

DEEP SLEEP BLEND

Of all the blends that we have formulated and have recommended to people for sleep, we keep going back to this one. Tried and true, it has proven an invaluable nighttime staple to help our Natural Living Family enjoy deep, restful sleep.

30 drops lavender essential oil
20 drops Roman chamomile essential oil
10 drops vetiver essential oil

continues

SUPPLIES

Small glass jar with cap

1. Drop the essential oils into the jar, cap, and shake to mix thoroughly.
2. Use as directed in the following recipes.

DEEP SLEEP SPRITZER

10 drops organic 190-proof grain alcohol

10 drops Deep Sleep Blend (page 65)

10 drops witch hazel

Distilled water, as needed

SUPPLIES

1-ounce spray bottle

1. Mix the grain alcohol, essential oil blend, and witch hazel in the spray bottle.
2. Fill with distilled water and shake gently to mix well.
3. Spray on your pillow and sheets 5 minutes before going to bed for an aroma-therapy sleep treatment.

NOTE: *This water-based formula will last for a couple of weeks. We've used it for as long as two months and have not noticed bacterial overgrowth, which can happen with any water-based product. This may not be obvious at first, but the smell will become rancid, and you will notice a change in color if it is contaminated.*

DEEP SLEEP EVENING BATH

10 drops Deep Sleep Blend (page 65)

1 tablespoon jojoba oil

1 cup plain Epsom salts

¼ cup unfiltered, raw apple cider vinegar

SUPPLIES

Medium glass bowl

1. Mix the essential oil blend and jojoba oil in a glass bowl.

2. Add the Epsom salts and vinegar and mix thoroughly.

3. Fill your bathtub with the warmest water you can stand.

4. Slowly pour the mixture into the running water.

5. Soak your whole body for 20 to 30 minutes.

6. Exit the bath slowly by first sitting up, then kneeling, and finally standing to prevent feeling faint.

DEEP SLEEP MASSAGE OIL

16 drops Deep Sleep Blend (page 65)

2 ounces carrier oil or Mama Z's Oil Base (page 25)

SUPPLIES

Medium glass bowl

Lidded glass jar or lotion dispenser

1. Drop the essential oil blend into a glass bowl.

2. Add the carrier oil and mix thoroughly.

3. Right before bed, give yourself and your loved ones a soothing foot, shoulder, and/or neck massage. (The mixture is also safe for kids and pets.)

4. Store in a glass jar or lotion dispenser.

DEEP SLEEP ROLL-ON BLEND

12 drops Deep Sleep Blend (page 65)

Carrier oil of choice—jojoba and fractionated coconut oil absorb quickly and
  work best—as needed

SUPPLIES

10 ml glass roller bottle

1. Drop the essential oil blend into your roll-on bottle.

2. Fill the bottle with a carrier oil and shake well.

continues

3. Massage your neck, shoulders, hands, wrists, feet, and ankles with the oil before bed. (The mixture is safe for kids and pets.)

4. While spending a few minutes giving yourself a gentle massage, reflect on the day and focus on at least one thing that you are grateful for.

DEEP SLEEP DIFFUSER BLEND

6 drops Deep Sleep Blend (page 65)

SUPPLIES

Diffuser

1. Fill your diffuser with purified water as directed in the manufacturer's instructions.

2. Add the essential oil blend.

3. Turn on the diffuser 10 to 20 minutes before you go to bed, setting it to run through the night.

DEEP SLEEP INHALER

20 drops Deep Sleep Blend (page 65)

SUPPLIES

Precut organic cotton pad

Aromatherapy inhaler

1. Place a cotton pad in the inhaler tube.

2. Drop the essential oil blend directly onto the cotton pad in the tube. Alternatively, you can drop the blend into a glass bowl, roll the cotton pad in the oils to absorb them, and then insert it into the inhaler tube using tweezers.

3. While in bed, open the inhaler and take deep breaths of the vapors from the tube for about 2 minutes.

2. Ylang Ylang

Do you have trouble getting to sleep rather than staying asleep? If so, try ylang ylang. A study from the Human Cognitive Neuroscience Unit at the UK's University of

Northumbria found that ylang ylang essential oil slowed down the brain's processing speed among participants, so ylang ylang might a be a useful oil to diffuse before bed if you experience racing thoughts while you're trying to fall asleep.

Ylang ylang (along with sandalwood) is a known harmonizer, meaning it is an adaptive, whatever-you-need kind of oil and can help the body meet the needs that it's facing.

Application: Try our Harmony Diffuser Blend for a clear, harmonizing escape from anxious thoughts and stress so you can close out the day writing in your gratitude journal with peace of mind.

HARMONY DIFFUSER BLEND

2 drops orange essential oil

2 drops frankincense essential oil

1 drop sandalwood essential oil

1 drop ylang ylang essential oil

SUPPLIES

Diffuser

1. Fill your diffuser with purified water as directed in the manufacturer's instructions.

2. Add the essential oils.

3. Turn on the diffuser 10 to 20 minutes before you go to bed, setting the diffuser to run through the night.

3. Roman Chamomile

If you've been dealing with insomnia for a while, maybe you've tried sipping a cup of chamomile tea to help you sleep. Although this is beneficial, you may find Roman chamomile essential oil to be more effective.

Like many essential oils, this one has a long history of use. For more than two thousand years, Roman chamomile has been used for cosmetic purposes such as shampoo, deodorant, and perfume. The Greeks treated fevers and female health conditions with it. The Romans used it for flavoring foods, building courage, fighting disease, and increasing life span. Early American settlers administered it to treat pain, poor digestion, and allergies.

Today, Roman chamomile essential oil is used for an array of health issues. It is particularly helpful in treating sleep disorders. When you inhale the oil, hormones that induce stress are lowered, bringing on relaxation. As demonstrated in a 2006 study, the effects of inhaling the oil promoted sleep with calmness and drowsiness among healthy volunteers.

Application: Add 2 drops of this oil to some sweet almond oil for a pre-bedtime massage. Or diffuse 3 or 4 drops of Roman chamomile in your bedroom as you prepare for sleep. If you want an extra-strength sleep aid, make our Bee-Powered Sleepy Tea.

BEE-POWERED SLEEPY TEA

Makes 1 serving

Organic chamomile tea (1 tea bag or 2 teaspoons loose-leaf tea)

1 cup boiling water

1 teaspoon raw honey

1 dose full-spectrum CBD (follow manufacturer's instructions for dosage)

1 drop Roman chamomile essential oil

2 tablespoons unsweetened vanilla almond milk or coconut milk (optional)

1. In a mug or teapot, steep the tea and boiling water for 5 minutes.
2. In separate mug, mix together the honey, CBD, and essential oil.
3. Remove the tea bag or strain the tea, pour it into the mug, and add milk, if desired.
4. Take this remedy an hour before you go to bed to promote deep sleep.

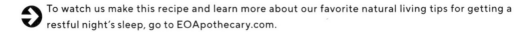 To watch us make this recipe and learn more about our favorite natural living tips for getting a restful night's sleep, go to EOApothecary.com.

4. Sweet Marjoram

This oil contains several compounds that may aid sleep, while inducing emotional calming and muscle relaxation. A 2017 study evaluated sweet marjoram aromatherapy massage given to nurses who worked on a night shift.

The nurses removed all accessories and electronics and then relaxed, lying down, in an aromatherapy room for five minutes with slow music in the background. Then they received a head, shoulders, and neck massage for twenty-five minutes using a 2 percent dilution of sweet marjoram and sweet almond oil. Afterward, the nurses drank a cup of warm water and were instructed to rest for an additional thirty minutes. As you'd expect, this routine was like taking a sleeping pill! Compared to the control group, the aromatherapy massage helped the nurses enjoy a "significant increase" in sleep quality and a decrease in sleep disturbances and daytime dysfunction.

The reason we like this study is because it highlights the significance of creating a ritual to improve sleep quality. Calming music, rest, aromatherapy massage, drinking warm water—these are all rituals, which are simply sequences of repeatable acts. They all played a part in the success that sweet marjoram has on improving sleep quality and suggest that, if we really want to change our sleep pattern for the better, we need to put in some work and intentionally make it happen.

Application: Take a moment and design what your ideal sleep routine will look like. Consider adding a sweet marjoram foot and shoulder rub as part of the formula; make a soothing massage oil by simply mixing 12 drops of sweet marjoram essential oil with 1 ounce of your favorite carrier oil!

5. Valerian

When you've tossed and turned all night, you'll probably try just about anything to get some sleep. Valerian to your rescue.

Known for its sedative effect, valerian herb is oftentimes paired with hops in the dried supplement industry because they are especially effective when used together, and sleep experts regularly recommend this strategy.

Distilled from a tall, flowering grassland plant, the essential oil that's extracted from valerian contains natural chemicals that inhibit the enzyme-induced breakdown of the calming neurotransmitter gamma-aminobutyric acid (GABA) in the brain, resulting in sedation. Although some conflicting studies exist, most research shows that taking valerian can reduce the amount of time it takes to fall asleep by fifteen to twenty minutes. Valerian has also been shown to greatly improve sleep quality in postmenopausal women.

Taking valerian might also improve the sleep quality of people who are withdrawing from the use of sleeping pills.

Application: Modify the Deep Sleep Blend (page 65) by replacing vetiver with valerian, and enjoy an alternate to the evening bath, massage oil, roll-on, diffuser, and inhaler recipes above.

6. Rose

Do your children have trouble getting to sleep? Try rose essential oil. A study from Iran showed that children exposed to rose oil reduced resistance to sleep, nightmares, waking in the night, and difficulty waking in the morning. The children inhaled five drops of rose oil on a cotton ball before sleep for twenty minutes over two weeks.

Application: Diffuse rose before bed by pairing it with one of these enchanting blends:

- 2 drops frankincense, 2 drops myrrh, 1 drop rose
- 2 drops patchouli, 2 drops vetiver, 1 drop rose
- 4 drops sandalwood, 2 drops rose
- 3 drops bergamot, 2 drops orange, 1 drop rose
- 4 drops lavender, 1 drop sweet marjoram, 1 drop rose
- 2 drops ylang ylang, 2 drops neroli, 2 drops rose

7. Vetiver

Quickly becoming a popular and in-demand oil, vetiver has sleep-inducing properties that can be incredibly powerful. Native to India and cultivated in other tropical areas, the herb is rich in sesquiterpenes that help calm your emotions and improve mental well-being.

Using vetiver oil in a diffuser while you sleep could help improve your breathing patterns. A small 2010 study measured the response of thirty-six people with sleep apnea who were exposed to differing aromas during their sleep. Vetiver oil increased the quality of exhalation and decreased inhalation when sleeping-study participants detected it. This could mean vetiver oil might help people who snore heavily (a sign of sleep apnea).

Application: Make our Deep Sleep Blend (page 65) and the accompanying recipes to enjoy vetiver-powered sleep!

8. Cedarwood

For centuries, cedarwood has been used to treat skin and hair conditions, but growing evidence suggests it may also be effective for insomnia. Derived from the bark of cedar trees, this essential oil contains cedrol, which has been found to produce a sedative effect, making it useful for occasional bouts of insomnia. There are a few types of cedarwood you'll generally see on the market, referred to as atlas cedarwood and Himalayan cedarwood, that come from China, Morocco, Nepal, and the United States. Even though people swear by one over the other, we have found them to be so similar that it's truly a matter of preference when it comes to our purposes of making blends for chronic diseases.

A small study showed that when cedarwood was placed on the pillows of older adults with dementia, the participants slept longer and were less likely to experience early morning awakening.

Not just for your home sauna, cedarwood's earthy scent blends well with other wood oils and resins.

Application: Try our Earthy Wood Blend (page 74) for serene, meditative sleep.

EARTHY WOOD BLEND

20 drops cedarwood essential oil

20 drops Douglas fir essential oil

10 drops pine essential oil

10 drops sandalwood essential oil

SUPPLIES

5 ml bottle with cap

1. Mix the essential oils in a 5 ml bottle.
2. Use as an alternative to the Deep Sleep Blend (page 65) in the recipes above.

9. Sandalwood

Sourced from various types of sandalwood trees, sandalwood essential oil contains aromatic compounds thought to be beneficial to health—and it shows promise as a sleep aid. The various types of sandalwood that you'll generally find on the market come from Australia, East India, and Hawaii. Though, like cedarwood, some people swear by one over the other, we have found them to be so similar that it's truly a matter of preference.

According to a 2007 animal study published in the *Japanese Journal of Psychopharmacology*, researchers noted that the oil contains beta-santalol, which had a mild sedative effect in lab rats when inhaled. The compound decreased waking time and increased rapid eye movement (REM), consistent with deep sleep.

As for human use, this oil was tested at an Indonesian orphanage, where many adolescents had difficulty sleeping. The results showed that while only 13.6 percent of these children reported sound sleep before aromatherapy, that number improved to 45.5 percent afterward.

Application: For massage purposes, add between 9 and 18 drops of sandalwood oil to an ounce of carrier oil. Sandalwood oil can be inhaled after sprinkling a few drops onto a cotton ball or by using a diffuser. Sandalwood oil can also be added to your bathwater for a calming soak.

TO CPAP OR NOT TO CPAP

One of the most common questions we field from our online community in terms of sleep is whether or not essential oils are safe to use with a CPAP machine.

The quick answer to this question is no, for two reasons.

First, commonly used to treat obstructive sleep apnea, continuous positive airway pressure (CPAP) therapy utilizes a hose and mask (or nosepiece) to deliver a constant and steady flow of air pressure. CPAP machines are not designed to withstand the potentially corrosive nature of essential oils. As we mentioned in earlier chapters, never use essential oils in plastic containers unless they are specially designed for such use, and CPAP parts can be damaged if they come in contact with essential oils.

Simply put, just don't do it.

Second, using essential oils with CPAP therapy poses more safety concerns than potential benefits. In the words of one CPAP manufacturer, "Putting essential oils in your CPAP machine is not safe. It does not matter if you put them in the machine itself, in the hose, on the mask, in the filter, or the CPAP humidifier."

The device propels air into your respiratory tract to keep your breathing steady while you sleep and, while using it, you end up inhaling air and steam. To treat sleep apnea, a considerable amount of air pressure is required to open your airway. According to an interview with Dr. Andrew Weil, Dr. Randy Horwitz from the Arizona Center for Integrative Medicine warns, "If you add essential oils to the CPAP machine, the device could propel droplets of the oil deep into your lungs [and] even a small amount might cause lung irritation."

One proposed solution we've seen online is to place aromatherapy pads or a diffuser near the air intake on the CPAP machine. In theory, as the machine draws in the air, it also draws in the volatile organic compounds without any of the oil entering the machine.

We don't recommend it. Yes, it protects the machine from harm, but there's zero research to substantiate the therapeutic efficacy of this approach. In fact, the volatile organic compounds (VOCs) can still irritate your lungs if you employ this method.

What's the solution for people with sleep apnea?

We recommend diffusing some sleepy-time essential oils thirty to sixty minutes before bedtime and massaging your favorite calming blend into your feet, shoulders, and neck before you sleep.

Other essential oils that promote better sleep quality include bergamot, lemon, mandarin orange, bitter orange, patchouli, angelica root, ravensara, juniper berry, cumin, sweet thyme, clary sage, Melissa (lemon balm), basil, may chang, and myrtle. Combining popular and complementary oils can provide synergistic effects. For example, a blend of lavender, sweet marjoram, and ylang ylang may reduce insomnia as well as stress, anxiety, and blood pressure, contributing to a better night's sleep. We see this over and over again in the medical literature.

Getting a better night's sleep is arguably the most overlooked but effective way to keep your body healthy. With quality sleep, you'll be able to recuperate and regenerate beautifully from long days full of stressors and worries. Let essential oils help you get the sleep you need!

If, after trying a few of the strategies in this chapter, you are still not enjoying the sleep that you need to feel rested and energized when you wake up in the morning, then there is probably a deeper issue that needs to be addressed. Most likely you have some anxiety and stress in your life that needs to be managed, and it is with that in mind that we move on to the next chapter.

Chapter 5

Stress and Anxiety

One immutable truth of life is that none of us can escape stress. We are exposed to stress every day in many ways. Of course, it's a necessary reaction to threats—physical, emotional, existential—and it's both natural and even healthy to experience it from time to time. When stress or anxiety is occasional, we are often able to cope with it in ways that reduce its hold on us. But when stress is unrelenting or we are not able to turn down our reactiveness to its presence, it can be overwhelming. And unhealthy. Indeed, stress is a contributing cause of most chronic diseases.

THE NUMBER ONE KILLER, REALLY?

The argument can be made that emotional stress is actually the number one underlying cause of death worldwide.

In the United States, for instance, it is a primary contributing factor to the six leading causes of death: accidental injuries, cancer, cirrhosis of the liver, coronary heart disease, respiratory disorders, and suicide. It has been reported that 75 to 90 percent of all doctor's visits and as much as 90 percent of illness and disease are stress related. According to the National Institute of Mental Health, chronic, unresolved stress can damage our immune, digestive, and reproductive systems and disrupt sleep. That's why long-standing stress has been linked to chronic diseases such as cardiovascular disease, hypertension, diabetes, depression, obesity, menstrual problems, acne, eczema, and mental health disorders like anxiety and panic attacks.

We see this in other nations as well. According to the Meridian Stress Management Consultancy, nearly 180,000 people in the United Kingdom die each year from some form of stress-related illness.

EMBRACING EMOTIONAL STRESS

It's important to keep in mind that not all stress is bad. In fact, it can be quite healthy for us!

Case in point: weightlifting and resistance training. While exercising, you physically stress and break down muscle fibers by causing small tears or "microtraumas." In turn, your body responds by healing those tears and making wounded muscles larger to prevent further injury. As you continue to train, your body continues to build muscle tissue as protection layer upon layer, thus building your strength and physique.

In the same way, we need to experience emotional stress periodically to become stronger and more resilient so we can successfully weather the inevitable storms of life. Traffic jams, arguments with your spouse, losing a loved one, a bad day at work, a failed business opportunity, and occasional money problems are all normal acute stressors that (if handled properly) will make us stronger in the end.

We're sure you've heard the phrase "God will not give you more than you can handle," right? Well, we wholeheartedly believe in that sentiment and in the idea that "micro-stressors" throughout our lives protect us from becoming overburdened and help train us to be resilient and mature so we can be a source of hope and strength for others.

STRESS VERSUS ANXIETY

From the outside looking in, it can be tough to differentiate between stress and anxiety. Think of it this way: stress is caused by a challenge, or stressor, to your system. It is generally a short-term experience. Anxiety, on the other hand, is a reaction to the stressor, involving feelings of apprehension, worry, or fear and is often accompanied by a sense of impending doom. Anxiety doesn't fade after the stressor is gone. It lingers for a bit and can cause significant harm to relationships, family, our work, and other important areas of life.

It's difficult to measure "stress," as it is more of a subjective feeling, but anxiety is much more palpable. Usually accompanied by physical symptoms, such as a racing heart or knots in your stomach, anxiety symptoms vary in intensity depending on the stressor. Panic attacks are one such symptom and generally climax at ten minutes or less and then begin to subside.

It's important to know if you suffer from an anxiety disorder or panic attacks because, due to the intensity of the symptoms, they tend to mimic a plethora of unrelated health conditions like heart disease, thyroid problems, and breathing disorders. This is one of the primary reasons people suffering from panic attacks often visit the emergency room or their doctor's office, convinced they have a life-threatening issue.

If you've ever experienced significant stress, anxiety, or panic attacks, rest assured you're not alone. Anxiety—the most common of all mental disorders—currently affects 40 million Americans age eighteen and older and 264 million people globally. And according to a recent American Psychological Association survey, one-third of adults report feeling nervous or anxious (36 percent), irritable or angry (35 percent), and fatigued (34 percent) due to their stress.

Yes, it's normal (and healthy) to experience stress occasionally, and feeling anxious from time to time is okay. What gets people in trouble is when the "acute" becomes "chronic."

Excessive, prolonged worry and anxiety will wear you down physically, emotionally, mentally, and spiritually. The tell-tale sign that you have a more advanced problem requiring extra attention is when anxious feelings interfere with your day-to-day activities. This may indicate that you are dealing with something more serious: a generalized anxiety disorder.

THE CONVENTIONAL MEDICAL APPROACH TO STRESS

We must say that we are pleasantly surprised by the conventional medical recommendations to folks who are trying to manage stress. The Mayo Clinic, for example, offers this well-balanced approach:

- Don't feel that you have to figure it out on your own. Seek help and support from family and friends, whether you need someone to listen to you, help with childcare, or a ride to work when your car's in the shop.
- Many people benefit from practices such as deep breathing, tai chi, yoga, meditation, or being in nature.
- Set aside time for yourself. Get a massage, soak in a bubble bath, dance, listen to music, watch a comedy—whatever helps you relax. Maintaining a healthy lifestyle will help you manage stress.
- Eat a healthy diet, exercise regularly, and get enough sleep.
- Make a conscious effort to spend less time in front of a screen—television, tablet, computer, and phone—and more time relaxing. Stress won't disappear from your life.
- Stress management needs to be ongoing. By paying attention to what causes your stress and practicing ways to relax, you can counter some of the bad effects of stress and increase your ability to cope with challenges.

Five Missing Gems

There are only five things that we'd add to those stress management recommendations:

1. Aromatherapy (more on that below)
2. Limited or completely absent alcohol, caffeine, and nicotine

3. Reduced electromagnetic frequency (EMF) exposure
4. Regular emotional detoxification
5. Prayer or daily spiritual reflection

We cover all of these strategies in our book *The Essential Oils Diet.* Go to EssentialOilsDiet.com to learn more.

The concern we have with the conventional medical approach, however, occurs when chronic stress develops into anxiety.

Because people with an anxiety disorder are three to five times more likely to go to the doctor and six times more likely to be hospitalized for psychiatric disorders than those who do not suffer from anxiety, the push to take pharmaceuticals can be overwhelming to an already vulnerable group of people.

The current pharmaceutical approach to treating anxiety generally includes one of the following three drugs:

- **Antidepressants.** Neurotransmitter-altering drugs, including selective serotonin reuptake inhibitors (SSRIs) such as Prozac, Paxil, and Zoloft, take up to six weeks to get desired results.
- **Benzodiazepines.** Habit-forming sedatives presumably used only on a short-term basis, commonly prescribed benzodiazepines include Xanax and Valium.
- **Beta-blockers.** Often used for heart conditions, beta-blockers such as Inderal are used off-label to treat anxiety.

Other approaches include anticonvulsant and antipsychotic drugs—each of which has mild to severe side effects.

ARE YOU TOO STRESSED OUT?

One of the most dangerous things about stress is that many people don't even realize when they are stressed out. People adapt to their environments and become numb to the microtraumas that they experience day in and day out. They develop resistance, as a defense mechanism, kind of like how people need to increase the amount of pain pills, for example, to get the relief they are looking for because the dose they used to take doesn't work anymore.

Not sure if you're stressed too much? Or not sure if the stress you're under is damaging to your body? Here are some clues:

- Chronic aches and pains
- Constipation or diarrhea
- Forgetfulness
- Headaches and migraines
- Lack of energy or focus
- Low libido and sexual problems
- Nausea and upset stomach
- Stiff jaw or neck
- Sleeping too much or too little
- Use of alcohol or drugs to relax
- Weight loss or gain

If you have thoughts of suicide, please call your local suicide hotline or get in touch with your natural health-care provider or qualified counselor at once.

THE ESSENTIAL OILS APPROACH TO STRESS AND ANXIETY

As with each of the chronic diseases that we discuss in this book, an ounce of prevention is worth more than a pound of cure.

Essential oils offer a supportive and powerful way to manage these issues and keep them from challenging your system. They have a direct effect on the parts of the brain that control anxiety, stress, mood, and fear. In addition, exposure to specific essential oils can help slow down a racing heart and regulate blood pressure, both of which are affected by stress and its aftermath.

Below is a rundown of the essential oils the medical literature suggests are best for stress relief, anxiety, and overall mental wellness.

STOP Before you start implementing these essential oils for stress and anxiety, be sure to review the known drug interaction chart in Appendix B and consult with your physician if you're currently taking any medications. Also, don't forget that using essential oils while living a "fast food" lifestyle is like taking one step forward but two steps back! In other words, for essential oils to help you enjoy abundant health and wellness—free from chronic disease—it is vital to use them within the context of a healthy lifestyle. Go to Appendix A for our favorite "Disease-Busting Healthy Lifestyle Hacks" to learn more!

1. Lavender

One of the best-known and most-researched essential oils for stress management, lavender has been used medicinally and in religious rituals for more than 2,500 years. Rich in linalyl acetate and linalool, this time-tested oil relieves mild anxiety, produces relaxation, and soothes the nerves. It is believed to work by impacting the limbic system, the part of the brain that controls our emotions.

As a fascinating 2009 study suggests, lavender is an excellent antianxiety therapy. In this clinical trial, volunteers watched both neutral and anxiety-provoking film clips. Those who took lavender capsules beforehand experienced less anxiety and lower heart rates compared to volunteers given a placebo.

Also, we know from other studies that lavender can ease the stress of going to the dentist or getting shots at the doctor's office. Even babies exposed to the scent of lavender tend to cry less.

Widely available, affordable, and very tolerable, lavender should be your go-to essential oil for treating stress and anxiety.

Application: The next time you feel stressed or anxious, try ending your day with a lavender-powered detox bath. It will be a super-relaxing experience!

RESTFUL EVENING DETOX BATH

Adapted from *The Healing Power of Essential Oils*

3 drops lavender essential oil
2 drops Roman chamomile essential oil

continues

2 drops ylang ylang essential oil

1 drop lemon essential oil

1 tablespoon jojoba oil

1 cup plain Epsom salts

¼ cup unfiltered, raw apple cider vinegar

SUPPLIES

Medium glass bowl

1. Mix the essential oils and jojoba oil in a glass bowl.

2. Add the Epsom salts and vinegar and mix well.

3. Fill your bathtub with the warmest water you can stand.

4. Slowly pour the mixture into the running water.

5. Soak your whole body for 20 to 30 minutes.

6. Exit the bath slowly by first sitting up, then kneeling, and finally standing to prevent feeling faint.

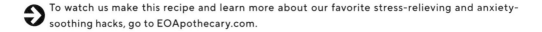 To watch us make this recipe and learn more about our favorite stress-relieving and anxiety-soothing hacks, go to EOApothecary.com.

2. Ylang Ylang

For a really tranquil mood when you're under pressure or facing a big challenge, lie back, close your eyes, and slowly and deeply breathe in the relaxing fragrance of ylang ylang. Extracted from the flower petals of the tropical ylang ylang tree, native to the Philippines and Indonesia, it is known for its sweet floral scent. In fact, its dual name literally means "flower of flowers."

Because ylang ylang acts directly through the olfactory system of your brain, you can immediately feel positive improvement in your mood once you take a whiff of it. Research has found that the oil's mild sedative effects lower stress responses like high blood pressure and a rapid heartbeat. Ylang ylang is a bona fide natural agent against mild anxiety and depression.

Application: Make a simple 2 percent body oil by mixing 12 drops of ylang ylang essential oil with 2 tablespoons of your favorite carrier oil; apply over your body, rubbing it in, after bathing.

3. Geranium

Here's another mood-booster for creating a sense of peace, calm, and readiness for a stressful day: geranium essential oil, derived from the leaves of *Pelargonium graveolens*, a plant species native to South Africa. It is widely used as an ingredient in perfumes and cosmetics because of its appealing floral scent.

That same scent makes geranium oil a wonderful aromatherapy agent, especially for treating anxiety. A 2017 study examined the effects of geranium aroma on anxiety among eighty patients who had suffered heart attacks (which could definitely cause ongoing stress, worry, and anxiety).

The patients were divided into either a geranium or a placebo group and asked to inhale an aroma for twenty minutes a day on two consecutive days. The patients who inhaled the geranium aroma had significantly lower anxiety scores than those in the placebo group. The researchers concluded that "inhalation aromatherapy with geranium essential oil is recommended as an easy-to-use intervention to reduce anxiety among patients with AMI [acute myocardial infarction—the medical term for heart attack]." If this oil can help people who have had heart attacks, it is certainly a potent weapon against stress and anxiety.

Application: Make our Floral-Powered Stress Roll-On.

FLORAL-POWERED STRESS ROLL-ON

5 drops geranium essential oil

4 drops clary sage essential oil

4 drops lavender essential oil

3 drops ylang ylang essential oil

Carrier oil of choice—jojoba and fractionated coconut oil absorb quickly and
    work best—as needed

continues

SUPPLIES

10 ml glass roller bottle

1. Drop the essential oils into the roller bottle.
2. Fill the bottle with a carrier oil and shake well.
3. Apply over your pulse points and back of the neck when you want to circuit-break stress or anxiety.

LINALOOL AND LINALYL ACETATE

Linalool is known for its calming, sedative, anticonvulsant, and anxiolytic (anti-anxiety) properties. Chemically, it is a monoterpenoid—a major compound found in essential oils—and is widely used as an antimicrobial agent and a fragrance.

Linalyl acetate is a naturally occurring phytochemical and widely used flavoring found in many flowers and spice plants. It is a principal component in many of the essential oils that are known to help reduce stress and anxiety. Chemically, it is the acetate ester of linalool, and the two often occur together in nature.

Essential Oils Rich in Linalool

- Ho wood (95 percent)
- Rosewood (82.3 to 90.3 percent)
- Coriander seed (59.0 to 87.5 percent)
- Magnolia leaf or flower (78.9 percent / 69.9 percent)
- Bergamot mint (24.9 to 55.2 percent)
- Neroli (31.4 to 54.3 percent)
- Lavender (25.0 to 45.0 percent)
- Ylang ylang (0.8 to 30.0 percent)
- Petitgrain (20.8 to 25.2 percent)
- Bergamot (1.7 to 20.6 percent)
- Clary sage (9.0 to 19.3 percent)
- Geranium (0.5 to 13.8 percent)

Essential Oils Rich in Linalyl Acetate*

- Clary sage (45.3 to 73.6 percent)
- Petitgrain (47.4 to 58.0 percent)
- Lavender (25.0 to 46.0 percent)
- Bergamot (17.1 to 40.4 percent)
- Bergamot mint (34.0 to 57.3 percent)
- Sweet marjoram (7.4 to 10.5 percent)
- Neroli (0.6 to 10.0 percent)
- Cardamom (0.7 to 7.7 percent)

* Adapted from R. Tisserand and R. Young, *Essential Oil Safety: A Guide for Health Care Professionals,* 2nd ed., London: Churchill Livingstone, 2013, p. 588.

4. Bergamot

One of the great essential-oil success stories is bergamot, which is extracted from bergamot oranges that grow mostly in Italy. Rich in linalyl acetate and linalool, this essential oil has an invigorating citrus scent and is one of the basic constituents of many perfumes. First used in Italian folk medicine, bergamot oil has more recently been found to fight everything from germs to inflammation to certain cancers. One of its other amazing healing effects is its ability to ease anxiety.

According to a detailed review study published in 2015, both animal and human trials have found that bergamot helps relieve anxiety and improve mood. The primary constituent in bergamot is limonene, which has remarkable mood-boosting properties.

Application: Bergamot blends well with lime, so try adding 3 drops of lime and 3 drops of bergamot to your diffuser next time you want an uplifting, stress-busting experience.

5. Orange

After about ten minutes of aromatherapy with orange essential oil, we both feel that our bodies are less tense, our minds are no longer racing, and we feel calm. Extracted from the rinds of oranges, this essential oil is thus a great choice to relieve stress—and a couple of studies back us up on this.

In a 2013 study, Iranian researchers found that aromatherapy with orange essential oil reduced the pulse rate and stress hormone levels in children undergoing dental procedures (which can be scary and stressful to kids and adults alike!).

Another Iranian study published in 2015 reported that women in labor experienced less anxiety after inhaling orange essential oil than women in the control group who inhaled distilled water.

Budget-friendly orange oil has many other applications, such as boosting immunity and serving as a powerful disease-fighting antioxidant—so stock up on it.

Application: Make Mama Z's famous Joyful Body Oil.

MAMA Z'S JOYFUL BODY OIL

Adapted from The *Healing Power of Essential Oils*

¼ cup carrier oil or Mama Z's Oil Base (page 25)

2 drops lemon essential oil

2 drops orange essential oil

2 drops lime or Key lime essential oil

2 drops grapefruit essential oil

8 drops vanilla absolute, CO_2, or oleoresin

SUPPLIES

Small glass bowl

2-ounce glass bottle or salve jar with lid

1. Mix the carrier oil with the essential oils in a glass bowl, making sure the oils blend together thoroughly.

2. Use as a body moisturizer or rub on your belly, wrists, and temples as needed for an overall emotional pick-me-up.

3. Store in a glass container.

6. Bitter Orange

This one is less commercially popular, so you may not have heard of it. If not, let us introduce you to yet another citrus oil: bitter orange, derived from a fruit that has been employed for centuries in Asia as medicine and for holistic therapies. Bitter orange is used in Ayurvedic medicine as an aid to meditation and can be extremely helpful in easing stress and anxiety.

If you've ever faced surgery, you know the apprehension and anxiety that come with it. A study from Iranian researchers found that when patients were given bitter orange prior to a minor operation, they felt more relaxed, with much less anxiety.

Application: Diffuse 3 drops of bitter orange and 3 drops of Douglas fir essential oils for a unique, grounding experience that will certainly wake up your senses.

7. Neroli

Extracted from blossoms of the bitter orange tree, neroli has a delicate, sweet floral scent that is almost intoxicating. Like rose, neroli is an expensive oil because of the sheer amount of plant matter required to produce a single bottle. But many people feel the price is worth it. An interesting study out of Korea evaluated how inhaling neroli for just five minutes on five separate days affected sixty-three healthy post-menopausal women and discovered that it significantly lowered diastolic blood pressure and improved pulse rate and estrogen concentrations as well as lowering serum cortisol, which is a hormone marker for stress.

Another Korean study, involving fifty-six intensive care unit (ICU) patients, confirmed that neroli contains anxiolytic properties. Blending lavender, Roman chamomile, and neroli in a 6:2:0.5 ratio, the researchers uncovered that the patients experienced "significantly low anxiety" and improved sleep quality compared with those patients who were cared for with the standard hospital treatment.

Application: Prepare our Anxiety-Busting Body Oil for relief.

ANXIETY-BUSTING BODY OIL

12 drops lavender essential oil

4 drops Roman chamomile essential oil

1 drop neroli essential oil

2 ounces carrier oil of choice or Mama Z's Oil Base (page 25)

SUPPLIES

Medium glass bowl

Glass lotion dispenser or jar

1. Drop the essential oils into a bowl.
2. Add the carrier oil and mix thoroughly. Store in a glass container.
3. Use as a body oil after you shower and as a moisturizer throughout the day.

8. Thyme

You've probably used this member of the mint family to season meats, vegetables, soups, and stews. But thyme—particularly thyme oil—has also been used for centuries as a healing remedy. Thyme essential oil can boost the immune system, soothe symptoms of respiratory infections like the common cold, improve circulation, and remove toxins from the body.

Research continues to emerge that thyme essential oil is a powerful therapeutic for stress and anxiety. Like many essential oils, thyme oil works by stimulating smell receptors in the nose, which then transmit messages through the nervous system to the emotion-controlling limbic system in the brain. Thyme also contains a healing chemical called luteolin, which, according to numerous studies, can protect the brain for a calming benefit. Another natural chemical in thyme is carvacrol, cited in research as an antianxiety agent.

Application: Thyme essential oil has a very strong, pungent smell, so you'll definitely want to blend oils that complement its aroma. Try adding 2 drops spruce, 2 drops bergamot, 1 drop juniper berry, and 1 drop thyme into your diffuser when you want to bring the peaceful, calming outdoors into the comfort of your home.

9. Lemon Balm

Lemon balm—which is actually an herb (*Melissa officinalis*)—contains a number of active plant chemicals that are thought to affect brain health and function, but the most important is rosmarinic acid, which may have antianxiety effects. It helps increase the activity of gamma-aminobutyric acid (GABA) in the brain. GABA is an important calming neurotransmitter.

In one of the many studies published on lemon balm, Australian researchers examined the mood and cognitive effects of foods containing lemon balm. The herb was mixed into a beverage and into yogurt along with either natural or artificial sweeteners. Participants who consumed both mixtures reported feeling uplifted with less anxiety.

Application: For stress relief and anti-anxiety purposes, try putting 1 or 2 drops of lemon balm in a vegan gel capsule and taking it once a day after eating. Be sure to fill up your capsule with an edible carrier oil to ensure safety and efficacy. Lemon balm is also useful as a topical massage oil; just be sure not to exceed a 5 percent dilution in order to avoid irritation. You'll love its bright and uplifting aroma.

PROVEN TO EASE TENSION: HAND MASSAGES

Feeling frazzled but have no time for a full-body massage? Try a hand massage.

Hand massages using essential oils bring instant calm. That's a finding of a 2018 study published in *Mental Illness,* where Japanese investigators evaluated the anti-stress benefit of aromatherapeutic hand massages in twenty healthy women in their twenties.

The women were first given a baseline electrocardiogram to measure the activity of the autonomic nervous system, which regulates involuntary body functions such as heartbeat. Next, the women were asked to spend thirty minutes doing a math test (which can certainly induce stress in some people!).

Afterward, the researchers organized the women into five groups: (1) a control group, in which participants sat in the experimental room for ten minutes without any treatment; (2) massage with jojoba oil group, in which the palm, fingers, and back of the hand were massaged for ten minutes with jojoba oil only; (3) whole massage group, in which the palm, fingers, and back of the hand were massaged for ten minutes using an essential oil mixture of lemon, tuberose, and labdanum oils; (4) simplified massage group, in which only the palm and back of the hand were massaged using the essential oil mixture; and (5) inhalation group, in which the participants inhaled the smell of the essential oil mixture for ten minutes

Compared to massage without essential oil or inhalation, aromatherapeutic hand massage significantly increased parasympathetic nervous function and significantly decreased sympathetic nervous function. The parasympathetic nervous system is your "rest and digest" side, while the sympathetic nervous system function is your "fight or flight"—or stress-inducing—side. So, when under stress, treat yourself to a hand massage with essential oils and allow the fragrance to wash over you.

10. Lemongrass

To rejuvenate after a frazzled day at work, try lemongrass essential oil, extracted from the leaves and stalks of the lemongrass plant.

A 2015 study evaluated the antianxiety impact of aromatherapy using lemongrass oil. Forty men were assigned to one of the following groups: inhalation of lemongrass essential oil (test aroma: three or six drops), tea tree essential oil (control aroma: three drops), or distilled water (nonaromatic control: three drops). Immediately after inhalation, each volunteer underwent a stressful task. Those in the lemongrass group had the lowest level of anxiety during the task, and unlike the control groups, completely recovered from their anxiety in five minutes. The results suggest to us that lemongrass aromatherapy is a powerful choice for instant stress reduction.

Worth noting, too, is that high blood pressure is a common side effect of stress. Lemongrass to the rescue! A 2015 study evaluated the ability of lemongrass and sweet almond oils to reduce stress-related high blood pressure. Once a week for three weeks, volunteers were treated to massages using this oil combo; another group served as a control group. Those in the essential oil group had lower diastolic blood pressure (the bottom number in a blood pressure reading) than those in the control group. Systolic blood pressure (the top number) and pulse rate were not affected.

Application: One drop of lemongrass essential oil is a perfect addition to your favorite herbal tea. Be sure to mix it with a fatty substance like coconut milk first to dilute it. Also, try making our Stress-Relieving Herbal Inhaler.

STRESS-RELIEVING HERBAL INHALER

10 drops lemon balm essential oil

6 drops lemongrass essential oil

4 drops thyme essential oil

SUPPLIES

Precut organic cotton pad

Aromatherapy inhaler

1. Place a cotton pad in the inhaler tube.

2. Drop the essential oils directly onto the cotton pad inside the tube. Alternatively, you can drop the blend into a glass bowl, roll the cotton pad in the oils to absorb them, and then insert it into the inhaler using tweezers.

3. Secure the cap and store the inhaler in a desk drawer, purse, or glove compartment so you have it handy.

4. When anxious, emotionally stressed, or a panic attack hits, open the inhaler and take 10 deep breaths of the vapor from the tube.

5. Focus on your breathing as a meditation technique, and remind yourself that everything is going to all right and that you have the strength to overcome the situation that you're in.

11. Patchouli

Any discussion of stress-reducing essential oils would be incomplete without mentioning patchouli. Known in the literature to "relieve depression, stress, calm nerves, control appetite, and to improve sexual interest," patchouli oil is rich in sesquiterpenes, primarily patchoulol, which is widely used in perfumery products, soaps, and other cosmetic goods because of its skin-healing properties.

Musky, earthy, and with hint of spice, patchouli contains a strong smell that not everyone loves (some prefer spikenard or vetiver instead). But it blends well with resins like frankincense and florals like ylang ylang, which makes it a versatile oil in the battle against stress.

Application: Patchouli is delightful with other essential oils in a diffuser blend such as the one below.

GROUNDING DIFFUSER BLEND

2 drops patchouli essential oil

2 drops bergamot essential oil

1 drop frankincense essential oil

1 drop ylang ylang essential oil

SUPPLIES

Diffuser

1. Fill your diffuser with purified water as directed in the manufacturer's instructions.

2. Add the essential oils.

3. Turn on the diffuser during stressful moments or 5 minutes before you begin your prayer and meditation practice to permeate the room with the aroma.

4. Turn off the diffuser when done.

12. Rose

Extracted from rose petals, this essential oil has an enchanting floral scent and is a well-known relaxation agent. A meta-analysis (statistical study) of its power analyzed thirteen clinical trials of rose oil, in which it was administered via inhalation or used topically in humans. Five of the studies substantiated pain-relieving effects of rose oil. Five other studies described the physiological relaxation benefit of rose oil. Other clinical properties reported in the study were rose oil's antidepressant benefits, stress-relieving qualities, libido-boosting advantages, and antianxiety effects.

There's more: Throughout the centuries, women have used rose oil for a number of health concerns, including labor and delivery. And no wonder. Rose oil has been found to manage and reduce anxiety in pregnant women during labor. In 2014, a study randomly assigned 120 first-time moms into two groups. One group received an aromatherapy session and warm footbath with rose oil at the beginning of active and transitional phases of labor, while the other group had a footbath with plain water only. The rose oil group reported significantly lower anxiety levels. This reduction in anxiety is good not only for Mom but also for her newborn.

Application: Soak your feet in a basin filled with warm water and a few drops of rose essential oil, or enjoy it in a diffuser. Rose also blends well with bergamot and patchouli, and you can place 3 drops of each in your diffuser.

For the best stress-relieving outcome, don't forget that essential oils work synergistically, in that their efficacy is amplified when they are blended together. Start off by making the remedies above as your springboard, but don't fall into the trap that these are hard-and-fast recipes that you cannot modify. The key is to discover which oils work for you, and that may very well change over time as the stressors of your life change. If you can crack the stress and anxiety code early on, you will be infinitely less likely to fall into depression—one of the topics of the next chapter.

Chapter 6

Depression and Substance Abuse

Similar to what we shared in the last chapter regarding stress and anxiety, depression and substance abuse are not only symptoms of and risk factors for the other chronic conditions mentioned in this book, but also chronic illnesses themselves and a rising cause of death worldwide.

The mean life span in depressed patients, for example, is twenty-five to thirty years less than that of the general population, and the impact of depression on public health is on par with that of smoking and obesity. Globally, more than 264 million people of all ages suffer from depression.

Of the 20 million Americans (aged twelve and older) who battle a substance use disorder, nearly 75 percent also struggle with an alcohol use disorder. Collectively, smoking, alcohol, and illicit drug use kill 11.8 million people each year globally. This is more than the number of deaths from all cancers. When you consider the untold deaths due to prescription drug overdose and misuse, the numbers are shocking.

A staggering 9.2 million Americans have dual diagnoses, referring to having a mental illness, such as depression, and a substance use disorder at the same time. Developing a codependency of sorts, an estimated one-third of people with major depression disorder also have an alcohol problem. Also, people diagnosed with a mood disorder like depression are twice as likely to abuse substances as a person without a mood disorder. If this weren't sobering enough, people suffering from depression have approximately a 10 percent lifetime suicide risk. When combined with substance abuse, the suicide risk rises to about 25 percent.

These are clearly very serious issues, and our thoughts and prayers go out to all of the families affected.

MENTAL ILLNESS

With good mental health, you enjoy a relatively happy and healthy life. It helps you demonstrate resilience in the face of stress and cope well with adversities that come your way. Think of all the good things that come from maintaining a positive mental attitude and experiencing healthy emotions, from enjoying fruitful relationships to succeeding on the job, from fulfilling your purpose in life to simply being able to relax and enjoy a cup of tea in the morning with the birds chirping outside the kitchen window. Now flip that upside-down, smear all the good things you can think of with black paint, and you can get a picture of what mental illness is like.

Having a wide spectrum from mild to severe and debilitating, mental illness alters a person's thoughts, feelings, and behaviors in distinct ways and can literally be a life-or-death matter for someone. It demands our attention and the utmost respect.

Similar to most of the chronic diseases discussed in this book, most individuals who have a mental illness don't look like they are sick. You'd be surprised to discover who in your life has been affected. From neighbors to co-workers to people you sit next to at church or walk by in the grocery-store aisles, chances are you'd never recognize that someone was struggling with addiction, depression, or another one of the countless mental health disorders that plague our nation. Relatively speaking, few people with mental illness show signs of explicit symptoms, such as outbursts of anger, agitation, confusion, or withdrawal.

The fact that depression and substance abuse both fall under the diagnosis of mental illnesses is important for a few reasons. Namely, we have found that the essential oils approach for all mental health conditions is essentially the same: help people feel better, boost mood and mental function, and aid in balancing brain chemistry.

And, as described by the National Institute on Drug Abuse (NIDA), when you treat one, you also reduce the effects of the other.

Because mood disorders [like depression] increase vulnerability to drug abuse and addiction, the diagnosis and treatment of the mood disorder can reduce the risk of subsequent drug use. Because the inverse may also be true, the diagnosis and treatment of drug use disorders may reduce the risk of developing other mental illnesses and, if they do occur, lessen their severity or make them more amenable to effective treatment.

This, in turn, greatly decreases someone's likelihood of developing a chronic disease that's linked to smoking (i.e., all of them) because, as the NIDA points out,

more than 40 percent of the cigarettes smoked in this country are smoked by individuals with a psychiatric disorder, such as major depressive disorder, alcoholism, post-traumatic stress disorder (PTSD), schizophrenia, or bipolar disorder, [and] smoking by patients with mental illness contributes greatly to their increased morbidity and mortality.

If you currently suffer from a mental illness, or have in the past, you're certainly not alone. For tens of millions of people across the globe, good mental health is elusive, and they have difficulty getting through day-to-day life. In fact, depending on where you live, you have anywhere between a 10 and 50 percent chance of developing a mental health condition.

Of all the countries, the United States tops the charts. The statistics are staggering:

- 47.4 percent of all Americans will be diagnosed with a mental illness at some point in their lives.
- 42.6 percent of American adults received mental health services in the past year, with women representing the majority of cases.
- 49.5 percent of American children are affected by at least one mental health disorder.

The situation gets very sobering when you consider that suicide, which is often associated with mental illness, is the tenth leading cause of death the United States. and the second leading cause of death among people aged fifteen to thirty-four.

The use of prescription drugs to treat depression and substance abuse has soared to dangerous levels, and we have a deadly crisis on our hands. Fortunately, people are using natural remedies such as essential oils for better mental health, which is positive because we need to get back to our roots before mental health disorders affect us all!

SUICIDE IS NEVER THE ANSWER

The effects of suicide go beyond the person who acts to take his or her life. It has a lasting effect on family, friends, and communities.

It's important to recognize that suicide does not discriminate. It can touch anyone, anywhere, at any time. But certain factors determine whether or not someone is willing to take their own life, and the connection between suicide and chronic disease is shockingly relevant to our discussion:

- Depression, anxiety, and other mental health disorders
- Alcohol or drug use disorder (including prescription drugs)
- Family history of a mental health disorder
- Family history of an alcohol or drug use disorder
- Chronic illnesses and chronic pain
- Stressful life events, such as a job loss, financial problems, loss of a loved one, or the breakup of a relationship

If you or someone you know is contemplating suicide, get help right away, especially if there is a change in behavior, like withdrawing from family and friends and social isolation. If it is an emergency, dial your local emergency number. Or call your local suicide prevention hotline.

BRAIN CHEMISTRY AND ESSENTIAL OILS

Both addiction and depression disorders are associated with changes in brain chemistry. There is significant overlap in the parts of the brain that are disrupted, and thus medical treatments prescribed to help reduce symptoms are mainly antidepressants. Referred to as selective serotonin reuptake inhibitors (SSRIs), the most commonly prescribed antidepressants are fluoxetine (Prozac), sertraline (Zoloft), paroxetine (Paxil), fluvoxamine (Luvox), citalopram (Celexa), and escitalopram (Lexapro).

However, we should all be hugely concerned about the long list of documented dangerous side effects associated with these habit-forming, brain-altering drugs (which includes suicide) and, if possible, seek safer alternatives, such as aromatherapy. As a recent 2020 study so eloquently put it, "The use of essential oils, in relieving anxiety and depression, does not have the disadvantages associated with currently used drug therapies."

Nonetheless, if someone is at risk of taking her life or harming herself, she needs to do whatever she needs to stay alive. If that means going to the doctor and taking a prescription antidepressant, then so be it. But she needs to recognize that she may have gotten on a never-ending train that's running on a one-way track.

There is a common belief about antidepressants that once you start, you need to stay on them for the rest of your life. And there is plenty of valid anecdotal evidence that supports this assumption. Clinicians generally recommend staying on antidepressants for six to nine months before considering going off of them, with the caveat that, if you've had three or more recurrences of depression, you'll need at least two years to wean yourself off.

To complicate the issue, the most addictive drugs in our society are nicotine, alcohol, and illicit drugs such as cocaine and heroin. All three types of drugs alter brain chemistry and produce their high by stimulating the production of dopamine—a joy-producing brain chemical—in the pleasure centers of the brain. When dopamine levels are jacked up, you feel euphoric for as long as the high lasts.

But as you move from voluntary to compulsory use (addiction), the continued use of these drugs tends to dull dopamine receptors on brain cells and reduces their number. Consequently, cells don't recognize dopamine properly, leaving too much of it in the pleasure centers of the brain. Those centers eventually adapt to the drug, and the addict no longer feels satisfied—a condition known as tolerance—so increasingly larger doses of the drug are needed to produce the high. The addict develops not only a physical dependence on the drug but also a psychological one.

(But let us sprinkle some hope into the equation. With the use of essential oils to expedite the process, we've seen many people wean themselves off brain-altering medications for anxiety, depression, and substance abuse with great success!)

Unlike drugs, aromatherapy is not habit-forming and does not cause codependency, and there is compelling evidence that using certain essential oils can bring balance to your brain chemistry and help you beat depression and substance abuse for good.

The most effective and instant pathway is through inhalation. When you smell essential oils, the volatile organic compounds (VOCs) interact with nerve cells in the nose and trigger the olfactory system (sense of smell). In turn, this sets off a cascade of neural impulses that instantly impact your limbic system. Also known as the "primal brain" that is in control of our mood, memory, and emotions, the limbic system is made up of the hypothalamus, amygdala, thalamus, hippocampus, and other parts of the brain.

When applied topically or ingested, aromatic compounds enter the blood circulation system through the lungs and affect brain chemistry as they are carried by the blood to the brain.

CITRUS OILS TO THE RESCUE!

Which citrus oils can help with depression and substance abuse? All of them!

They are uplifting, happy smelling, and rich in d-limonene (or limonene for short), a chemical well researched for its antidepressant properties. Peer-reviewed research has already confirmed that bergamot, lemon, orange, and yuzu oils can help with depression, and we expect to see other citrus oils studied in the future. Limonene can also help with substance abuse and addiction. A recent study uncovered that limonene can greatly reduce drug addiction–related behaviors and dependence in lab rats. See page 108 for a list of limonene-rich oils.

An interesting study a few years back evaluated seventy-eight people in a hopeless situation (i.e., people were asked to solve an unsolvable social discrimination task). During this task, d-limonene and vanillin (the main component of vanilla) were diffused and the volunteers were asked to rate the aroma's quality (intensity, pleasantness, unpleasantness, familiarity, etc.) prior to and following the helplessness exercise. Fascinatingly, the more pleasant the participants judged the aroma in the room, the less effective the helplessness induction was in reducing happiness and the greater their increase in mood, thus suggesting that the prophylactic use of citrus oils and vanilla can help reduce the negative emotional ramifications of everyday stressors and depression-causing events!

Let this sink in for a moment, especially if you struggle with depression or substance abuse.

If you use essential oils as part of your daily routine (body care, diffusion, culinary doses, etc.), you will be less likely to suffer from depression, and when you do get down into the dumps, it won't be as bad as it might be without aromatherapy helping to keep your mood as elevated as possible.

Here are some ways that you can get started using essential oils to treat depression and substance abuse!

CITRUS DELIGHT BLEND

When it comes to boosting mood and banishing depression symptoms, there is no better approach than citrus oils. They are literally liquid antidepressants, which is why you'll see most essential oil companies blend several together with a sweet floral like vanilla to create an orange-vanilla reminiscent of those Creamsicles everyone loves! Try mixing equal parts of vanilla absolute (or vanilla CO_2) and all of the citrus oils that you have on hand for a truly uplifting aromatic experience.

10 drops orange essential oil
10 drops bergamot essential oil
10 drops clementine essential oil
10 drops grapefruit lemon essential oil
10 drops lemon essential oil

10 drops mandarin essential oil

10 drops tangerine essential oil

10 drops vanilla absolute, CO_2, or oleoresin

SUPPLIES

5 ml bottle

1. Drop the essential oils into a 5 ml bottle, cap, and shake to mix.

2. Depending on the type and source of vanilla that you use, it may overpower the citrus oils, so start with a few drops and blend until you find that perfect smell that perks you up and puts a smile on your face.

3. Use as directed in the following recipes.

NOTE: *Don't forget that citrus oils tend to be photosensitizers, so use them carefully if you're going to be out in the sun. For more safety tips, visit chapter 2.*

CITRUS DELIGHT SPRITZER

10 drops Citrus Delight Blend (page 102)

10 drops organic 190-proof grain alcohol

10 drops witch hazel

Distilled water, as needed

SUPPLIES

1-ounce spray bottle

1. Drop the oil blend, grain alcohol, and witch hazel in the bottle.

2. Fill with distilled water and shake gently to mix well.

3. This works great as a body spray or to freshen up your linens, carpet, car floor mats, bed sheets, or anywhere that you want an aromatic boost. (Be sure to test a small area first to prevent staining.)

NOTE: *This water-based formula will last for a couple of weeks. We've used it for as long as two months and have not noticed bacterial overgrowth, which can happen with any water-based product. It may not be obvious at first, but the smell will become rancid, and you will notice a change in color if it is contaminated.*

CITRUS DELIGHT MASSAGE OIL

16 drops Citrus Delight Blend (page 102)

2 ounces carrier oil or Mama Z's Oil Base (page 25)

SUPPLIES

Medium glass bowl

Lidded glass jar or lotion dispenser

1. Drop the essential oil blend into a glass bowl.
2. Add the carrier oil and mix thoroughly.
3. Apply after you shower as a moisturizer or as a body oil throughout the day.
4. This is also safe for kids and helps set them off to school in a great mood, but because of the d-limonene content, it's not safe to apply on pets in case they lick their fur.
5. Store in a glass jar or lotion dispenser.

CITRUS DELIGHT ROLL-ON BLEND

12 drops Citrus Delight Blend (page 102)

Carrier oil of choice—jojoba and fractionated coconut absorb quickly and work best—as needed

SUPPLIES

10 ml glass roller bottle

1. Drop the essential oil blend into your roll-on bottle.
2. Fill the roller bottle with a carrier oil, cap it, and shake well to mix.
3. Massage your neck, shoulders, hands, wrists, feet, and ankles with the oil when you need an emotional pick-me-up, mood boost, or support through addiction cravings.
4. While spending a few minutes giving yourself a gentle massage, reflect on the day and focus on at least one thing that you are grateful for.

NOTE: *This is also safe for kids and helps set them off to school in a great mood, but because of the d-limonene content, it's not safe to apply on pets in case they lick their fur.*

CITRUS DELIGHT DIFFUSER BLEND

6 drops Citrus Delight Blend (page 102)

SUPPLIES
Diffuser

1. Fill your diffuser with purified water as directed in the manufacturer's instructions.

2. Add the essential oil blend.

3. Turn on the diffuser first thing in the morning to set your day on a positive note or anytime you need an emotional pick-me-up, mood boost, or support through addiction cravings. This recipe works well in an aromatherapy necklace.

CITRUS DELIGHT INHALER

20 drops Citrus Delight Blend (page 102)

SUPPLIES
Precut organic cotton pad
Aromatherapy inhaler

1. Place a cotton pad in the inhaler tube.

2. Drop the essential oil blend directly onto the cotton pad inside the tube. Alternatively, you can drop the blend into a glass bowl, roll the cotton pad in the oils to absorb them, and then insert it into the inhaler tube using tweezers.

3. Secure the cap and store the inhaler in a desk drawer, purse, or glove compartment so you have it handy.

4. When you feel a little run down emotionally, want a mood boost, or need help with addiction cravings, open the inhaler and take 10 deep breaths of the vapor from the tube.

CITRUS DELIGHT COOLER

Serves 2

1 cup ice

16 ounces organic orange juice

8 ounces unsweetened vanilla-flavored almond or coconut milk

3 to 4 dropperfuls vanilla-cream-flavored liquid stevia (to taste)

4 drops Citrus Delight Blend (page 102)

¼ cup frozen pineapple chunks

¼ cup frozen mango pieces

1. Put the ingredients into a blender in the order listed above.

2. Blend until smooth.

3. Drink when you want a tasty, healthy mood boost and some support to overcome unhealthy food or drug cravings.

 To watch us make this recipe and learn more about how to harness the power of citrus oils to banish depression and unhealthy cravings, go to EOApothecary.com.

CITRUS DELIGHT CAPSULE

Makes 1 dose

4 drops Citrus Delight Blend (page 102)

Organic virgin coconut oil or extra-virgin olive oil

SUPPLIES

Pipette

Size 00 vegan gel capsule

1. Using a pipette, drop the essential oil blend into the bottom half (the longer, narrower one) of the capsule. Fill this half to the brim with coconut or extra-virgin olive oil.

2. Fit the wider top half of the capsule over the bottom half and secure it snugly.

3. Immediately swallow the capsule with water after breakfast (see Note). Take daily and monitor your symptoms.

NOTE: *Do **not** make and store these capsules for future use. Also, this is not a long-term solution, and using it for more than four weeks at a time is not advisable. Be sure to switch up your protocol monthly and consult with your health-care provider first if you're currently taking medications. Discontinue if adverse reactions occur.*

THE POWER OF D-LIMONENE

The most powerful plant-based compound in nature is arguably d-limonene. An article in the *Alternative Medicine Review* sums up its therapeutic prowess perfectly:

- It does not pose a mutagenic, carcinogenic, or nephrotoxic risk to humans.
- It has been used clinically to dissolve cholesterol-containing gallstones.
- It has been used for relief of heartburn and gastroesophageal reflux (GERD).
- It has well-established chemopreventive (the ability to slow or prevent the progression of cancer) activity against many types of cancer.

Additionally, we know that d-limonene is a superpower in several other ways:

- **It boosts immunity.** D-limonene is a potent antioxidant and anti-inflammatory agent.
- **It reverses liver and pancreas damage.** D-limonene has been shown to reverse the effects of a high-fat diet in rats and restore the damage done to their liver and pancreas that was inflicted by the diet.
- **It kills pathogens and acts as a preservative.** D-limonene can extend the shelf life of prepared foods by keeping fungal infestation and toxic aflatoxin threats at bay. Aflatoxins and carcinogens are a family of toxins produced by certain fungi that are found on agricultural crops such as maize (corn), peanuts, cottonseed, and tree nuts.
- **It aids in weight loss.** D-limonene suppresses appetite and can promote weight loss and fat burning.
- **It decreases stress.** D-limonene is nature's stress reliever and anxiolytic.
- **It promotes restful sleep.** D-limonene can help promote a better night's

sleep by activating adenosine A_{2A} receptors, which are suspected to induce sedative effects.

An interesting fact about d-limonene suggests that we should topically apply blends containing citrus oils on regular basis: it is a known "absorption promoter or accelerant for improving transdermal drug delivery and works by penetrating the skin to reversibly decrease barrier resistance," meaning that it helps facilitate the healthy components of your topical preparations (i.e., nutrients from carrier oils and other essential oils compounds) into the bloodstream for an amplified effect!

Essential Oils Rich in D-limonene

In addition to the citrus family, several other essential oils are rich sources of d-limonene. Here's how they compare:

- Orange (83.9 to 95.9 percent)
- Grapefruit (84.8 to 95.4 percent)
- Tangerine (87.4 to 91.7 percent)
- Lemon, expressed (56.6 to 76.0 percent)
- Celery seed (68.0 to 75.0 percent)
- Mandarin (65.3 to 74.2 percent)
- Tangelo (73.2 percent)
- Lemon, distilled (64.0 to 70.5 percent)
- Dill seed (35.9 to 68.4 percent)
- Elemi (26.9 to 65.0 percent)
- Palo santo (58.6 to 63.3 percent)
- Yuzu (63.1 percent)
- Lime, expressed (51.5 to 59.6 percent)
- Lime, distilled (55.6 percent)
- Fir needle, silver (54.7 percent)
- Bergamot, expressed (27.4 to 52.0 percent)
- Caraway (36.9 to 48.8 percent)

MORE ESSENTIAL OILS FOR DEPRESSION AND SUBSTANCE ABUSE

Truth be told, any essential oil can help with depression and substance abuse because of the subjective nature of the power of smell. The aromatic approach is the most subjective and largely depends on someone's personal preference and history.

For some people who have had negative or traumatic experiences around a certain aroma, the scent could exacerbate the situation greatly. We see this with people who have dealt with abuse or trauma, and it can trigger depression or post-traumatic stress disorder (PTSD).

On the converse, a positive memory and feeling can be elicited by smelling a familiar fragrance. Maybe you have fond memories of family get-togethers at Thanksgiving time and eating pumpkin pie. So, smelling a roasted turkey or cinnamon, cloves, or nutmeg can make you feel at ease and happy.

While it can be a long-term process, recovery from addiction is possible, but it usually requires multiple approaches—including the use of essential oils and other holistic therapies, like detoxification, dietary therapy, and counseling.

Thankfully, the world of medicine is evolving and adapting to more holistic methods of treatment and care. One such adaption is the use of essential oils and aromatherapy to affect you positively and help you feel better psychologically while trying to eliminate addiction.

In this section, we will explore the top essential oils for depression and addiction recovery and how they help you. When using them, be sure to listen to your body and keep track of how each makes you feel.

Note: There are several oils that could have made this list, but for the sake of space, we tried to include some of the more interesting studies and oils that you may not be familiar with. These can also help with depression and addiction, and we encourage you to experiment with them as well:

- Coriander
- Rose
- Rosemary
- Thyme
- Ylang ylang

STOP Before you start implementing these essential oils for depression and substance abuse, be sure to review the known drug interaction chart in Appendix B and consult with your physician if you're currently taking any medications. Also, don't forget that using essential oils while living a "fast food" lifestyle is like taking one step forward but two steps back! In other words, for essential oils to help you enjoy abundant health and wellness—free from chronic disease—it is vital to use them within the context of a healthy lifestyle. Go to Appendix A for our favorite "Disease-Busting Healthy Lifestyle Hacks" to learn more!

1. Linalool-Rich Oils

What if you don't enjoy the smell of citrus oils? No problem, linalool and beta-pinene to the rescue!

Like d-limonene, linalool is an essential oil compound that has been shown to help with depression and substance abuse. It has the ability to affect gamma-aminobutyric acid (GABA), a neurotransmitter that slows and can balance brain activity and reduce symptoms of depression as well as anxiety, autism, panic, and schizophrenia. Compounds that target the GABA system can also help in the treatment of addiction, because GABA receptors modulate substance reward and reinforcement behaviors.

For a list of essential oils rich in linalool, see chapter 5, page 86.

Application: Try this linalool-powered remedy for on-the-go depression relief.

LINALOOL-POWERED INHALER

5 drops clary sage essential oil

5 drops geranium or rose geranium essential oil

3 drops lavender essential oil

3 drops ylang ylang essential oil

2 drops neroli essential oil

2 drops rosewood essential oil (see Note)

SUPPLIES

Precut organic cotton pad

Tweezers (optional)

1. Place a cotton pad in the inhaler tube.

2. Drop the essential oils directly onto the cotton pad inside the tube. Alternatively, you can drop the blend into a glass bowl, roll the cotton pad in the oils to absorb them, and then insert it into the inhaler using tweezers.

3. Secure the cap and store the inhaler in a desk drawer, purse, or glove compartment so you have it handy.

4. When you feel a little run down emotionally, want a mood boost, or need help with addiction cravings, open the inhaler and take 10 deep breaths of the vapor from the tube. This recipe works well in an aromatherapy necklace.

NOTE: *Include sustainably harvested rosewood essential oil if you get your hands on some! Read more about concerns on rosewood's sustainability in chapter 12 (page 225).*

2. Galbanum

Galbanum is an aromatic gum resin that Hippocrates supposedly used as medicine and Pliny praised for its extraordinary curative powers. The essential oil also happens to be the richest source of beta-pinene, a chemical known to have antidepressant effects and the ability to help with addiction cravings through interaction with the monoaminergic system. A monoaminergic drug is a chemical that changes the amount of serotonin, dopamine, norepinephrine, epinephrine, and/or histamine available in the brain.

Galbanum blends well with frankincense and is even prescribed in the Bible as a sacred incense:

Then the Lord said to Moses, "Take fragrant spices—gum resin, onycha, and galbanum—and pure frankincense, all in equal amounts, and make a fragrant blend of incense, the work of a perfumer. It is to be salted and pure and sacred." (Exodus 30:34–35)

Application: Our Sacred Incense Diffuser Blend (page 112) is an aromatic delight!

SACRED INCENSE DIFFUSER BLEND

3 drops frankincense essential oil

3 drops galbanum essential oil

SUPPLIES

Diffuser

1. Fill your diffuser with purified water as directed in the manufacturer's instructions.

2. Add the essential oils.

3. Turn on the diffuser during your spiritual practices to create a peaceful, meditative environment. It can also be used throughout the day to enhance mood, promote positive emotions, and help balance brain chemistry when addiction cravings become a problem.

3. Frankincense

Referred to as the "king of oils" for good reason, frankincense is touted by essential oil enthusiasts across the globe for its immune-boosting, anticancer, anti-inflammatory, and hormone-balancing properties. We can also add mood boosting and antidepressant to that list.

Aromatherapy hand massage using a blend of bergamot, frankincense, and lavender (1:1:1 ratio) diluted to 1.5 percent with sweet almond oil was evaluated several years ago on hospice patients with terminal cancer. Not only did this simple week-long, five-minute-per-day intervention improve their depression, but the mixture diminished their pain levels as well!

Application: Use our adapted recipe from this study to harness the mood-balancing and pain-relieving properties of the "king of oils."

ROYAL MASSAGE OIL

6 drops bergamot essential oil

6 drops frankincense essential oil

6 drops lavender essential oil

2 ounces sweet almond oil or your favorite carrier oil

SUPPLIES

Medium glass bowl

Lidded glass jar or lotion dispenser

1. Drop the essential oils into a glass bowl.
2. Add the carrier oil and mix thoroughly.
3. Give yourself a hand or foot massage using this oil, or swap out massages with a friend to enhance your mood, reduce pain, and enjoy a balancing escape from the stressors of life and substance abuse.
4. Store in a glass jar or lotion dispenser.

4. Clary Sage

A famed women's health remedy, clary sage oil demonstrates mood-enhancing activity even when the mood is altered due to hormonal changes associated with menopause. Specifically, it has been shown to influence brain chemistry to help restore more normal levels of key brain chemicals like dopamine, which are responsible for addiction and depression.

Application: Clary sage and the oils in the Linalool-Powered Inhaler (page 110) can easily be converted into a diffuser remedy by putting 1 drop of each in your diffuser next time you want a mood boost or help through addiction cravings.

5. Rose Geranium

Technically referred to as *Pelargonium roseum*, rose geranium is similar to but different from its close cousin *Pelargonium graveolens* (i.e., "geranium"). A wonderful pairing with clary sage, rose geranium has been used for hundreds of years for all things related to women's health, including relief from pain, stress, anxiety, and depression.

Recently tested on animals via injection, rose geranium oil was discovered to have an even greater impact on these health issues than previously thought, as well as through a different neurological pathway than GABA transmission or the others discussed so far: serotonin. For people on SSRIs, this is a huge finding and suggests that rose geranium can possibly help wean someone off antidepressants under the scope of a medical professional.

Application: Rose geranium and the oils in the Linalool-Powered Inhaler (page 110) can easily be converted into a capsule remedy by putting 1 drop of each in a vegan gel capsule and taking it once a day after eating. Be sure to fill up your capsule with an edible carrier oil to ensure safety and efficacy.

6. Plai

The aroma of plai root essential oil is strikingly similar to eucalyptus with additional spicy notes. A cousin to ginger and favorite with massage therapists, plai is traditionally used to soothe achy muscles and help deep tissue wounds heal. A study investigated how plai affects mood and stress among healthy male volunteers and observed that the essential oil produced an immediate improvement on mood states "by easing the negative emotions and enhancing positive emotions, especially feelings of pleasure and contentment."

Application: Plai blends well with rosemary, another powerhouse that regulates several neurotransmitters related to depression and substance abuse (dopamine, norepinephrine, serotonin and acetylcholine). Try mixing 3 drops of plai with 3 drops of rosemary essential oil in your diffuser for a spicy, aromatic remedy.

7. Black Pepper

We probably use black pepper every day on our foods, but people seldom know how useful its essential oil can be. For example, dip a toothpick in it and chew on the toothpick to reduce cravings for cigarettes, alcohol, or marijuana. Black pepper oil can also help you fight withdrawal symptoms and keep you calm throughout. It works by elevating levels of the feel-good neurotransmitter serotonin in your brain (similar to what most mood-boosting prescription drugs do).

Since 1994, we have known that inhaling black pepper essential oil reduces smoking withdrawal symptoms. In 2013, researchers confirmed this when they conducted a small study on an American college campus. Daily nicotine users inhaled one drop of black pepper or angelica essential oil for two minutes whenever they felt cravings. Both oils reduced the cravings and extended the time until nicotine was used again, with black pepper reducing the cravings more and angelica helping volunteers delay use longer.

Application: Try our Quit Sticks to help you quit the habit. Chewing on a toothpick satisfies the oral fixation that many smokers need to fulfill, and the essential oils can help with withdrawals. The Cut-Your-Cravings Diffuser Blend (page 116) is another good one to use for ongoing support.

QUIT STICKS

15 drops angelica essential oil

15 drops black pepper essential oil

5 drops grapefruit essential oil

5 drops peppermint essential oil

5 drops orange essential oil

5 drops cinnamon bark essential oil

Edible carrier oil (see Note)

SUPPLIES

1-ounce glass measuring cup or shot glass

continues

50 to 75 wooden toothpicks (enough to fill your glass)

Clean plate or baking sheet

Lidded glass toothpick container

1. Drop the essential oils into the measuring cup.

2. Fill the cup three-quarters full with the carrier oil and stir well.

3. Place the toothpicks in the cup and let them soak overnight.

4. Remove the toothpicks and let them dry on a clean plate or baking sheet. Store the remaining oil mixture in a glass jar for future use.

5. When addiction cravings arise, suck on a toothpick for as long as you need until the cravings go away.

6. Store in a lidded glass toothpick container for future use.

NOTE: *Use an edible carrier oil that won't harden, such as extra-virgin olive oil, grapeseed oil, or avocado oil.*

CUT-YOUR-CRAVINGS DIFFUSER BLEND

2 drops angelica essential oil

2 drops black pepper essential oil

2 drops peppermint essential oil

1 drop cinnamon bark essential oil

SUPPLIES

Diffuser

1. Fill your diffuser with purified water as directed in the manufacturer's instructions.

2. Add the essential oils to the water.

3. When addiction cravings occur, turn on the diffuser, sit down, and relax for a few minutes. Be sure to take intentional, slow, deep breaths.

4. Turn off the diffuser when your cravings cease.

BE PATIENT AND TRUST THE PROCESS

As long as you're not noticing any direct adverse reactions to these remedies, it is advisable that you continue using them as directed, even if you don't *feel* better at first!

Unlike blood pressure, glucose levels, or weight loss, depression and addiction cravings are largely subjective and based on *feelings*. Sometimes people enjoy instant relief. Other times, it takes time. Essentially the mind needs to catch up with the body.

Note, this is not the placebo effect. It's real science.

It is a well-known fact that aromatherapy cannot produce one effect on the mind and the opposite effect on the body. They have to coincide. In other words, your mind will follow what your body is experiencing at the physiologically level.

Thus, when you inhale citrus oils, your body responds by producing dopamine (the "happy hormone"). You may not notice this at first, but if you're consistent, your mood will elevate and you'll feel happier than what you felt before you inhaled the citrus oils.

There are clearly so many potent essential oils to help deal with depression and addiction—and they do so in countless ways, from easing the mind, reducing cravings, and alleviating stress and anxiety, to restoring physical health. At the end of the day, all of these will help you in treatment and recovery, and our prayers are with you to find the answer(s) that you're looking for!

Chapter 7

Chronic Fatigue Syndrome and Fibromyalgia

Imagine an illness that seems to come out of nowhere, leaving you desperately tired and feeling sick, weak, and depressed. Your muscles and joints hurt for no reason, your brain feels like it's in a thick fog, and it's impossible to concentrate. You notice that you're getting headaches a lot, and, even though you get enough sleep at night, you still wake up feeling tired. And the cycle continues day after day after day.

You go to the doctor and she diagnoses you with chronic fatigue syndrome (CFS). She tells you that there's no cure and no known treatment, so she prescribes you some things for the symptoms that are bothering you most. Antidepressants and painkillers most likely top the list, because they can help you sleep a bit better and relieve some pain.

Now, imagine a scenario where you go to a different doctor to get a second opinion, and this new physician diagnoses you with fibromyalgia. She, too, prescribes you some things for the symptoms that are bothering you most. Again, antidepressants and painkillers are recommended.

Sound crazy?

Welcome to the world of chronic fatigue and fibromyalgia.

UNDERSTANDING CHRONIC FATIGUE

Also referred to as systemic exertion intolerance disease (SEID) or myalgic encephalomyelitis (ME), chronic fatigue syndrome has come to be recognized as a very real medical problem—one that causes major difficulties for its victims. Yet the true cause is still a mystery. The Centers for Disease Control and Prevention estimates that this disabling and complex illness affects between 836,000 and 2.5 million Americans.

Sudden onset sometimes follows a gastrointestinal, respiratory, or other acute viral infection. Some cases develop after emotional or physical traumas, such as a serious accident, bereavement, or surgery. Still other cases take longer to develop with no obvious trigger.

Because it was known to appear after the flu or another illness, it was once thought to be brought on by the Epstein-Barr virus, which triggers mononucleosis. But more recently, medical experts and researchers believe that CFS does not have a single cause but may be a combination of viral infections, allergies, hormonal imbalance, and psychological factors all acting on the immune system.

Currently, women are four times more likely than men to be diagnosed with CFS, although both men and women can develop the disease, as can children. However, people aged forty to fifty-nine are more frequently diagnosed with the illness. Contrary to what you may see online, CFS is not currently considered an autoimmune disorder.

As with fibromyalgia, there are currently no medical tests to confirm you even have chronic fatigue. A CFS diagnosis is based on symptoms, which are similar to those of many other illnesses and conditions, so it oftentimes becomes a judgment call by the physician. Technically, to be diagnosed with CFS, you must have suffered from new and persistent fatigue for at least six months. The existence of any other disease, infection, malignancy, or condition that may produce similar symptoms, as well as the use of drugs, medications, or chemicals, must be ruled out by a physician.

You must also have had eight of the following symptoms for at least six months:

- Mild fever or chills
- Sore throat

- Painful lymph nodes (such as glands on the sides of the neck)
- Unexplained general body weakness
- Muscle discomfort or pain
- Unusual headaches
- Difficulty sleeping
- Aches and pains that travel from joint to joint
- Fatigue for twenty-four hours or more after levels of exercise that used to be tolerated
- Any of these complaints: forgetfulness, excessive irritability, confusion, difficulty thinking, inability to concentrate, depression

UNDERSTANDING FIBROMYALGIA

Fibromyalgia is a chronic condition in which there is widespread musculoskeletal pain, fatigue, and sleep, mood, and memory issues. The defining characteristic is tenderness in localized areas. Because it often is accompanied by chronic fatigue, there is significant overlap between CFS prevention and treatment strategies.

As with CFS, women are more likely to develop fibromyalgia, and symptoms oftentimes begin after an infection, physical trauma, surgery, or significant psychological stress, or as a result of autoimmune disorders like rheumatoid arthritis and lupus. Many people who have fibromyalgia also have anxiety, depression, irritable bowel syndrome (IBS), tension headaches, and temporomandibular joint (TMJ) disorders.

Fibromyalgia is a symptom-based diagnosis—just like CFS—meaning, you cannot *prove* it exists. Unlike cancer where you can determine the presence of malignant cells, diabetes where you can measure blood glucose levels, or hypertension where you can evaluate blood pressure, there is no test to determine if someone has fibromyalgia. The criteria have changed over the years, and they will most likely continue to change as doctors learn more about this condition. Currently, to be diagnosed with fibromyalgia, someone needs to present with these three symptoms:

1. *Widespread pain.* To be considered "widespread," the pain must occur above

and below your waist, on both sides of your body. The pain is generally described as a constant dull ache that has lasted for at least three months.

2. *Fatigue.* People with fibromyalgia often wake up tired, in spite of getting an adequate amount of sleep. Their sleep is often disrupted by pain, and many patients have other sleep disorders, such as restless legs syndrome and sleep apnea.

3. *Cognitive difficulties.* Commonly referred to as "fibro fog," fibromyalgia patients have an uncanny inability to focus and concentrate.

While there is no cure for fibromyalgia, a variety of medications are prescribed in an attempt to help control symptoms. Exercise, relaxation, and stress-reduction measures are known to help.

IMPORTANCE OF FORGIVENESS

"Bearing with one another and, if one has a complaint against another, forgiving each other; as the Lord has forgiven you, so you also must forgive."

—Colossians 3:13

When's the last time you checked your heart?

Earlier, in chapter 5, we discussed the importance of stress management and emotional detoxification. Also important is forgiveness (including self-forgiveness), especially when it comes to beating disease, especially CFS and fibromyalgia!

Research has been done at length and confirmed that "learning to become more forgiving may be a complementary treatment to cope with the ongoing stress, frustration, and negative emotions that result from these two conditions." Forgiveness interventions have also been shown to reduce fibromyalgia symptoms in female volunteers!

Studies have found people who regularly forgive others reap huge rewards in their health. Lowering the risk of heart attack, improving sleep and cholesterol levels, and reducing pain, blood pressure, and levels of anxiety, depression, and stress are just a few examples.

Research specifically points to an increase in the forgiveness/health connection as we age. "There is an enormous physical burden to being hurt and disappointed," says Karen Swartz, MD, director of the Mood Disorders Adult Consultation Clinic at The Johns Hopkins Hospital. Anger and chronic feelings of being wronged put you into a sympathetic fight-or-flight state, which increases heart rate and blood pressure and dampens the immune response. This puts you at risk of developing virtually every chronic disease discussed in this book!

The description that researchers give us of *forgiveness* involves "overcoming resentment and withholding retaliation in the context of injustice and responding to an offender with benevolence." We once heard that harboring unforgiveness or holding grudges in your heart is like drinking poison and expecting the other person to get hurt.

If for no other reason, do it for yourself—no matter what someone has done to you. You're worth it!

 To watch us demonstrate a forgiveness therapy session, go to EOApothecary.com.

THE ESSENTIAL OILS APPROACH TO CHRONIC FATIGUE AND FIBROMYALGIA

Although there is really no specific "cure" or treatment for CFS and fibromyalgia, sometimes antidepressants, painkillers, and stimulant drugs are prescribed, but only in an attempt to improve symptoms. However, many patients fail to respond satisfactorily to these drugs or suffer nasty side effects from them. Therefore, the control of chronic fatigue and pain remains a challenge for doctors and patients alike. Thankfully, essential oils can help—and bring relief and a sense of normalcy to everyday life.

Here are some symptoms to look for—and the essential oils that work best for each one. We recommend starting off with a 2 percent dilution of each oil or blend to be applied over problem areas or over your chest and neck if fatigue is your primary concern. (See the dilution chart on pages 26–28.)

- Morning stiffness: arnica, German chamomile, ginger, lavender, peppermint
- Sleep disturbances: lavender, Roman chamomile

- Tingling or numbness in hands and feet: eucalyptus, frankincense, geranium, lavender
- Headaches, including migraines: copaiba, eucalyptus, laurel leaf
- Irritable bowel syndrome: coriander seed, Melissa (lemon balm), peppermint, spearmint
- Problems with thinking and memory: cedarwood, vetiver
- Painful menstrual cycles: clary sage, fennel, marjoram
- Other pain syndromes: German chamomile, orange, wintergreen

Relieving these symptoms can further slow the fatigue and pain cycle, which helps people suffering from CFS and fibromyalgia become more mobile and lets them sleep better; this, in turn, can limit further fatigue and pain. Here are some other strategies you can use to help.

 Before you start implementing these essential oils for chronic fatigue and fibromyalgia, be sure to review the known drug interaction chart in Appendix B and consult with your physician if you're currently taking any medications. Also, don't forget that using essential oils while still living a "fast food" lifestyle is like taking one step forward but two steps back! In other words, for essential oils to help you enjoy abundant health and wellness—free from chronic disease—it is vital to use them within the context of a healthy lifestyle. Go to Appendix A for our favorite "Disease-Busting Healthy Lifestyle Hacks" to learn more!

TOP ESSENTIAL OILS FOR CHRONIC FATIGUE

Essential oils are being considered as potential new treatments for fatigue because CFS has been linked to infectious diseases. Fortunately, essential oils possess many antibacterial, antimicrobial and antiviral properties that can help strengthen the immune system and return it to balance. Also, some essential oils help decrease cell-destructing oxidation in the body—a benefit that may prevent physical fatigue.

These powerful essential oils are considered some of the most consistently effective natural therapies for the symptoms of CFS. When used, they address the problem at many different levels.

1. Peppermint

Want to instantly perk up? Take a whiff of peppermint essential oil.

When volunteers with mental exhaustion and burnout were asked to inhale either a mixture of essential oils (peppermint, basil, and helichrysum) or rose water (the control), the essential oils group felt a significant reduction of their fatigue symptoms over a three-week period. The researchers noted, "The results suggest that inhaling essential oils may reduce the perceived level of mental fatigue/burnout."

As an added bonus, research has shown that simply consuming one drop of peppermint oil every day promotes deep breathing and can even improve exercise performance—meaning that you can work out longer without tiring if taking peppermint oil.

Chronic fatigue has been linked to a gut infection known as small intestinal bacterial overgrowth (SIBO), and peppermint oil can help, as it has long been known to soothe inflammation in the gastrointestinal system. Researchers have noted that peppermint improved symptoms through its antimicrobial activity in the small intestine.

Application: Try a culinary approach and make our EO-Powered Matcha Latte every day for a week. The natural boost you'll get from the matcha green tea can do wonders when paired with peppermint. In addition, make the peppermint-powered inhaler and body oil recipes below for a quick pick-me-up!

EO-POWERED MATCHA LATTE

Serves 2

1 tablespoon matcha green tea powder

1 cup unsweetened vanilla-flavored almond milk

1 cup unsweetened vanilla-flavored coconut milk

2 cups boiling purified water

4 dropperfuls vanilla- or coconut- flavored liquid stevia

4 to 5 drops essential oil (see Note)

½ teaspoon freshly ground pink Himalayan salt

½ teaspoon ground Ceylon cinnamon (optional)

1. Combine the matcha powder, almond and coconut milks, boiling water, stevia, essential oil, salt, and cinnamon (if using) in a blender. Do not heat milks prior to using.
2. Blend for 30 seconds, until frothy.
3. Pour into two 16-ounce glasses. Sprinkle more cinnamon on top, if desired.
4. Serve immediately.

NOTE: *Try the following blends to give your matcha an EO-powered boost!*
- 2 drops peppermint and 2 drops cinnamon bark essential oils (good for weight loss, appetite suppression, and balancing blood sugar)
- 2 drops caraway and 2 drops fennel essential oils (good for digestion and inflammation)
- 2 drops turmeric, 1 drop black pepper, 1 drop clove bud, and 1 drop ginger essential oils (an adaption of our Easy Golden Milk recipe on page 266—good for digestion and inflammation)
- 2 drops orange and 2 drops lemon essential oils (good for boosting mood and rich in antioxidants)

GET-UP-AND-GO INHALER

7 drops peppermint essential oil
7 drops orange essential oil
5 drops rosemary essential oil

SUPPLIES
Precut organic cotton pad
Aromatherapy inhaler

1. Place a cotton pad in the inhaler tube.
2. Drop the essential oils directly onto the cotton pad inside the tube. Alternatively, you can drop the blend into a glass bowl, roll the cotton pad in the oils to absorb them, and then insert it into the inhaler using tweezers.
3. Secure the cap and store the inhaler in a desk drawer, purse, or glove compartment so you have it handy.

continues

Chronic Fatigue Syndrome and Fibromyalgia   125

4. First thing in the morning or when you need a pick-me-up, open the inhaler and take 10 deep breaths of the vapor from the tube.

GET UP-AND-GO BODY OIL

15 drops orange essential oil

10 drops peppermint essential oil

5 drops rosemary essential oil

2 ounces carrier oil of choice or Mama Z's Oil Base (page 25)

SUPPLIES

Medium glass bowl

Lidded glass jar or lotion dispenser

1. Drop the essential oils into a bowl.
2. Add the carrier oil and mix thoroughly.
3. Use as a body oil after you shower and as a moisturizer throughout the day.

GET-UP-AND-GO ROLL-ON

8 drops orange essential oil

5 drops peppermint essential oil

3 drops rosemary essential oil

Carrier oil of choice—jojoba and fractionated coconut oil absorb quickly and work best—as needed

SUPPLIES

10 ml glass roller bottle

1. Drop the essential oil blend into your roll-on bottle.
2. Fill the bottle with carrier oil, cap it, and shake well.
3. Apply over pulse points and the back of your neck as needed.

GET-UP-AND-GO CAPSULE

Makes 1 dose

2 drops peppermint essential oil

1 drop orange essential oil

1 drop rosemary essential oil

Organic virgin coconut oil or extra-virgin olive oil

SUPPLIES

Pipette

Size 00 vegan gel capsule

1. Using a pipette, drop the essential oils into the bottom half (the longer, narrower one) of the capsule. Fill this half to the brim with coconut or extra-virgin olive oil.

2. Fit the wider top half of the capsule over the bottom half and secure it snugly.

3. Immediately swallow the capsule with water after breakfast (see Note). Take daily and monitor your symptoms.

NOTE: *Do not make and store these capsules for future use. Also, this is not a long-term solution, and using it for more than four weeks at a time is not advisable. Be sure to switch up your protocol monthly and consult with your health-care provider first if you're currently taking medications. Discontinue if adverse reactions occur.*

2. Rosemary

Traditionally thought of as the oil of remembrance, rosemary oil is well-known for its stimulating effect on the central nervous system. It's a fantastic brain stimulant effective for fatigue, depression, and lethargy.

In a 2012 study, researchers administered to volunteers an electroencephalogram (EEG), a test that records the electrical signals of the brain. The results showed significant increases in blood pressure, heart rate, and respiratory rate after inhaling rosemary oil. After the inhalation, subjects were found to have become more active and stated that they felt "fresher." The EEG also showed a reduction in the power of alpha brain waves (a sign of relaxation) and an increase in beta brain waves (sign of alertness). Extremely effective for exhaustion, rosemary works harmoniously with other oils listed here, too.

Great care should be taken for people currently on hypertension medication because of rosemary's tendency to increase cardiovascular risk factors (blood pressure, heart rate, and respiratory rate). We discuss this more in chapter 12.

Application: Make our Get Moving Diffuser Blend to enjoy the energizing power of rosemary oil!

GET MOVING DIFFUSER BLEND

2 drops rosemary essential oil

2 drops bergamot essential oil

2 drops peppermint essential oil

SUPPLIES

Diffuser

1. Fill your diffuser with purified water as directed in the manufacturer's instructions.

2. Add the essential oils.

3. Turn on the diffuser first thing in the morning or when you need a pick-me-up.

4. Turn off the diffuser when done.

3. Lavender

If it seems as if lavender is our go-to oil for almost everything, you're right. With its harmonizing effect on the nervous system and ability to relieve muscular aches and pains, lavender is excellent for certain symptoms of CFS.

A few years ago, Ukrainian researchers evaluated how inhaling bitter orange, geranium, lavender, rosemary, and sandalwood essential oils (along with their combinations) helped 17 patients with CFS. With a population of 42 million, it's of interest to note that 250,000 people in Ukraine suffer from CFS, which is disproportionately higher than in the United States. This is obviously a source of concern for them, and thankfully aromatherapy is helping.

Of all the different combinations, it seems that the blend of lavender and rosemary oil (1:2 ratio) has the most positive impact. Other blends that do well are lavender, geranium, and sandalwood (1:1:1 ratio) and lavender and geranium (1:1 ratio), with lavender obviously being the common denominator. Patients' symptoms improved, including better sleep and less anxiety.

Validating, once again, the importance of essential oil synergy, the researchers made it a point to note that the blends worked much faster than a single oil and helped produce a positive impact for several days after the study ended.

Lavender oil is a multifunctional and flexible oil that is useful for relieving an array of symptoms caused by CFS.

Application: Make personal inhalers with the lavender-based blends from the Ukrainian study and see which one works best for you.

SOOTHING CFS INHALER

OPTION #1: 7 drops lavender and 14 drops rosemary essential oils

OPTION #2: 7 drops each of lavender, geranium, and sandalwood essential oils

OPTION #3: 10 drops each lavender and geranium essential oils

SUPPLIES

Precut organic cotton pad

Aromatherapy inhaler

1. Place a cotton pad in the inhaler tube.

2. Drop the essential oils for one option directly onto the cotton pad inside the tube. Alternatively, you can drop the blend into a glass bowl, roll the cotton pad in the oils to absorb them, and then insert it into the inhaler using tweezers.

3. Secure the cap and store the inhaler in a desk drawer, purse, or glove compartment so you have it handy.

4. When you feel a little run-down mentally or need a pick-me-up, open the inhaler and take 10 deep breaths of the vapor from the tube.

4. Citrus Oils

Fatigue can often stem from a mental health struggle, and mood is a big piece of energy. We know that chronic stress and depression can lead to chronic fatigue, and we also know that citrus essential oils such as orange, lemon, lime, neroli, petitgrain, bergamot, and grapefruit are linked to boosting mood.

With their fresh, sharp citrus aroma, these oils are excellent for clearing the mind and fighting fatigue as they strengthen, revitalize, and refresh the nervous system.

In 2018, a group of researchers studied the problem of central fatigue (CF), a condition that shares many of the same symptoms as CFS but has its root in central nervous system dysfunction. They looked into the impact that essential oils had on rats with CF. Nine essential oils, including lemon, bitter orange, and grapefruit among others, were blended with distilled water and inhaled by the rats. The test animals demonstrated increased physical function and endurance after therapy.

We see similar results in studies evaluating sweet orange and bergamot oils as well.

As one of the most stimulating oils available, bergamot is used by people suffering from fatigue and exhaustion, as well as anxiety, depression, and sleep disorders (all of which can cause fatigue). It can also rebalance your circadian rhythms, boost your energy, and stimulate the production of key neurotransmitters. Bergamot was tested on forty-one healthy women and, compared to the control group, volunteers who enjoyed fifteen minutes of diffusing bergamot oil while resting significantly improved scores for physical and mental fatigue. They also displayed less tension, reduced anger, and less confusion.

Citrus oils also have a wide range of uses and blend well with many other oils. Try different varieties for different effects.

Application: In addition to making citrus oils part of your daily diffuser routine, Try drinking a glass of Dr. Z's Citrus Soda Pop (page 267) every day for two weeks and monitor your energy levels.

5. Oregano

Often referred to as nature's antibiotic, oregano is a top solution for all things related to infection: bacterial, fungal, and viral. Because CFS sometimes can be triggered after a viral attack, oregano oil may be a good choice if you can link chronic fatigue to an infection.

The active ingredient in oregano oil is carvacrol. Also found in thyme and bergamot (as well as several other plants), carvacrol possesses a wide range of biological activities, including antimicrobial, antioxidant, and anticancer applications. In fact, carvacrol's antimicrobial activity is higher than that of other compounds present in essential oils.

Oregano essential oil also has extremely high levels of antioxidants that help protect the body from chronic conditions, and its protective powers make it a superior choice to help your immune system to heal.

Application: If you suspect you have a bacterial, fungal, or viral infection that may be the cause of CFS, consider trying this Triple-Threat Infection-Fighting Protocol. These essential oils are all extremely potent at fighting a variety of infections that drugs are ineffective at managing (including MRSA, a staph infection that is highly resistant to antibiotics) and are safe to consume, and you may find the relief that you've been praying for!

TRIPLE-THREAT INFECTION-FIGHTING PROTOCOL

Makes 1 dose

2 drops tea tree essential oil

1 drop oregano essential oil

1 drop lemongrass essential oil

1 drop thyme essential oil

Organic extra virgin-coconut oil or extra-virgin olive oil

continues

Pipette

Size 00 vegan enteric-coated capsule

1. Using a pipette, drop the essential oils into the bottom half (the longer, narrower one) of the capsule. Fill this half to the brim with organic extra-virgin coconut or extra-virgin olive oil.

2. Fit the wider top half of the capsule over the bottom half and secure it snugly.

3. Immediately swallow the capsule with water after breakfast and/or dinner (see Note). Take once or twice daily and monitor your symptoms.

NOTE: *Do **not** make and store these capsules for future use. Also, this is not a long-term solution, and using it for more than four weeks at a time is not advisable. Be sure to switch up your protocol monthly and consult with your health-care provider first if you're currently taking medications. Discontinue if adverse reactions occur.*

6. Thyme

Thyme essential oil has a strong, earthy aroma, and its main component—thymol—is one of the most studied essential oils, thanks to its ability to cleanse harmful microbes. It may also reduce fatigue. In a 2016 study, researchers induced fatigue in the brains of mice, then injected them with thymol. This produced anti-fatigue activity in their brains. The researchers suggested that this activity may have been caused by thymol's anti-inflammatory and nerve-activating properties.

Thyme oil may also boost immunity and has antidepressant capabilities, making it a powerful choice to alleviate the symptoms of CFS.

Application: Try the Triple-Threat Infection-Fighting Protocol (page 131).

7. Helichrysum

A beautiful annual flower, helichrysum is from the daisy family and is named for its appearance—not unlike a burst of sunshine! Also known by the name immortelle, helichrysum essential oil uses are more aptly considered a gift to us, with age-reversing capabilities and healing factors packaged in a delightful, bright flower.

In 2013, volunteers with mental exhaustion and burnout were given an aromatherapy inhaler with a blend of peppermint, basil, and helichrysum; this intervention's benefits were compared with those of rose water (the control). The essential oils group felt a significant reduction in their fatigue symptoms over a three-week period. Given these attributes, helichrysum, in concert with other oils, may contribute to the relief of CFS symptoms.

Application: Here's an easy-to-make homemade adaption of the protocol the researchers used in this study.

IMMORTELLE ENERGY INHALER

10 drops helichrysum essential oil

5 drops basil essential oil

5 drops peppermint essential oil

SUPPLIES

Precut organic cotton pad

Aromatherapy inhaler

1. Place a cotton pad in the inhaler tube.

2. Drop the essential oils directly onto the cotton pad inside the tube. Alternatively, you can drop the blend into a glass bowl, roll the cotton pad in the oils to absorb them, and then insert it into the inhaler using tweezers.

3. Secure the cap and store the inhaler in a desk drawer, purse, or glove compartment so you have it handy.

4. When you feel a little run down mentally or need a pick-me-up, open the inhaler and take 10 deep breaths of the vapor from the tube.

➜ To watch us make this recipe and learn more about our favorite ways to promote natural energy, go to EOApothecary.com.

THE TOP ESSENTIAL OILS FOR FIBROMYALGIA

As more people fail to respond satisfactorily to drugs prescribed for fibromyalgia symptoms, aromatherapy continues to top the list of natural alternatives. Relieving these symptoms can further help to slow the pain cycle, which helps people suffering from fibromyalgia become more mobile and sleep better, which can limit further pain.

1. Camphor

Similar to eucalyptus and peppermint in its ability to heal and reduce pain, camphor should be in every fibromyalgia patient's medicine cabinet. One of the largest studies to date investigated the benefit of a proprietary blend of camphor, eucalyptus, lemon, orange, rosemary, and peppermint essential oils along with aloe vera gel on 133 patients with fibromyalgia symptoms. It was reported that every person enjoyed pain relief, better sleep, and even improved grip strength.

Application: Use this adaption of the research study formula for speedy, effective fibromyalgia pain relief.

FIBRO RELIEF OINTMENT

2 ounces aloe vera gel

2 ounces organic virgin coconut oil, melted

20 drops lemon essential oil

20 drops orange essential oil

15 drops camphor essential oil

15 drops peppermint essential oil

10 drops eucalyptus essential oil (any species will do)

10 drops rosemary essential oil

SUPPLIES

Food processor or blender

Lidded glass storage container

1. Blend the aloe vera get, organic virgin coconut oil, and essential oils in a food processor or blender until smooth.

2. Once well mixed and smooth, transfer the mixture to a storage container, cover, and keep in a cool place (like the fridge) so the coconut oil remains hardened.

3. Apply twice daily over any trigger points and achy muscles.

2. Basil

Basil oil is used all over the world to treat disorders of the central nervous system, including anxiety, epilepsy, and pain. Its essential compound, linalool, is known for its analgesic (pain-reducing) properties.

In 2015, researchers set out to prove whether topical application of basil essential oil could reduce chronic muscle pain caused by fibromyalgia in mice and compared it to the standard prescription medication, tramadol. They discovered that basil oil had the better pain-reducing impact. Researchers noted that basil essential oil "can be an interesting alternative for the development of new therapeutic options for the treatment of chronic painful conditions, as fibromyalgia."

Migraines are common to fibromyalgia patients, and, during a triple-blind clinical trial evaluating 144 migraine patients, it was discovered that a 6 percent topical application of basil essential oil reduced the intensity and frequency of migraine attacks.

Consuming basil essential oil is safe and has protective, anti-inflammatory, and antimicrobial benefits as well.

Application: Blending well with minty oils, enjoy a 6 percent basil dilution by adding 30 drops of basil essential oil and 5 drops of wintergreen essential oil with 1 ounce of Mama Z's Oil Base (page 25) and apply at the first sign of a flare-up.

3. Pine

Many people, including CFS and fibromyalgia sufferers, experience adrenal fatigue, the burnout of your adrenal glands due to chronic stress. Your adrenals are two small glands that sit above your kidneys and are part of your endocrine system. They are responsible for producing a large number of hormones that are crucial in our day-to-day functions.

One of the major hormones your adrenals regulate is cortisol, also referred to as the stress hormone. Normally, a certain amount of cortisol release is a good thing, as it helps regulate our circadian rhythm. However, if too little cortisol is released (i.e., hypocortisolism) during times of chronic stress, it can burden your adrenals.

This is where pine essential oil can help because it has cortisol-like effects on the body.

Previously stressed adrenals increase the risk of developing CFS and fibromyalgia syndrome. This is a paradox unique to CFS and fibromyalgia, because cortisol levels normally rise in response to inflammation, pain, and psychological and emotional stress factors. However, in CFS and fibromyalgia, cortisol levels tend to fall. According to some experts, "As a result of this paradoxical response, it is likely that people with CFS and FMS [fibromyalgia syndrome] suffer more because they have inadequate anti-inflammatory and analgesic adrenal hormones."

Application: Try blending frankincense and orange essential oils with pine for powerful pain relief and an earthy-smelling escape from fibromyalgia symptoms. Mix 7 doses topical CBD (see manufacturer's instructions for dosage) with 15 drops each pine, frankincense, and orange essential oils and 2 ounces Mama Z's Oil Base (page 25). Apply over sore muscles and trigger points twice daily for one week and see how you respond.

4. Linalool-Rich Oils

Linalool is a natural compound found in many essential oils that contain well-known anti-inflammatory and antinociceptive (pain-relieving) properties.

In multiple animal studies, treatment with soothing linalool, for instance, has shown us that the compound produces a "significant reduction" of mechanical hyperalgesia (heightened pain upon moving) and chronic noninflammatory muscle pain. When you see the long list of essential oils that contain copious amounts of linalool, it's no surprise that many of these are regarded as natural painkillers! Refer to chapter 4 for the full list of essential oils that are rich in linalool.

Application: Try the following four linalool-powered remedies to tackle fibromyalgia.

FLOWER-POWER BODY OIL

5 drops clary sage essential oil

5 drops neroli essential oil

5 drops lavender essential oil

3 drops ylang ylang essential oil

2 drops geranium essential oil

2 tablespoons carrier oil of your choice

SUPPLIES

Medium glass bowl

Lidded glass jar or lotion dispenser

1. Drop the essential oils into a bowl.
2. Add a carrier oil and mix thoroughly.
3. Use as a body oil after you shower and as a body moisturizer throughout the day.

CITRUS SPICE FIBRO CAPSULE

Makes 1 dose

2 drops coriander seed essential oil

1 drop bergamot mint essential oil

1 dose full-spectrum CBD (follow manufacturer's instructions for dosage)

Organic virgin coconut oil or extra-virgin olive oil

SUPPLIES

Pipette

Size 00 vegan gel capsule

continues

1. Using a pipette, drop the essential oils and CBD into the bottom half (the longer, narrower one) of the capsule. Fill this half to the brim with organic extra-virgin coconut or extra-virgin olive oil.
2. Fit the wider top half of the capsule over the bottom half and secure it snugly.
3. Immediately swallow the capsule with water after breakfast and/or dinner (see Note). Take once or twice daily and monitor your symptoms.

NOTE: *Do **not** make and store these capsules for future use. Also, this is not a long-term solution, and using it for more than four weeks at a time is not advisable. Be sure to switch up your protocol monthly and consult with your health-care provider first if you're currently taking medications. Discontinue if adverse reactions occur.*

FIBRO FIX DIFFUSER BLENDS

OPTION #1
2 drops bergamot mint essential oil
2 drops coriander seed essential oil
2 drops petitgrain essential oil

OPTION #2
2 drops bergamot mint essential oil
1 drop geranium essential oil
1 drop lavender essential oil
1 drop ylang ylang essential oil

SUPPLIES
Diffuser

1. Fill your diffuser with purified water as directed in the manufacturer's instructions.
2. Add the essential oils for one option.
3. Turn on the diffuser when fibromyalgia symptoms flare up.
4. Turn off the diffuser when done.

CITRUS FLOWER ROLL-ON

5 drops magnolia flower essential oil

3 drops petitgrain essential oil

3 drops bergamot essential oil

2 drops neroli essential oil

Carrier oil of choice—jojoba and fractionated coconut oil absorb quickly and
    work best—as needed

SUPPLIES

10 ml glass roller bottle

1. Drop the essential oil blend into your roll-on bottle.
2. Fill the bottle with carrier oil and shake well.
3. Apply over trigger points and sore muscles as needed.

Essential oils are a vital piece of the fatigue-fighting puzzle. For best results, use them in conjunction with other natural therapies, such as eating healthier, improving sleep, and minimizing stress. With a comprehensive approach, you have a better chance of regaining your energy and transforming your life.

Chapter 8

Libido and Erectile Dysfunction

T ruth or dare: Did you skip to this chapter without reading the first few chapters of the book? If you did, don't worry, your secret is safe with us. In fact, we wouldn't be surprised if this chapter ends up with the most dog-ears, highlighting, and notes in the entire book!

Why?

Because last year we were pleasantly surprised to learn that our most popular blog post was "Essential Oils for Sex." Not only was it the number one most-visited post out of the hundreds that are on our site, but a majority of the people reading it came from a search engine like Google, Bing, or Yahoo. This means that a considerable amount of people are actively searching for the phrase "essential oils for sex" online.

This caught us by surprise, because we rarely receive questions about sex from our Natural Living Family readers and members. Sex is a very private thing, and we had no idea that so many people in our online community needed help between the sheets.

If you suffer with a chronic disease, you most likely have had or will have problems with your sex drive. With low libido and erectile dysfunction topping the list of sexual dysfunctions, the fact is anyone with chronic disease is at risk of developing some sexual dysfunction. For reasons that we don't quite understand just yet, men with diabetes and women who suffer from chronic fatigue and pain syndromes like fibromyalgia, arthritis, and osteoporosis seem to be affected most.

Before we talk about the best essential oils for sex, the first thing to understand is that you are not alone. For men, low libido often results in erectile dysfunction, which ranges in prevalence from 5 percent in younger men to 25 percent in men over sixty-five. In women, low libido is common in all stages of life because of fluctuating hormones. Chronic illnesses just complicate and compound the issue.

Suffering from low libido periodically or chronically is nothing to be ashamed of. Bringing your concerns into the open with your partner can start the path toward health, intimacy, and resolution—along with positive lifestyle changes. This chapter will help you on your journey back to intimacy.

ESTROGEN AND VAGINAL DRYNESS

As estrogen levels ebb and flow during a woman's lifetime, so does her risk of developing vaginal dryness and experiencing painful sex. Thyroid conditions, too much exercise, menopause, anorexia, pituitary gland problems, and chemotherapy are just a few of the common causes of low estrogen.

Estrogen helps the vagina remain lubricated with a thin layer of clear fluid, which keeps the vaginal walls elastic, healthy, and thick. When estrogen drops, this natural healing lubricant is reduced, thus making the vaginal wall thinner and less elastic. For this condition, technically referred to as vaginal atrophy, many doctors prescribe a topical estrogen cream to help reduce pain and friction throughout the day.

It is important to avoid all conventional store-bought douches, bubble baths, lotions, and scented soaps, because the chemicals in these products can exacerbate the issue. Instead, we recommend making your own lubricant not just for sex but for your day-to-day activities, as vaginal dryness can be painful even if you're simply walking!

When making a lubricant, be sure to only use gentle oils at a max 0.5 to 1 percent dilution. As long as you use the safe oils we recommend in the proper dilutions, there are no safety issues that you need to be concerned with. Use as you would any store-bought lubricant. Here's a recipe that you may find helpful.

GENTLE LUBRICANT

3 drops geranium essential oil

3 drops lavender essential oil

3 drops Roman chamomile essential oil

3 drops ylang ylang essential oil

2 ounces Mama Z's Oil Base (page 25) or organic virgin coconut oil

SUPPLIES

Medium glass bowl

Lidded glass jar or lotion dispenser

1. Drop the essential oils into the bowl.
2. Add the oil base and mix well. Cover and store in a lidded jar or lotion dispenser.
3. Massage into the labia before and after sexual intercourse and as needed.
4. You may also find it helpful to lubricate before and after putting in a tampon or after swimming and showering.

THE ESSENTIAL OILS APPROACH TO LIBIDO

Enjoying sex is part of the abundant life that we preach about so much. With gentle and relaxing aromas, essential oils can play a unique role in helping you do this. Get creative to see how you can boost your libido with them and how they can enhance your time between the sheets!

The following essential oils have been proven to help, giving you and your partner an additional way to rekindle the romance in your home.

STOP Before you start implementing these essential oils for libido and erectile dysfunction, be sure to review the known drug interaction chart in Appendix B and consult with your physician if you're currently taking any medications. Also, don't forget that using essential oils while living a "fast food" lifestyle is like taking one step forward but two steps back! In other words, for essential oils to help you enjoy abundant health and wellness—free from chronic disease—it is vital to use them within the context of a healthy lifestyle. Go to Appendix A for our favorite "Disease-Busting Healthy Lifestyle Hacks" to learn more!

SENSUAL BLEND

Making your own get-in-the-mood blend is as easy as choosing four or five of these oils and blending them together in different ratios until you find "the one": vanilla, cinnamon bark, patchouli, bergamot, orange, neroli, geranium, clary sage, lavender, sandalwood, ylang ylang, rose, and jasmine. We know how expensive and hard to find jasmine and rose can be, so try this blend as your base to get you started.

15 drops orange essential oil

10 drops bergamot essential oil

10 drops neroli essential oil

10 drops lavender essential oil

10 drops ylang ylang essential oil

5 drops sandalwood essential oil

5 drops geranium essential oil

5 drops jasmine absolute essential oil (see Note)

5 drops patchouli essential oil

5 drops rose essential oil (see Note)

7 drops vanilla absolute, CO_2, or oleoresin (see Note)

SUPPLIES

5 ml glass bottle

1. Mix the essential oils in a 5 ml bottle. Cap and shake well.

2. Use as directed in the following recipes.

NOTE: *Simply omit jasmine, rose, and vanilla absolute essential oils if you do not have them. No other modifications need to be made.*

SENSUAL INHALER

20 to 25 drops Sensual Blend (page 143)

SUPPLIES

Precut organic cotton pad

Aromatherapy inhaler

1. Place a cotton pad in the inhaler tube.

2. Drop the essential oils directly onto the cotton pad inside the tube. Alternatively, you can drop the blend into a glass bowl, roll the cotton pad in the oils to absorb them, and then insert it into the inhaler using tweezers.

3. Secure the cap and store the inhaler in a desk drawer, purse, or glove compartment so you have it handy.

4. When you want to rev up the engines on your libido, open the inhaler, take 10 deep breaths of the vapor from the tube, and think about love, romance, and "happy thoughts" related to sex.

SENSUAL DIFFUSER BLEND

6 drops Sensual Blend (page 143)

SUPPLIES

Diffuser

1. Fill your diffuser with purified water as directed in the manufacturer's instructions.

2. Add the essential oil blend.

3. Turn on the diffuser for 10 to 20 minutes to "set the mood," letting the essential oils permeate the room. Keep the diffuser running as long as you need.

SENSUAL BODY AND MASSAGE OIL

36 drops Sensual Blend (page 143)

2 ounces carrier oil of your choice or Mama Z's Oil Base (page 25)

SUPPLIES

Medium glass bowl

Lidded glass jar or lotion dispenser

1. Drop the essential oil blend into a bowl.
2. Add a carrier oil and mix well.
3. Use as a body oil after you shower to moisturize and as a sensual massage oil.

SENSUAL ROLL-ON

20 drops Sensual Blend (page 143)

Carrier oil of choice—jojoba and fractionated coconut oil absorb quickly and work best—as needed

SUPPLIES

10 ml glass roller bottle

1. Drop the essential oils into the roller bottle.
2. Fill the bottle with your carrier oil of choice and shake well.
3. Apply over pulse points and the back of your neck as a sensual perfume.

SENSUAL BATH

6 to 10 drops Sensual Blend (page 143)

1 tablespoon jojoba oil

1 cup plain Epsom salts

¼ cup unfiltered, raw apple cider vinegar

SUPPLIES

Medium glass bowl

continues

1. Mix the essential oil blend and jojoba oil in a glass bowl.
2. Add the Epsom salts and cider vinegar and mix well.
3. Fill your bathtub with the warmest water you can stand.
4. Slowly pour the mixture into the running water.
5. Enjoy a sensual bath with your partner for 20 to 30 minutes.
6. Exit the bath slowly by first sitting up, then kneeling, and finally standing to prevent feeling faint.

SENSUAL BODY SPRAY

36 drops Sensual Blend (page 143)

10 drops organic 190-proof grain alcohol (or the highest proof alcohol you can get)

½ ounce witch hazel extract or organic hydrosol of your choice

Distilled water or rose hydrosol (a product obtained from steam distillation of fresh/dried rose petals)

SUPPLIES

2-ounce glass spray bottle

1. Drop the essential oil blend into the spray bottle, add the alcohol and witch hazel, and shake well to mix.
2. Fill the remainder of bottle with water or hydrosol.
3. Spritz on skin or hair as desired, shaking well before each use.

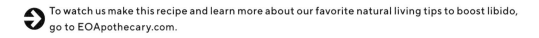 To watch us make this recipe and learn more about our favorite natural living tips to boost libido, go to EOApothecary.com.

BETWEEN THE SHEETS SPRAY

1 ounce organic witch hazel extract or rose hydrosol

36 drops Sensual Blend (page 143)

Distilled water

SUPPLIES

2-ounce glass spray bottle

1. Drop the essential oil blend in the spray bottle, add the witch hazel extract or hydrosol, and shake well to mix.

2. Fill the remainder of the bottle with water or rose hydrosol.

3. Spritz on sheets, the couch, or your lingerie 10 to 15 minutes before "to set the mood," shaking the bottle well before each use. Be sure to test fabrics first to make sure it doesn't stain.

NOTE: *The essential oils in this solution are not properly dissolved because there is no alcohol used, so be sure to shake it well to physically disperse the oil in the mixture before spraying. This also means that this recipe has a shorter shelf life than a solution made with alcohol. Be sure to use it up within one month. Making smaller batches helps prevent waste.*

1. Rose

Known for centuries as an aphrodisiac, it's no surprise that rose oil is a libido booster—and today's science supports that claim. In a 2015 study, rose oil was shown to improve sexual dysfunction in male patients who were taking medication for depression. Not only that, but the men claimed their symptoms of depression were reduced as well.

As a pricey oil, however, rose is most efficiently used in blends or heavy dilutions.

Application: Blend this fragrant oil with bergamot and patchouli for a wonderfully stimulating aroma. Add 3 drops bergamot, 2 drops patchouli, and 1 drop rose essential oils to your diffuser.

2. Jasmine

A precious oil derived from delicate flower petals, jasmine has proven itself in studies. Researchers tested alertness and "behavioral arousal" after a topical application of jasmine oil. The participants were found to be more refreshed, with their senses on alert.

This amazing oil is ideal to use in a sensual massage oil with your partner. Researchers in Thailand found that diluted jasmine oil applied on the stomach increased sexual arousal in forty healthy adult women. It also had a stimulating and uplifting effect on the volunteers, making this a beautiful floral oil to improve romantic encounters with your partner.

Application: More companies are selling pre-diluted jasmine essential oil and absolute roll-ons to help make this rare, expensive product more accessible to the general public. Here's an easy hack to get the most out of your money and make some jasmine-based blends to spice up your love life.

RARE OIL ROLL-ON HACK

10 ml pre-diluted jasmine, neroli, or rose roll-on

4 to 6 drops of 2 different essential oils (see Note)

Carrier oil of choice—jojoba and fractionated coconut oil absorb quickly—as needed

SUPPLIES

5 (10 ml) roll-on bottles

1. Pour 2 ml of the pre-diluted oil into each empty roll-on bottle. Now you have 5 roll-on bottles that are ready to be "enhanced" with other libido-stimulating oils.

2. Add 2 or 3 drops of each essential oil to each of the roll-on bottles to find that "perfect" blend for you and your partner!

3. Fill the roller bottle with your carrier oil of choice and shake well.

NOTE: *Oils that blend well with jasmine include bergamot, clary sage, clove bud, ginger, grapefruit, lemon, lime, magnolia, mandarin, neroli, orange, palmarosa, patchouli, petitgrain, rose, sandalwood, tangerine, and ylang ylang.*

3. Clary Sage

An important one for women's health, clary sage essential oil contains many components known for their anti-inflammatory and calming benefits, including linalool (a major component of lavender oil) and linalyl acetate (along with excellent anti-inflammatory benefits on the skin, it also contains a natural chemical called sclareol, which has an impact on the way cancer cells proliferate that could help induce apoptosis, or cancer cell death).

As for sexuality, a 2014 study undertook the question of menopause-symptom relief and essential oils. The research found that simply inhaling hormone-balancing clary sage essential oil had an antidepressant effect on menopausal women. When libido is low due to hormonal shifts like menopause, clary sage is a balancer that may bring some relief.

Application: For a women's health blend like no other, clary sage mixes well with florals like geranium, jasmine, lavender, magnolia, and rose. Start off by placing 1 drop of each floral oil you have on hand in your diffuser, and then experiment with roll-ons and body oil at a 2 percent total dilution for a gentle, healing aroma. See pages 26–28 for our dilution chart.

4. Ylang Ylang

Ylang ylang has a reputation as an aphrodisiac throughout the aromatherapy world and is one of the best essential oils for increasing arousal and improving sex.

But, in fact, the effect ylang ylang has on the body is actually not to boost the libido. But it does reduce anxiety, which can get in the way of lovemaking. By that token, ylang ylang can help set the mood.

Ylang ylang is also a known harmonizer, which means it helps your body reach balance (homeostasis), and it is a wonderful addition to any "love" blend.

Application: Use by diffusion, inhalation, or diluted into a 2 percent solution with a carrier oil to create a massage oil for both men and women. Ylang Ylang also mixes well with florals and resins like copaiba, frankincense, and myrrh. See pages 26–28 for our dilution chart.

5. Neroli

This essential oil, derived from orange blossoms, is a precious and very useful oil. In one clinical trial, researchers found that the "inhalation of neroli oil helps relieve menopausal symptoms, increase sexual desire, and reduce blood pressure in post-menopausal women," making it another helpful option when libido is low due to hormones or stress.

A systematic review of the literature suggests that it's best to blend neroli with other oils for a more enhanced experience. When combined with fennel, geranium, lavender, and rose, for example, neroli "significantly improved" sexual desire and intimacy in postmenopausal women. It's interesting to note that a significant change in estrogen levels wasn't detected in volunteers, and they didn't report vaginal dryness symptoms improving. This suggests the importance for safe, nontoxic lubrication during sex.

Application: Neroli is also a rare, expensive oil, and like jasmine and rose, we're seeing more companies sell neroli in a pre-diluted roll-on form. Try our Rare Oil Roll-On Hack (page 148). Oils that blend well with neroli include Roman chamomile, clary sage, copaiba, coriander, frankincense, geranium, ginger, grapefruit, jasmine, juniper, lavender, lemon, mandarin, myrrh, orange, palmarosa, petitgrain, rose, sandalwood, and ylang ylang.

6. Fennel

The essential oil derived from fennel seeds has been reputed to promote menstruation, facilitate birth, ease the symptoms of menopause, and increase libido.

Note that in the study referenced above, fennel was used as part of the neroli blend to enhance sexual desire and helped reduce intimacy avoidance. We see this in other studies where fennel is used as a stand-alone therapy to boost libido.

Application: Mix 3 drops each of fennel, geranium, lavender, neroli, and rose essential oils with 1 ounce of Mama Z's Oil Base (page 25) for an after-shower, libido-boosting moisturizer or massage oil.

7. Lavender

As you'd expect, the soporific, parasympathetic-inducing prowess of lavender oil makes this a wonderful addition to any healthy sex protocol.

A review of the literature suggests the effectiveness of using lavender in all three ways (ingestion, inhalation, topical) not only to increase sexual desire but also to help improve sleep, depression, anxiety, and psychological and physical symptoms that can complicate low libido and erectile dysfunction.

We associate lavender oil with relaxation, so it's interesting to consider using it for arousal. However, that's just what the *Journal of Menopausal Medicine* suggested in a recent review of the effects of lavender on menopausal and elderly women. In three separate trials, women using lavender in oil or capsule form felt a significant improvement in sexual desire. They also reported improvements in sexual function, depression, anxiety, and physical symptoms and claimed to feel more relaxed and happy.

So be sure to have this amazingly flexible oil on hand for romantic evenings at home!

Application: Try taking 2 or 3 drops of lavender oil in a vegan gel capsule daily after dinner for a week to see if you can spice up your love life at night. Be sure to fill up your capsule with an edible carrier oil to help ensure safety and efficacy.

8. Cinnamon Bark

Let's end with one for the guys out there who love pumpkin pie. The spice blend that gives your favorite dessert its powerful flavor also doubles as an aphrodisiac. And, yes, this is backed up by research!

Dr. Alan Hirsch, director of Chicago's Smell and Taste Treatment and Research Foundation, tested forty odors and discovered that a mixture of lavender and pumpkin pie got the biggest rise in libido in men aged eighteen to sixty-four. This particular aroma was found to increase penile blood flow by an average of 40 percent. Hirsch's theory is that "the odors acted to reduce anxiety. By reducing anxiety, it acted to remove inhibitions."

What's in pumpkin pie spice? Like curry, there's no set recipe, but you'll generally find allspice, anise, cinnamon, cloves, ginger, and nutmeg in the mix.

We want to highlight cinnamon bark here, because it's a known aphrodisiac, recognized for increasing libido and counteracting erectile dysfunction. It was used by the ancient Egyptians in love potions.

This essential oil works by stimulating circulation, even to genital areas. This means it can help you manage or prevent erectile dysfunction issues caused by blood vessels and flow that functions improperly.

There are not any human studies evaluating cinnamon bark oil and libido, but, in 2019, scientists from Turkey and Croatia looked into the effect of injecting cinnamaldehyde, the main component of the oil, into mice and found that it helped improve erectile dysfunction. Until we have some human studies, don't give up on cinnamon bark oil as a potent aphrodisiac. Its pleasant aroma is a great addition to a romantic evening.

Furthermore, although we don't have studies on the essential oils specifically, research on clove, ginger, and nutmeg extracts all show sexual-enhancing properties in male animals.

Application: Make a pumpkin pie spice blend by mixing 1 drop anise, 1 drop clove bud, 1 drop cinnamon bark, 1 drop ginger, and 1 drop nutmeg essential oils into your diffuser to help you (or your partner) get into the mood!

You are not alone in dealing with libido issues. Men and women of all ages have faced this problem and found hope and renewal. There is no shame in admitting the frustration and in seeking a natural solution! Along with openness, sharing, and healthy lifestyle choices, add essential oils and enjoy the renewal that takes place in your relationship.

Advanced Strategies and Protocols for Chronic Disease

I n this section, we cover how essential oils can help naturally prevent and manage the most prevalent chronic diseases, which also happen to make up the vast majority of preventable deaths in the world.

For many reading this book, you may be in a life-or-death situation and are frantically looking for natural solutions because standard medical care has failed you. Please note that we're praying for you. We cannot stress enough how much respect we have for your situation, and we have put the utmost care into each and every recommendation in the following pages. We hope and pray that you find the solution(s) that you're looking for!

With that said, keep in mind that before you start implementing these essential oils for chronic disease remedies, it is vital to use them within the context of a healthy lifestyle.

While writing this section, it became glaringly obvious to us how consistent and redundant the recommendations are for each of these diseases. Stop smoking, don't drink too much alcohol, exercise, manage stress and feeling over-whelmed, get at least seven hours of sleep a night, eat the right foods, and so forth. All of these are risk factors for each and every one of the diseases mentioned in this section. Thus, instead of repeating the same recommendations over and over again, we created our favorite "Disease-Busting Healthy Lifestyle Hacks," which you can find in Appendix A.

→ To help you along the journey, we have created a series of demo videos on preparing several of the essential oil remedies and recipes featured in the *Essential Oils Apothecary*. Each of the videos contains extra insights into the strategies and information covered in this book. You can access these free videos at EOApothecary.com.

Chapter 9

Alzheimer's and Dementia

When it comes to using essential oils to promote brain health and manage Alzheimer's disease (AD), a recent literature review sums it up best:

> *EOs are effective against almost all currently known pathological targets of AD. EOs also possess neuroprotective, anti-aging potentials and are effective in dementia, epilepsy, anxiety and other neurological disorders. . . . Special focus must be on the edible EOs, which are either part of diet or used as spices will be more useful.*

Hence, essential oils can be referred to as *nootropics* ("smart drugs") or cognitive enhancers: drugs, supplements, and other substances that improve cognitive function, particularly executive functions, memory, creativity, or motivation.

It is with this in mind that we present the following strategy on how to safely and effectively approach Alzheimer's disease and dementia.

DEMENTIA AND ALZHEIMER'S DISEASE

The very word *dementia* frightens most people. Dementia is a condition that leaves you a shell of yourself, and people are lost long before they actually die.

If someone you love is diagnosed with dementia, it means he or she has a progressive and sometimes chronic brain condition in which the ability to remember, think, reason, interact socially, and perform self-care is lost. And we are finding that practically everyone we meet knows someone who is battling dementia or caring for a relative affected by it. We've been staggered by how commonplace it is—which is why we must start talking about it more often and look at natural ways to prevent it from occurring.

Dementia is not a single disease but a term for a cluster of overall symptoms covering a wide range of specific brain disorders. More formally defined as a chronic or persistent mental processing disorder, dementia is caused by brain disease or injury and marked by memory disorders, personality changes, and impaired reasoning. Alzheimer's disease accounts for roughly 60 to 80 percent of all dementia cases.

Named after Dr. Alois Alzheimer, who discovered it in 1906, this is an irreversible dementia in which you lose your mind—literally. If someone you know has Alzheimer's, you'll notice symptoms such as memory loss, behavior changes, and difficulty doing everyday tasks. The symptoms are mild at first but worsen over time and include the following:

- Being forgetful (It is generally normal, for example, to lose our keys. Someone with AD might not only lose keys but also forget what keys and other everyday objects are.)
- Being confused about time, date, or place
- Experiencing problems speaking or writing
- Showing poor judgment
- Exhibiting mood and personality changes (agitation being the hallmark sign)

In Alzheimer's disease, a protein called beta amyloid peptide builds up both outside brain cells, forming brain-cell-killing plaques, and inside brain cells, causing fibrous tangles. It's thought that these clumps damage healthy neurons and the fibers connecting them.

Although not all causes of AD have been identified, it has been reported that 70 percent of all Alzheimer's cases are attributable to genetics, whereas the remaining

30 percent are caused by environmental triggers like viruses, free-radical activity, head trauma, and chemical exposure to toxic metals like aluminum and copper, pesticides and insecticides, industrial chemicals and flame retardants, and air pollutants. At any given time, Alzheimer's is ranked between the third and sixth leading cause of death.

GET A LITTLE DIRTY ONCE IN A WHILE

Research from the Oxford journal *Evolution, Medicine, and Public Health* has found a strong link between overly sanitized, wealthier countries and a higher rate of Alzheimer's. Conducted across 192 countries, this study suggests that the lack of bacteria creates a poorly developed immune system, which puts your brain at risk for inflammation.

This is a strong indication that we shouldn't be using antibacterial products. Good old-fashioned soap and water is fine.

And think twice before using that hand sanitizer after opening the car door; exposure to microorganisms—both good and bad—is vitally important for the body to develop proper immune responses.

If you're in a situation where you feel it's necessary to use hand sanitizer, be sure to make your own with essential oils, which will help preserve the healthy bacteria balance on your skin. See page 47 for our Quick and Easy Hand Sanitizer recipe!

Start a garden, get your hands dirty, and enjoy some healthy bacteria from the ground.

And don't forget to load up on probiotics rich in soil-based organisms and fermented foods, which all contribute to a healthy bacteria balance.

ACETYLCHOLINESTERASE INHIBITORS AND ESSENTIAL OILS

The sad reality is that today there is no known cure for AD and the cognitive decline that affects millions with dementia across the globe; palliative care and attempts to manage symptoms are the only treatments.

Of those diagnosed with mild cognitive impairment, roughly half will develop dementia within five years. Not only is there no cure but "there are currently no FDA approved medications that can *stop that progression*," according to researchers at Boston's Beth Israel Deaconess Medical Center. So, once the train leaves the station, there's no slowing it down until it reaches its destination. And, in this case, that's generally Alzheimer's disease and eventually an untimely death.

Thus, the only potential benefits of AD medications are to control the patient's agitation, aggression, and/or psychotic symptoms. To add insult to injury, the use of these pharmacological agents has considerable limits: their effectiveness is generally experienced only in the first few weeks of treatment. Their efficacy greatly diminishes in the long term, and they present significant side effects.

Subsequently, there is growing interest in aromatherapy as a natural alternative because of the unique quality of essential oils to achieve the same outcome as the gold standard in AD medication: acetylcholinesterase inhibitors.

The primary medical approach for AD is to prescribe these drugs. More commonly referred to as cholinesterase inhibitors, they block the activity of an enzyme in the brain known as cholinesterase, which is responsible for breaking down the neurotransmitter acetylcholine.

Low levels of acetylcholine are devastating for nerve impulse function and cause mental impairment, both hallmarks of Alzheimer's disease. Cholinesterase inhibitors (such as donepezil, rivastigmine, and galantamine) are thus used to reduce the action of cholinesterase, thereby making more acetylcholine available to nerve cells in the brain.

Side effects of these drugs include death, vomiting, falling, dizziness, nausea, confusion, pneumonia, diarrhea, hallucinations, malaise, convulsions, rapid heart rate and other heart problems, loss of consciousness, decreased appetite, and unhealthy weight loss.

On the other hand, essential oils have been observed to inhibit acetylcholinesterase with no reported side effects! For instance, cinnamaldehyde and cinnamyl acetate, two primary components in cinnamon bark essential oil, have shown nearly an 80 percent inhibitory activity on cholinesterase.

There are other essential oils known for their anticholinesterase activity:

- Australian and black pine
- Basil
- Bergamot
- Key lime leaf
- Lavender
- Lemon balm
- Lemon myrtle
- Orange, bitter
- Oregon ash
- River red gum
- Rosemary
- Sage
- Spanish sage
- Thyme

THYME OIL AND CARVACROL

A study in 2007 evaluated the cholinesterase inhibitory properties of thyme essential oil and its primary components: linalool, thymol, carvacrol, and their derivatives. They discovered that linalool was least effective, thymol was second from last, and carvacrol topped the charts, being ten times stronger than thymol.

This shouldn't surprise us, as carvacrol, the primary component of oregano essential oil, has been acknowledged for its neuroprotective prowess in the medical literature for years.

Essential Oils Rich in Carvacrol

- Oregano (61.6 to 83.4 percent)
- Marjoram, wild (76.4 to 81.0 percent)
- Savory, winter (46.5 to 75.0 percent)
- Savory, summer (43.6 to 70.0 percent)
- Thyme (20 to 70 percent)
- Black seed (0.5 to 4.2 percent)

If you're looking to replace cholinesterase inhibitors for yourself or for a loved one for whom you care, consider consulting with your physician about using the following essential oils remedies.

CHOLINESTERASE-INHIBITING CAPSULE

Makes 1 dose

1 drop Melissa (lemon balm) essential oil

1 drop sage essential oil

1 drop thyme essential oil

1 drop oregano essential oil

Organic virgin coconut oil or extra-virgin olive oil

SUPPLIES

Pipette

Size 00 vegan gel capsule

1. Using a pipette, drop the essential oils into the bottom half (the longer, narrower one) of the capsule. Fill this half to the brim with organic extra-virgin coconut or extra-virgin olive oil.

2. Fit the wider top half of the capsule over the bottom half and secure it snugly.

3. Immediately swallow the capsule with water after breakfast and/or dinner (see Note). Take once or twice daily and monitor your symptoms.

NOTE: *Do not make and store these capsules for future use. Also, this is not a long-term solution, and using it for more than four weeks at a time is not advisable. Be sure to switch up your protocol monthly, and consult with your health-care provider first if you're currently taking medications. Discontinue if adverse reactions occur.*

CHOLINESTERASE-INHIBITING ROLL-ON

4 drops oregano essential oil

3 drops marjoram essential oil

3 drops thyme essential oil

3 drops sage essential oil

Carrier oil of choice—jojoba and fractionated coconut oil absorb quickly—as needed

SUPPLIES

10 ml glass roller bottle

1. Drop the essential oils into the roller bottle.
2. Fill the roller bottle with your carrier oil of choice and shake well.
3. Apply over pulse points and the back of your neck once daily.

CHOLINESTERASE-INHIBITING BODY OIL

10 drops bitter orange essential oil

4 drops lemon myrtle essential oil

4 drops Spanish sage essential oil

4 drops Melissa (lemon balm) essential oil

2 ounces carrier oil of choice or Mama Z's Oil Base (page 25)

SUPPLIES

Medium glass bowl

Lidded glass jar or lotion dispenser

1. Drop the essential oils into the bowl.
2. Add the carrier oil and mix thoroughly. Store in glass container.
3. Use as a body oil after you shower and as a moisturizer throughout the day.

CHOLINESTERASE-INHIBITING INHALER

10 drops bergamot essential oil

6 drops rosemary essential oil

4 drop bitter orange essential oil

SUPPLIES

Precut organic cotton pad

Aromatherapy inhaler

1. Place a cotton pad in the inhaler tube.

2. Drop the essential oils directly onto the cotton pad inside the tube. Alternatively, you can drop the blend into a glass bowl, roll the cotton pad in the oils to absorb them, and then insert it into the inhaler using tweezers.

3. Secure the cap and store the inhaler in a desk drawer, purse, or glove compartment so you have it handy.

4. When you feel a little run down mentally or want a brain boost, open the inhaler and take 10 deep breaths of the vapor from the tube.

CHOLINESTERASE-INHIBITING DIFFUSER BLEND

2 drops rosemary essential oil

2 drops bitter orange essential oil

2 drops bergamot essential oil

SUPPLIES

Diffuser

1. Fill your diffuser with purified water as directed in the manufacturer's instructions.

2. Add the essential oils.

3. Turn on the diffuser when you want a mental pick-me-up.

4. Turn off the diffuser when done.

A NOTE ABOUT ANOSMIA

A common question we receive regarding Alzheimer's comes from people with anosmia (impaired or no sense of smell), which is a common comorbidity of dementia. Essentially, people want to know if they're wasting their time with aromatherapy and whether essential oils will help if they cannot smell the volatile organic compounds (VOCs). The answer to this is yes, still use your oils for two reasons.

First, inhaling essential oils can stimulate olfactory cells, cause nerve rebirth, and regenerate a sense of smell for some people. No one can predict who will get their sense of smell back, but suffice it to say that inhaling diffused essential oils for a few minutes a day cannot hurt. It can only help, so why not give it a try?

Second, for those who still cannot smell even after being exposed to essential oils, don't worry, you're still going to benefit. For people with anosmia, the emotional (psychological) effects will most likely not take place, but the mental and physical (physiological) effects still do—meaning the body will still react to aromatherapy in the usual ways, but the mind will not.

This is because of how we are "wired." When we inhale essential oils, there are two reactions: a physiological one, which is hardwired in our brain and body, and a psychological one, which isn't hardwired and varies from person to person, depending on their emotional state.

So, even if you suffer from anosmia, keep using your oils!

THE ESSENTIAL OILS APPROACH TO ALZHEIMER'S

Of all the senses, the sense of smell is the most evocative, with the power to stimulate the brain—and to do it quickly. It's no wonder, then, that the healing art of aromatherapy is being used more and more to boost brainpower. Certain oils can rev up your mental powers, and these oils are discussed below, along with their applications.

STOP Before you start implementing these essential oils for Alzheimer's and dementia, be sure to review the known drug interaction chart in Appendix B and consult with your physician if you're currently taking any medications. Also, don't forget that using essential oils while living a "fast food" lifestyle is like taking one step forward but two steps back! In other words, for essential oils to help you enjoy abundant health and wellness—free from chronic disease—it is vital to use them within the context of a healthy lifestyle. Go to Appendix A to our favorite "Disease-Busting Healthy Lifestyle Hacks" to learn more!

1. Rosemary

No discussion about brain health and cognitive function would be complete without first discussing rosemary, the "herb of remembrance." Touted for centuries to help improve memory, the cognitive enhancing power of 1,8-cineole (a component of rosemary oil) has been well documented in the medical literature.

Only recently, however, has the scientific community begun to examine rosemary essential oil and its chemical constituents (specifically the terpenes) as a natural therapy for Alzheimer's disease, as it has been observed to inhibit neuronal cell death, significantly reduce inflammation, and strengthen attention span.

Application: Make our Focus and Clarity Inhaler for on-the-go mental alertness when you need it most!

FOCUS AND CLARITY INHALER

From *The Healing Power of Essential Oils*

10 drops rosemary essential oil

5 drops pine essential oil

5 drops may chang essential oil (*Litsea cubeba*)

SUPPLIES

Precut organic cotton pad

Aromatherapy inhaler

1. Place a cotton pad in the inhaler tube.
2. Drop the essential oils directly onto the cotton pad inside the tube. Alterna-

tively, you can drop the blend into a glass bowl, roll the cotton pad in the oils to absorb them, and then insert it into the inhaler using tweezers.

3. Secure the cap and store the inhaler in a desk drawer, purse, or glove compartment so you have it handy.

4. Whenever you need a quick boost of mental clarity, open the inhaler and take a few deep breaths through your nose with your eyes closed. Repeat as often as needed.

2. Ginger (CO_2)

As mentioned above, beta-amyloid deposit buildup causes the formation of senile plaques (an important pathological marker of AD), which cause apoptosis (programmed cell death) in neurons through oxidative stress. It has been found that 6-gingerol, a pungent phytochemical rich in antioxidants found in CO_2 ginger extract, can actually protect against this oxidative cell death in the brain.

Additionally, 6-gingerol can restore levels of the important immune system antioxidant glutathione that has been depleted by beta amyloid, which can contribute to overall brain health

Application: Try taking 3 or 4 drops of CO_2 ginger extract in a vegan gel capsule once a day for one month to see if dementia symptoms subside. Be sure to fill up your capsule with an edible carrier oil to help ensure safety and efficacy.

3. Lemon

Shown to have cholinesterase-inhibiting ability, components in lemon oil also contain the strong ability to improve memory and dopamine levels when the brain has been impaired by chemicals and pharmaceuticals.

One exciting study out of Japan evaluated what the researchers referred to as the "curative effects" of aromatherapy on twenty-eight elderly patients, seventeen of whom had AD. Compared to a control group with no exposure to essential oils, a 2:1 ratio blend of rosemary and lemon oils was diffused near patients from 9 a.m. to 11 a.m. every day for twenty-eight days. As anticipated by the researchers, this blend activated the sympathetic nervous system and strengthened concentration, memory, and personal orientation.

Application: In addition to adding lemon and rosemary to your diffuser, try this inhaler recipe for on-the-go support.

CITRUS HERB INHALER

13 drops rosemary essential oil

7 drops lemon essential oil

SUPPLIES

Precut organic cotton pad

Aromatherapy inhaler

1. Place a cotton pad in the inhaler tube.

2. Drop the essential oils directly onto the cotton pad inside the tube. Alternatively, you can drop the blend into a glass bowl, roll the cotton pad in the oils to absorb them, and then insert it into the inhaler using tweezers.

3. Secure the cap and store the inhaler in a desk drawer, purse, or glove compartment so you have it handy.

4. Open the inhaler and take a few deep breaths through your nose with your eyes closed first thing in the morning to help you start your day with mental focus and clarity.

4. Lavender

In the same Japanese study referenced above, researchers administered lavender and orange aromatherapy to help with overall cognitive function, personal orientation, and to promote rest and sleep. For twenty-eight days, a 2:1 blend of lavender and orange oils was diffused near patients from 7:30 p.m. to 9 p.m. every evening.

As expected, this blend activated the parasympathetic nervous system, calmed the patients' nerves, and also strengthened personal orientation and cognitive function.

Additionally, all of the volunteers (including those with AD), showed "significant improvement" in cognitive function after aromatherapy. As we see time and time again in research trials, no negative side effects were observed or reported during the study.

Application: Lavender can be directly inhaled, used as a massage oil, or sprayed on your bedsheets to promote sweet sleep. In addition to adding lavender and orange to your diffuser, try this inhaler recipe for on-the-go support.

CALM AND REFRESH INHALER

13 drops lavender essential oil

7 drops orange essential oil

SUPPLIES

Precut organic cotton pad

Aromatherapy inhaler

1. Place a cotton pad in the inhaler tube.

2. Drop the essential oils directly onto the cotton pad inside the tube. Alternatively, you can drop the blend into a glass bowl, roll the cotton pad in the oils to absorb them, and then insert it into the inhaler using tweezers.

3. Secure the cap and store the inhaler in a desk drawer, purse, or glove compartment so you have it handy.

4. Open the inhaler and take a few deep breaths through your nose with your eyes closed before bed to help you settle down and enjoy a restful night of deep sleep.

LAVENDER FOR AGGRESSION

Two extremely challenging and heart-wrenching symptoms of Alzheimer's and dementia are agitation and disruptive behavior. To watch a patient or loved one deteriorate mentally in front of your eyes is one thing, but to care for them day after day in spite of being mistreated is a sacrifice only health-care and family caretakers can relate to.

Once soporific lavender oil enters the scene, however, the situation tends to drastically change and aggressive behavior fades away, especially in the context of an aromatherapy hand massage. One study tested as low as a 2 percent dilution with great results.

As there is clear evidence that people with dementia have impaired olfactory abilities, researchers suggest that topical application (i.e., hand massage) is the best way to treat aggression.

5. Turmeric

As turmeric's popularity explodes, more researchers are looking to turmeric essential oil for its promise in healing and preventing neurological disorders. One study evaluating turmerone, the principal component of turmeric, suggested that inhaling it could help regenerate stem cells in the brain. Scientists have also demonstrated that this compound may reduce neuroinflammation and related memory impairment.

Another substance in turmeric is curcumin. It has a potent ability to prevent the formation of beta-amyloid plaques, which are a hallmark of Alzheimer's disease. Turmeric extract thus represents a hopeful approach for preventing, delaying, and also treating the progression of AD. Note: You will not find curcumin in turmeric essential oil, so you'll have to consume a CO_2 extract to enjoy its benefits.

Application: Use a personal aromatherapy inhaler with 10 drops of turmeric, 5 drops of frankincense, and 5 drops of lime essential oils.

6. Rose

Well-known for its soothing and emotionally uplifting aroma, rose essential oil creates a sense of relaxed well-being and can help take the edge off stress-related situations. We understand that it can sometimes be hard to find, and when it's available, it's usually very pricey, so try to purchase a blend that includes rose as an ingredient.

If you can get your hands on a bottle of pure rose that fits your budget, get damask rose (*Rosa damascena*); it's also known as rose otto. Pre-clinical in vitro research confirms that it has noteworthy anti-cholinesterase activity. Interestingly, phenylethyl alcohol, its main component, contained the highest anti-cholinesterase effect when compared to the other main components of rose (citronellol, geraniol, and nerol).

Phenylethyl alcohol also occurs in neroli—another floral essential oil with a wide variety of emotional and mental healing benefits.

Application: Make this Floral Bouquet Brain Oil for an intoxicating aroma to reduce mental angst and help promote brain health at the neurotransmitter level.

FLORAL BOUQUET BRAIN OIL

Makes 1 or 2 applications

1 ounce carrier oil of your choice

4 drops ylang ylang essential oil

3 drops geranium essential oil

3 drops neroli essential oil

2 drops rose essential oil

SUPPLIES

Small glass bowl

Lidded glass jar or lotion dispenser

1. Mix the carrier oil and essential oils thoroughly in a bowl.

2. Use as a neck, shoulder, and scalp massage oil. It also works great as a moisturizer; apply to damp skin after a shower.

3. Store any leftover oil in a glass jar or lotion container.

7. Thyme

In addition to being a cholinesterase inhibitor, thyme is one of the most researched essential oils on the planet. It is a profound antimicrobial essential oil with antifungal, antibacterial, and anti-inflammatory properties that are on par with many drugs on the market.

As discussed above, a high-fat diet and obesity are definitive risk factors for developing AD. According to a recent study, however, daily oral dosages of thyme oil for four weeks may help these risk factors. After being fed a high-fat diet for eight weeks, rats consuming thyme mixed with sunflower oil improved blood sugar and lipid levels as well as memory. It also broke up the formation of beta-amyloid plaques.

Application: Start by taking 2 or 3 drops of thyme essential oil in a vegan gel capsule once a day for one month. Be sure to fill up your capsule with an edible carrier oil to help ensure safety and efficacy.

8. Coriander Seed

Switching gears to more symptom-based management, coriander seed was employed for medicinal and culinary purposes in ancient Babylonia. The plant is mentioned in biblical passages, and it was discovered in the tombs of pharaohs.

The primary component in coriander seed essential oil is linalool, which makes up about 40 to 85 percent of the essential oil. It's actually one of the richest sources of linalool of all the essential oils readily available on the market. According to scientists in Columbia, ingesting linalool can reverse brain tissue damage, restore cognitive and emotional function, produce an effective anti-inflammatory response, and is a candidate to prevent and treat Alzheimer's naturally.

Inhaling coriander seed essential oil, on the other hand, reduces anxiety, depression oxidative stress, and is another candidate for Alzheimer's therapy.

Application: Mix 2 drops each of coriander seed, lavender, and ylang ylang essential oils in your diffuser next time you want to chill out and relax, or whenever you need help managing stress or anxiety.

9. Fennel

Fennel is grown throughout Europe and North America, and its essential oil is derived from crushed fennel seeds. It has many healing benefits, from boosting circulation to soothing digestion to fighting colds.

Wouldn't you love to have laser-sharp focus as you go through the day? There's also strong evidence that fennel can help you get it! A Japanese study published in 2002 found that inhaling fennel essential oil stimulated sympathetic nerve system activities and adrenaline levels. Both actions increase focus and concentration.

A study from Romania a few years ago uncovered that inhaling fennel oil greatly reduced the anxiety and depression that resulted from beta-amyloid plaques in rats with AD. Fennel essential oil is also another great choice for reducing anxiety and depression in Alzheimer's patients.

Application: Make our Sweet Chill-Out Diffuser Blend.

SWEET CHILL-OUT DIFFUSER BLEND

2 drops fennel essential oil

2 drops ginger CO_2 extract

2 drops bitter orange essential oil

SUPPLIES

Diffuser

1. Fill your diffuser with purified water as directed in the manufacturer's instructions.

2. Add the essential oils.

3. Turn on the diffuser when you are ready to relax and release stress or anxiety.

4. Turn off the diffuser when done.

10. Peppermint

A whiff of peppermint oil is thought to invigorate the mind, so aromatherapists often recommend it to people who need mental stimulation while performing their jobs. Some very promising research suggests that peppermint oil stimulates the brain and may increase its capacity to retain facts and boost recall.

In a double-blind, placebo-controlled study, twenty-four volunteers consumed single doses of encapsulated placebo and one or two drops of peppermint oil. When performing demanding mental tasks, the peppermint group enjoyed increased mental function, reduced mental fatigue, and overall better mental performance. Another study evaluated 144 people and discovered that peppermint oil significantly improved memory, mood, and motivation in volunteer subjects, compared to those exposed to ylang ylang or no aroma at all.

Application: Put 20 drops of peppermint essential oil in your aromatherapy inhaler for a power-packed memory, mood, and energy boost.

12. Lemon Balm (Melissa)

Grown originally in Mediterranean areas, this member of the mint family was a food for bees. Even today, beekeepers rub the leaves of this herb over beehives to encourage the insects' productivity.

Known to help calm anxiety, lemon balm was tested on seventy-two patients who lived in a health-care facility. In this study, lemon balm oil or a placebo was added to lotion and massaged twice a day, every day for four weeks on the face and arms of subjects with severe dementia and frequent agitation. Those who received the lemon balm lotion had less agitation and, more importantly, improved quality of life than those who did not.

Application: Make a 2 percent Melissa-powered body oil by mixing 12 drops of lemon balm essential oil with 1 ounce of Mama Z's Oil Base (page 25) and ask a loved one to give you a hand massage.

SPECIAL BLENDS FOR THE ELDERLY

In addition to being more at risk of developing Alzheimer's and dementia, the elderly often suffer from a wide variety of symptoms that aromatherapy can help with. There is significant overlap here with many common issues that AD patients struggle with; you can find a handy guide to help you in one of our go-to reference books, *Aromatherapy for Health Professionals*, 4th edition.

TREATING AILMENTS COMMON TO THE ELDERLY

CONDITION	ESSENTIAL OILS	APPLICATION	NOTES
		(Use 2% dilution for all topical applications)	
Poor appetite	Bergamot, lime	Inhalation, hand massage	Blend equal parts and use before mealtime to stimulate the appetite.
	Caraway, fennel, spearmint, nutmeg, ginger	Inhalation, hand massage	Use as single oil treatment, or mix 2 or 3 for a blended treatment.
Bereavement	Lavender, frankincense, lemon	Inhalation, hand massage	Blend equal parts and use when emotional support is needed.
	Geranium, frankincense, rose	Inhalation, hand massage	Blend equal parts and use when emotional support is needed.
Circulatory issues	Cypress, fennel, lemon, orange (bitter), rosemary, sage	Lower leg massage, footbaths	Use as single oil treatment, or mix 2 or 3 for a blended treatment.
Constipation	Fennel, rosemary, ginger, orange (bitter or sweet), spearmint	Abdominal massage	Use as single oil treatment or mix 2 or 3 for a blended treatment. Massage in clockwise direction.
Depression	Thyme	Hand massage	Rub on back of hand.
	Roman chamomile, manuka, may chang, spearmint, sweet marjoram	Inhalation, hand massage	Use as single oil treatment or mix 2 or 3 for a blended treatment.

CONDITION	ESSENTIAL OILS	APPLICATION	NOTES
Digestion (slow, sluggish)	Black pepper, coriander, nutmeg, sage	Abdominal massage	Use as single oil treatment or mix 2 or 3 for a blended treatment. Massage in clockwise direction.
Diverticulitis	German chamomile, juniper berry, Melissa, myrrh, orange (bitter), rosemary	Abdominal massage	Use as single oil treatment or mix 2 or 3 for a blended treatment. Massage in clockwise direction.
Headaches, migraines, general pain	Basil, lavender, peppermint, Roman chamomile, sweet marjoram	Massage, inhalation	Use as single oil treatment or mix 2 or 3 for a blended treatment. For headaches, massage over the temples and back of neck. Otherwise, massage over problem area/ painful joints.
	Peppermint	Cold compress	Apply to forehead or back of neck.
	Sweet marjoram	Warm compress	Use for migraines due to restricted blood flow.
Insomnia	Bergamot, lavender, lemon, neroli, orange, Roman chamomile, sweet marjoram, ylang ylang	Bath, inhalation, massage	Only use 1 or 2 drops for inhalation; too much can cause agitation.
Memory loss	Clove, may chang, rosemary, peppermint, sage	Inhalation	Use as single oil treatment or mix 2 or 3 for a blended treatment.

CONDITION	ESSENTIAL OILS	APPLICATION	NOTES
Respiratory problems	Eucalyptus, frankincense, myrtle, niaouli, silver fir, hyssop, lavender, peppermint, ravensara, sweet thyme	Cheek and neck massage, inhalation	Use as single oil treatment or mix 2 or 3 for a blended treatment.
Skin (dryness, wrinkles)	Clary sage, helichrysum, Roman chamomile, rose, sandalwood	General topical application	Use thicker carrier oils like avocado oil, calendula, evening primrose, and wheat germ

To watch us make compresses—which are extremely useful for a variety of applications—and to learn more about our favorite ways to soothe headaches and migraines, go to EOApothecary.com.

Watching a friend or family member suffer from a neurodegenerative disease, such as Alzheimer's or dementia, creates powerful and negative feelings. Although our knowledge of the brain is currently growing by leaps and bounds, we still know so little about brain health. But we do know that lifestyle changes, including the use of essential oils, can help—and may go a long way toward relieving symptoms.

Chapter 10

Bone and Joint Disorders

You'll never see bone and joint disorders listed as a top-ranked cause of death—and for some reason the CDC doesn't consider them chronic diseases, even though other agencies like the WHO do. Nonetheless, they are responsible for taking the lives of hundreds of thousands of people every year and are on the rise in epidemic proportions.

Of these disorders, two of the most common are arthritis, which is joint inflammation, and osteoporosis, a bone-wasting disease. Both can be very painful and debilitating. Fortunately, essential oils, along with lifestyle changes, have been well studied and can provide you with much-needed relief for these conditions.

UNDERLYING FACTORS OF LEADING CAUSE OF DEATH

In the elderly population, falls in particular are extremely dangerous. In fact, falls are the leading cause of fatal and nonfatal injuries for older Americans.

From a global perspective, falls are the second leading cause of accidental injury deaths, with nearly 650,000 individuals dying every year.

What are the most common underlying causes of falls?

Arthritis and osteoporosis!

In a nutshell, osteoporosis weakens bones, which makes them more likely to break and less likely to heal. Arthritis weakens the joints and makes walking less stable, thus causing more falls. Arthritis and osteoporosis are interlinked, where one can cause the other condition to worsen and the vicious cycle of instability and likelihood to fall increases exponentially as someone ages.

It's shocking that this hasn't gained more attention in the medical community. As Lyn March, MD, PhD, Liggins Professor of Rheumatology and Musculoskeletal Epidemiology Medicine, Northern Clinical School, the University of Sydney, points out, "Health professionals have been aware for some time that having a hip fracture when you are older increases your risk of dying in one to two years after the fracture, but we have not been so aware that other fractures could increase this risk as well." This is especially troublesome because the risk of falling increases exponentially as someone ages. Seeing how deaths from accidental injuries are the seventh leading cause of death among older adults worldwide, and that falls are responsible for the majority of those deaths, this is a life-or-death topic that needs to be addressed!

When you connect the dots, it is clear how dangerous and potentially deadly bone and joint disorders can be in the context of accidental injuries and falls:

- One-third of all fall-related deaths are attributed to osteoporosis and low bone-density disorders.
- People with rheumatoid arthritis are at increased risk for osteoporosis and subsequent fractures.
- Rheumatoid arthritis patients are also more prone to falls and fractures because of swollen and tender lower-extremity joints, fatigue, and use of psychotropic medications.

Though there is no proven way to completely prevent arthritis and osteoporosis, several strategies can be employed to delay the onset, limit the severity, and even slow the progression. Before we cover these strategies, it's important to get a better understanding of each condition first.

JOINT DISORDERS

Arthritis is a general term for conditions that affect the joints and describes approximately one hundred different diseases that cause pain in the joints, bones, and surrounding tissues. Customarily, we refer particularly to osteoarthritis or rheumatoid arthritis when we discuss the topic.

- Osteoarthritis is known as degenerative joint disease (DJD) because it is primarily related to aging. It occurs when cartilage—the cushioning surface on bones—wears away. Without cartilage, bone rubs against bone, resulting in pain, stiffness, and swelling.
- Rheumatoid arthritis (RA) is an autoimmune condition. In a sort of bodily "friendly fire," it occurs when your body's immune system turns on the tissues of the body. These attacks target the synovium, a soft, fluid-producing tissue in your joints that nourishes cartilage and lubricates your joints. The exact cause of the immune system's attacks is unknown, although genetic factors are involved and increase a person's risk of developing RA.
- RA is inflammatory, whereas DJD is not.
- In total, both affect nearly one in ten adults in the United States and far too many children.

Studies have shown an increased risk of bone loss and fracture in people with rheumatoid arthritis for a number of reasons. The glucocorticoid medications often prescribed for the treatment of rheumatoid arthritis, for instance, can trigger significant bone loss. Additionally, arthritis causes loss of joint function and pain, which oftentimes leads to inactivity, thus increasing osteoporosis risk.

Medical studies also show that bone loss in rheumatoid arthritis can occur as a direct result of the disease itself, with the bone loss being most pronounced in areas immediately surrounding the arthritic joints. Of special concern is that women, who are already at increased risk for osteoporosis, are more likely than men to be affected by rheumatoid arthritis.

BONE LOSS DISORDERS

Bone loss disease includes osteopenia and osteoporosis. Both are varying degrees of bone loss, as measured by bone mineral density, a marker for how strong a bone is and the risk that it might break.

Osteoporosis is a very serious bone disease in which the bones lose their mass and weaken. It affects twenty-five million Americans and leads to dangerous fractures of the hip, spine, and wrist. Many discover the condition only when they break something. Considered primarily a disease of women, the accelerated bone loss of osteoporosis is common after menopause as a result of declining estrogen.

Osteopenia is reduced bone mass of lesser severity than osteoporosis. If osteoporosis were likened to type 2 diabetes, osteopenia would be likened to prediabetes. If you think of bone mineral density as a downward slope, normal would be at the top and osteoporosis at the bottom. Osteopenia, which affects about half of Americans over age fifty, would fall somewhere in between.

In normal bone activity, cells called osteoclasts absorb old bone, creating cavities in existing bone. These cavities are then filled with old bone through the work of other cells called osteoblasts. Osteoporosis results from an imbalance between osteoblastic and osteoclastic functions—when the deposition of new bone does not keep pace with the absorption of old bone. The result is a decrease in the density of the bone, making it more brittle and susceptible to fracture. Your bone mass reaches its peak at about age thirty-five. After that, if you don't pursue various lifestyle measures, you can lose bone density.

Symptom relief is the most immediate and pressing need for arthritis and osteoporosis sufferers. Struggling against an illness defined by its diverse instances of pain isn't easy, which is why so many people resort to non-steroidal anti-inflammatory drugs (NSAIDs) like aspirin (Bayer, Bufferin, Excedrin), ibuprofen (Advil, Motrin IB), and naproxen (Aleve). Far too many physicians recommend them without second thought. Not to mention, most people don't realize that natural therapies are as effective—if not more so.

This is key: the medications tied to pain relief commonly given to arthritis patients are not only completely ineffective at managing the root cause of the disease, but they also are riddled with side effects. Even the US Food and Drug Administration (FDA) admits that "NSAID medicines may increase the chance of a heart attack or stroke that can lead to death." It's not a good idea to rely entirely on medication as the only treatment for arthritis or osteoporosis.

THE ESSENTIAL OILS APPROACH TO CHRONIC BONE AND JOINT DISEASE

The research literature is quite clear that aromatherapy and using specific essential oils for bone and joint disorders is exceptionally effective and the key is to focus on reducing inflammation. With that said, there is a special aromatherapy arthritis pain blend that has been proven clinically to top others.

Traditionally, several essential oils have been used for arthritic pain relief. One of the most promising studies was published in 2005 by Korean researchers who evaluated how arthritis patients were affected by this special blend: eucalyptus, lavender, marjoram, rosemary, and peppermint (in proportions of 2:1:2:1:1).

These oils were blended with a carrier oil mixture composed of sweet almond oil (45 percent), apricot oil (45 percent), and jojoba oil (10 percent) and then diluted to 1.5 percent (roughly 9 drops of essential oils per 1 ounce of carrier). After applying the blend topically, the results were outstanding: "Aromatherapy significantly decreased both the pain score and the depression score of the experimental group compared with the control group" with no side effects reported!

Make the recipe on page 181 for a month's supply of the formula these researchers used in their study.

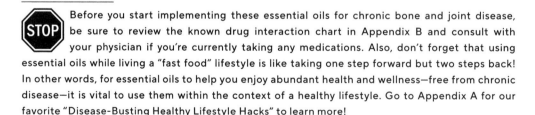

Before you start implementing these essential oils for chronic bone and joint disease, be sure to review the known drug interaction chart in Appendix B and consult with your physician if you're currently taking any medications. Also, don't forget that using essential oils while living a "fast food" lifestyle is like taking one step forward but two steps back! In other words, for essential oils to help you enjoy abundant health and wellness—free from chronic disease—it is vital to use them within the context of a healthy lifestyle. Go to Appendix A for our favorite "Disease-Busting Healthy Lifestyle Hacks" to learn more!

PAIN-FREE BONE AND JOINT OINTMENT

30 drops eucalyptus essential oil

30 drops sweet marjoram essential oil

16 drops lavender essential oil

16 drops peppermint essential oil

16 drops rosemary essential oil

1 ounce shea butter

4 ounces sweet almond oil

4 ounces apricot oil

1 ounce jojoba oil

SUPPLIES

Medium glass bowl

Lidded glass jar or lotion dispenser

1. Drop all of the essential oils into a bowl.
2. Add the shea butter along with the almond, apricot, and jojoba oils and mix well.
3. Rub over sore bones and arthritic joints daily for four weeks and monitor symptoms.
4. Store in a glass jar or lotion dispenser.

TOP ESSENTIAL OILS FOR ARTHRITIS

When discussing essential oils for arthritis, we must emphasize their anti-inflammatory benefits, as inflammation is the primary cause of pain in people suffering from arthritis.

1. Frankincense

Alpha-pinene and linalool, two of the top constituents of frankincense essential oil, are widely recognized as anti-inflammatories. Frankincense has also been shown to help with tissue remodeling, which suggests a cellular rejuvenation ability that can possibly help slow down the progression of bone and joint disorders.

By and large, it doesn't matter which species of frankincense you use, as alpha-pinene and linalool are primary components of all of the ones that are readily on the market today. One of our favorite strategies is to buy several frankincense varieties and mix them together for a "super frank blend." They create a synergistic cornucopia of healing properties and a delightful aroma. Use what you have available to you, and, if you can get your hands on a few different varieties, try them out to see which one(s) respond best for you!

Application: Try our Super Frank Blend pain-relieving recipes on achy joints and bones for relief.

SUPER FRANK BLEND

10 drops each of as many frankincense species as you can get (e.g., *Boswellia carterii, B. sacra, B. frereana, B. rivae, B. neglecta, B. papyrifera, B. serrata,* and *B. sacra*)

SUPPLIES
5 ml bottle

1. Mix the frankincense essential oils in a 5 ml bottle.
2. Use as directed in the following recipes.

SUPER FRANK ROLL-ON

10 drops Super Frank Blend (recipe above)
Carrier oil of choice—jojoba and fractionated coconut oil absorb quickly—as needed

SUPPLIES
10 ml glass roller bottle

1. Drop the essential oil blend into the roller bottle.
2. Fill the roller bottle with your carrier oil of choice and shake well.
3. Apply over sore joints and bones twice a day.

SUPER FRANK BODY OIL

15 drops Super Frank Blend (page 182)

1 ounce carrier oil of choice, such as jojoba oil, sweet almond oil, or Mama Z's
   Oil Base (page 25)

SUPPLIES

Small glass jar with a tight-fitting lid

1. Drop the essential oil blend into the glass jar.
2. Add the carrier oil and mix well.
3. Apply over sore joints and bones twice a day.

2. Copaiba

A powerful antioxidant regarded for its inflammation-soothing, anxiety-calming, and wound-healing properties, copaiba essential oil is extracted from the resin of a tropical tree native to South America. In fact, the healing efficacy of copaiba is so impressive that it includes a vast reduction in systemic inflammation and oxidative stress in arthritis studies evaluating rats.

If you don't find the relief that you're looking for from copaiba alone, consider using it along with ultrasound therapy. In 2017, researchers in Brazil set out to determine how copaiba essential oil compared with ultrasound therapy to alleviate pain and increase mobility and flexibility in patients suffering from knee osteoarthritis. Of the three therapies (copaiba oil, ultrasound alone, and copaiba with ultrasound), the most healing was the latter, combining copaiba with ultrasound therapy. This is logical, since ultrasound therapy is often used for treating chronic pain and promoting tissue healing.

One reason copaiba works so well is because it interacts with the endocannabinoid system similar to CBD. See chapter 17 (page 290) for more information.

Application: Start by taking 1 or 2 drops of copaiba in a vegan gel capsule once a day for one month. Be sure to fill up your capsule with an edible carrier oil to help ensure safety and efficacy. For extra strength, add a dose of full-spectrum CBD to the capsule, being sure to follow the manufacturer's instructions.

3. Lavender

When discussing the best essential oils for arthritis inflammation, lavender will generally make the short list.

As an anti-inflammatory oil, lavender can help to relieve the painful swelling and inflammation that arthritis, in its various forms, creates. Lavender is an analgesic as well, tackling arthritic pain from multiple angles. This was confirmed by a recent randomized control trial evaluating ninety patients with knee osteoarthritis, as lavender oil massage caused an immediate reduction in pain that continued one week after the intervention!

Because lavender can be used for anxiety and depression, it may also help relieve secondary issues that arise in the life of a person in chronic pain. Its gentle nature makes lavender a reliable choice for most people's use and application.

Application: The Inflammation-Soothing Roll-On and Capsule from Dr. Z's first book have been so popular at helping people with systemic inflammation, we suggest you try them. See the recipes on pages 185–186.

4. Caraway and Peppermint

Rheumatoid arthritis primarily affects the joints, but it can also cause systemic inflammation and symptoms throughout the body as the condition advances. This is when you'll need a total body approach to aromatherapy, which can only be accomplished through ingesting essential oils.

Research in 2006 evaluated the anti-inflammatory impact of caraway and peppermint essential oils both individually and blended together compared to a placebo in a group of animals suffering from a painful inflammatory gut disorder. Interestingly, neither oral peppermint nor caraway therapy for fourteen days was very effective alone at treating the pain or inflammation, but when combined, they reduced the condition by 50 percent!

We like this combo because caraway and peppermint are safe oils that are regularly used in capsules, and there is a lot of promise that they can synergistically work for systemic inflammation. When you add in lavender, the results are outstanding!

Application: Enjoy the anti-inflammatory synergy of caraway and peppermint by trying the roll-on body oil and capsule formulations below. We've had so many people tell us that these have worked wonders for them over the years that we wanted to share the recipes again.

INFLAMMATION-SOOTHING ROLL-ON

From *The Healing Power of Essential Oils*

5 drops caraway essential oil

5 drops peppermint essential oil

2 drops lavender essential oil

Carrier oil of choice—jojoba and fractionated coconut oil absorb quickly—as needed

SUPPLIES

10 ml glass roller bottle

1. Drop the essential oils into the roller bottle.
2. Fill the roller bottle with your carrier oil of choice and shake well.
3. Massage over your abdomen, chest, and back of neck twice daily for 4 weeks.

INFLAMMATION-SOOTHING CAPSULE

Adapted from *The Healing Power of Essential Oils*

Makes 1 dose

2 drops caraway essential oil

2 drops peppermint essential oil

1 dose full-spectrum CBD (follow manufacturer's instructions for dosage)

Organic virgin coconut oil or extra-virgin olive oil

SUPPLIES

Pipette

Size 00 vegan gel capsule

continues

1. Using a pipette, drop the essential oils and CBD into the bottom half (the longer, narrower one) of the capsule. Fill this half to the brim with organic extra-virgin coconut or extra-virgin olive oil.

2. Fit the wider top half of the capsule over the bottom half and secure it snugly.

3. Immediately swallow the capsule with water after breakfast and/or dinner (see Note). Take once or twice daily and monitor your symptoms.

NOTE: *Do not make and store these capsules for future use. Also, this is not a long-term solution, and using it for more than four weeks at a time is not advisable. Be sure to switch up your protocol monthly and consult with your health-care provider first if you're currently taking medications. Discontinue if adverse reactions occur.*

BLACK SEED OIL: THE PERFECT CARRIER FOR ARTHRITIS

Nigella sativa oil (or black seed oil) is a fixed oil that has been utilized in traditional medicine for over two thousand years, and its uses are virtually endless. When applied topically or orally, it is a wonderful remedy for back pain, joint issues, and RA. Specifically, studies have shown that it can reduce swollen joints and inflammation and modulate immune function in women with RA.

Application: Try using black seed oil instead of extra-virgin olive oil in your pain-relieving capsules. When making topical preparations, simply use black seed oil as the primary carrier.

5. German Chamomile

Not as widely used as its Roman cousin, German chamomile is nonirritating essential oil known for its calming, soothing, and anti-inflammatory effects. It should be no surprise, therefore, that researchers have discovered German chamomile use can significantly reduce the need for pain-relief medications.

One study applied diluted German chamomile essential oil over the knees of osteoarthritis patients three times a day for three weeks, and the use of acetaminophen to manage pain was significantly reduced. In fact, it appears that German chamomile helps reduce inflammation more effectively than your average NSAID. In addition to having a control group, some of the study participants received the NSAID diclofenac, and German chamomile oil fared better than the drug!

Application: Make a 5 percent dilution by mixing 30 drops of German chamomile with 1 ounce of black seed oil and apply over painful joints as needed.

6. Wintergreen

Wintergreen essential oil, another traditional analgesic that has helped countless arthritis patients, is also known as "liquid aspirin." Used with peppermint, it is particularly effective in reducing inflammation. The primary component of wintergreen oil is methyl salicylate, which is a compound closely related to acetylsalicylic acid (i.e., aspirin).

Wintergreen is as potentially dangerous as it is potent, however. It's one of the few oils on the market that you'll see with a childproof top, and for good reason. Ingesting it can be toxic, and applying more than a 3 percent dilution on the skin, according to aromatherapy safety guidelines, is beyond the max dermal dose.

A combination of wintergreen oil and peppermint oil is commonly used because it is believed to give far better pain relief than either wintergreen oil or peppermint oil alone.

Application: Make this bone and joint salve for wintergreen-peppermint-powered relief!

EXTRA-STRENGTH BONE AND JOINT SALVE

50 drops frankincense essential oil

50 drops peppermint essential oil

20 drops sweet marjoram essential oil

20 drops lavender essential oil

15 drops wintergreen essential oil

200 mg full-spectrum CBD

continues

2 ounces unrefined shea butter

2 ounces Mama Z's Oil Base (page 25)

SUPPLIES

Medium glass bowl

Lidded glass jar or lotion dispenser

1. Drop the essential oils into the bowl.
2. Add the CBD, shea butter, and oil base and mix thoroughly.
3. Apply a small amount as a moisturizer over your joints daily for 4 weeks and monitor for pain and other symptoms.
4. Store in a glass jar or lotion dispenser.

TOP ESSENTIAL OILS FOR OSTEOPOROSIS

Still experimental at this point, most of the research we have evaluating aromatherapy's efficacy to treat osteoporosis focuses on pain management, not on the root cause (i.e., bone-density loss). The same recommendations we shared above regarding arthritis pain apply to bone pain as well. See page 180 for recommendations if you're struggling with bone-density-related pain.

As more preclinical studies are being done on how essential oils can help with bone density, the strongest research we have suggests that ingesting monoterpenes can be used to inhibit bone resorption—the process by which osteoclasts break down bone tissue and release the minerals, causing calcium to enter the blood. This is important because abnormal increase in bone resorption causes osteoporosis and other bone loss diseases. Some essential oils highlighted in the literature for their osteoclastic-inhibiting ability are rosemary, sage, and thyme.

Studies on animals—virtually all preclinical evaluations at this point—cannot guide how we may prevent or treat a chronic disease like osteoporosis, but they do suggest that consistent, continual use of natural remedies can help. Most of the studies we see administer an exceptionally large dose to animals to stimulate the response that researchers are looking for. Obviously, we cannot transfer these dosing parameters to humans, as they can cause liver toxicity and other harmful effects to the body.

This is why the recommendations below focus on very low or "culinary" doses. There is a huge difference between adding a drop or two of essential oils to your morning latte and taking medicinal doses that reach ten to twenty drops per day!

1. Fennel

Postmenopausal osteoporosis is a well-known phenomenon associated with estrogen deficiency and rapid bone loss. It can also be greatly exacerbated if a woman has had an ovariectomy (removal of one of both ovaries). Rich in the cancer-fighting and inflammation-soothing chemical anethole, fennel oil has been shown to slow down this process in rats that consumed fennel oil every day for one month.

Application: For your morning pick-me-up, enjoy a cup of our EO-Powered Matcha Latte (page 124) using fennel.

2. Bergamot

Not only rich in antioxidants and monoterpenes (alpha-pinene, bergapten, limonene), bergamot essential oil is a wonderfully versatile remedy that can facilitate healing deep in your body. In long-term animal models, it has been shown to increase bone volume, decrease psoriatic plaques, increase skin collagen content, and promote hair growth. In fact, bergapten has been shown to slow the progression of diabetes-related osteoporosis.

Application: Enjoy a serving of Dr. Z's Citrus Oil Soda Pop (page 267) a few times a week.

3. Thyme

Thyme essential oil has many therapeutic values. It contains monoterpenes that are beneficial for optimum bone health. Among these are borneol, thymol, and thujanol.

A 2018 study observed the impact of thyme and rosemary oil for preventing calcium-deficient osteoporosis in rats. Compared to the control, thyme and rosemary oil supplementation significantly inhibited the development of bone loss, increased blood calcium and vitamin D$_3$ levels, improved bone mass density, and also reduced inflammation and oxidative stress. Of the two, thyme oil performed much better during the eight-week study.

Application: Start by taking 2 or 3 drops of thyme essential oil in a vegan gel capsule once a day for two months and monitor your bone density results with your doctor. Be sure to fill up your capsule with an edible carrier oil to help ensure safety and efficacy.

4. Pine

Essential oils of pine, juniper, sage, rosemary, dwarf pine, turpentine, and eucalyptus have been found to inhibit the breakdown and absorption of bone cells when added to food in animal studies. Pine oil specifically stood out as being able to protect from bone loss.

Application: Make our Bone-Strengthening Cream and apply it daily for one month, monitoring your symptoms.

BONE-STRENGTHENING CREAM

From *The Healing Power of Essential Oils*

7 drops juniper essential oil

7 drops sage essential oil

7 drops rosemary essential oil

7 drops eucalyptus essential oil

7 drops pine essential oil

1 ounce unrefined shea butter

2 ounces Mama Z's Oil Base (page 25)

SUPPLIES

Medium glass bowl

Lidded glass jar or lotion dispenser

1. Drop the essential oils into the bowl.

2. Add the shea butter and oil base and mix thoroughly.

3. Apply a small amount as a moisturizer over your joints daily for 4 weeks and monitor your pain and other symptoms.

4. Store in a glass jar or lotion dispenser.

→ To watch us make this recipe and get Mama Z's bone-healing protocol that helped our son's fractured clavicle heal in record time, go to EOApothecary.com.

As you can see, there are many ways to use natural therapies like essential oils to better enjoy your golden years. We enjoy recalling the story of Caleb in the Bible, who, at eighty years old, wanted to go into battle to get the land that God had promised him. How many people do you know at eighty with that much energy and vigor?

Do you want to be one of them?

Then go! Get your Promised Land! It is your birthright to enjoy abundant life, health, and wellness well into your eighties, nineties, and hundreds!

Chapter 11

Cancer Support

At this point, it's virtually impossible to be untouched by cancer. We all know someone whose life has been affected by cancer, whether ourselves, a loved one, a neighbor, or a co-worker. So feared is this disease that many are afraid to even utter its name, calling it instead the "Big C."

We're sure you've seen the headlines (if not, you soon will): *in the United Kingdom, one in two people will get cancer at some point in their lives.* And we can only expect to see the rest of the world follow suit unless everyone does an about-face on their lifestyle.

You may be surprised to learn that at least one-third of all cancer cases in the world are preventable, because they are linked to five behavioral and dietary risks: high body mass index, low fruit and vegetable intake, lack of physical activity, tobacco use, and alcohol use. Up until recently, tobacco use was the dominant risk factor for cancer, responsible for approximately 22 percent of cancer deaths globally. But now, obesity is poised to take the top spot, at least in America, as waistlines continue to expand while tobacco use plummets.

If you want to have a fighting chance at preventing and successfully treating cancer, we highly encourage you to revisit the chapters in this book that discuss how to do these four key things:

1. Get your weight and blood sugar in check.
2. Successfully manage stress and anxiety.
3. Greatly reduce (and even banish) depression and substance abuse.
4. Regularly enjoy at least seven hours of sleep every night.

If you do these four things, you'll put yourself in an infinitely better place to beat not only cancer but the other chronic illnesses mentioned in this book as well!

QUICK OVERVIEW ABOUT CANCER

Cancer is a global epidemic, and chemotherapy, radiation, and surgery have not solved the problem. Despite billions of dollars of medical research and interventions, cancer is still *the* major public health crisis in the United States and throughout the world. It is currently the second leading cause of death globally and is expected to shortly surpass heart disease as the world's leading cause of death. To put this into perspective, at the beginning of 2020, it was expected that 1,806,590 new cancer cases and 606,520 cancer deaths would occur annually in the United States. Globally, that's nearly 10 million deaths every year.

Cancer is not just one disease. There are many types, and it can start in any organ or tissue of the body, including the blood. The most common cancers (listed in descending order) are breast cancer, lung cancer, prostate cancer, colon and rectum cancer, melanoma, bladder cancer, non-Hodgkin lymphoma, kidney cancer, endometrial cancer, leukemia, pancreatic cancer, thyroid cancer, and liver cancer. Cancer mortality is higher among men than women, which is interesting since the most common cancer is breast cancer, and most people who get breast cancer are women. We can only expect that this is because men are far more likely than women to smoke, abuse alcohol, and be overweight and aren't as likely to change their lifestyles.

The disease typically begins when cells grow out of control and crowd out healthy cells. This makes it hard for the body to work the way it should. Some cancers spread very fast, while others spread more slowly. They are also treated in different ways. Some types of cancer are best treated with surgery, others appear to respond better to chemotherapy, and still others to radiation. Often two or more treatments are used.

The truth is there is no diet, no natural remedy protocol or chemotherapy strategy that will work every time. In other words, the answer for you will not necessarily be the answer for your loved ones. Focus needs to be placed on customizing protocols and strategies to fit each individual.

- Sometimes "beating cancer" is when someone finds emotional peace or mental stability during their crisis.
- Other times, "beating cancer" is when someone starts to sleep better, their pain goes away, or their desire to live returns.
- And for others, "beating cancer" is when someone "wins" the battle and ends up cancer-free.

Fortunately, cancer can be treated successfully for many people. And, as discussed above, it is largely preventable if the right lifestyle choices are made.

THE NEED FOR AN INTEGRATIVE APPROACH

It's common knowledge that cancer treatments don't always work and that they cause a slew of side effects, including cancer. We'll never forget when we read the side effects listed on Mama Z's father's skin cancer cream; that very cream formulated to treat his melanoma could cause cancer in other parts of his body!

It's important to realize that natural therapies can and, in our opinion, should be used in conjunction with conventional medicine unless obvious contraindications are present. It's not an all-or-nothing thing, meaning you don't have to choose between going conventional or "all natural." You can use both strategies. In fact, there's a name for this approach. It's referred to as "integrative oncology" and is defined as a patient-centered, evidence-informed field of cancer care that utilizes mind and body practices, natural products, and/or lifestyle modifications from different traditions alongside conventional cancer treatments. Integrative oncology aims to optimize health, quality of life, and clinical outcomes across the cancer care continuum and to empower people to prevent cancer and become active participants before, during, and beyond cancer treatment.

And, in our humble opinion, one of the most beneficial modalities a cancer patient can incorporate into their integrative treatment plan is aromatherapy. In the words of study published in the journal *BioMed Research International*:

> EOs have also been reported to improve the quality of life of the cancer patients by lowering the level of their agony. EOs-mediated therapy cannot be a substitute to the standard chemotherapy and radiotherapy but can be used in combination with cancer therapy to decrease the side effects of the drugs. Hence, EOs can be used for improving the health of the cancer patients and as a source of novel anticancer compounds.

In fact, research is increasingly showing that the use of EOs as dietary supplements and co-administration with drugs can enhance patients' response to treatment.

This last sentence is *really* important! Like we always say, everything is better with oils. Even chemo! Our personal recommendation is to work with an integrative oncologist who is knowledgeable about natural therapies like aromatherapy and will help find the right protocol for you.

→ If you'd like to learn more about integrative oncology, we invite you to watch our award-winning documentary to see how one brave young mom traveled the world customizing her own integrative cancer therapies. Visit HopeForBreastCancer.com for a free screening.

THREE THINGS YOU NEED TO KNOW

As more research is conducted validating the therapeutic efficacy of using holistic remedies as a viable prevention, treatment, and symptom management strategy for cancer patients, it's important to recognize that essential oils fit into cancer treatment in light of these three truths.

First, the research concerning essential oils and cancer suggests that aromatherapy can help prevent and treat cancer from growing at the cellular level. Additionally, and oftentimes overlooked, essential oils have been shown to be exceptionally effective at managing the side effects related to cancer itself and the side effects people suffer at the hands of many medical interventions.

Second, we need to put things into proper perspective and remember that the peer-reviewed articles we have that evaluate the ability of essential oils to prevent, stop, and even reverse the growth of various malignant lines are in vitro or animal studies. In other words, we don't have many live human trials, let alone cohort studies with hundreds or thousands of participants. We have studies that are testing human or animal cells in a petri dish or live lab rats. This is not to say that these studies are useless. The point we need to take from this is that using essential oils for cancer is still highly experimental. Nonetheless, a considerable amount of research has been evaluating the *chemotherapeutic* (i.e., the therapeutic use of chemical agents to treat disease, especially cancer) and *chemoprotective* (i.e., protecting the body from chemotherapy) efficacy of aromatherapy.

Third, there are what appears to be countless testimonials on the Internet from people claiming that essential oils have helped them manage symptoms and even beat a cancer diagnosis. Yes, we acknowledge this is anecdotal evidence at best, but the fact remains that it is not wise to dispute these testimonies, as many are legitimately documented medical cases that are ultimately going to be the basis for further research.

Still, with all of these considerations in mind, we need to be careful not to offer outrageous, irresponsible claims suggest essential oils can "cure" cancer. The jury is still out, and it will be so for some time.

Until then, we encourage you to study up, work with an integrative oncologist who is at least familiar with aromatherapy, and approach cancer through a variety of natural modalities.

THE ESSENTIAL OILS APPROACH TO CANCER

As you've learned thus far in this book, essential oils have been shown to help manage the many side effects and co-morbidities of cancer: anxiety, depression, fatigue, immune compromise, low libido, obesity, pain, stress, and more. They can also be used to fight cancer directly.

How exactly can they do this? Through a variety of mechanisms, according to a study published in the *BioMed Research International* journal,

> *EOs and their constituents act by multiple pathways and mechanisms involving apoptosis, cell cycle arrest, antimetastatic and antiangiogenic, increased levels of reactive oxygen and nitrogen species (ROS/RNS), DNA repair modulation, and others to demonstrate their antiproliferative activity in the cancer cell. The effect of EOs and their constituents on tumour suppressor proteins (p53 and Akt), transcription factors (NF-×B and AP-1), MAPK-pathway, and detoxification enzymes like SOD, catalase, glutathione peroxidase, and glutathione reductase has also been discussed.*

See pages 198–201 for a snapshot of just a fraction of the research that has been done suggesting that essential oils and their constituents can help fight cancer and protect the body from the harmful effects of chemotherapy and radiation. We mainly included the essential oils that you can readily find on the market. Additionally, there are dozens of other studies evaluating African basil, Brazilian peppertree, mojo berry or kenaf (also known as *Hibiscus cannabinus*), and a number of oils indigenous to native cultures that have been tested for the chemopreventive and chemotherapeutic efficacy.

CHEMOPROTECTIVE AND/OR CHEMOTHERAPEUTIC ESSENTIAL OILS

ESSENTIAL OIL	TYPE OF CANCER	SUBJECT
Basil (holy)	Mouth, leukemia, stomach	Mouse
	Mouth	Human
Basil (sweet)	Mouth	Human
	Leukemia	Mouse
Basil (pungent)	Skin	Mouse
Bay laurel	Breast	Human
Black pepper	Mouth	Human
	Leukemia	Mouse
Black seed	Colon	Rat
Caraway	Skin	Mouse
Cedarwood (Atlas)	Leukemia	Human
Cedarwood (Himalayan)	Leukemia	Human
Cinnamon	Fibroblast	Rat
Clove	Breast, cervical, esophageal, leukemia, lymphoma, prostate	Human
Cumin	Stomach	Mouse
Curry leaf	Breast	Human
Fir needle (Canada)	Various cell lines	Human
Frankincense (*Boswellia carterii*)	Bladder, breast, cervical, liver, skin, small cell (lung), urinary tract	Human
Frankincense (*Boswellia sacra*)	Breast	Human
Garlic	Cervix, leukemia, skin	Mouse
Grapefruit	Lung, forestomach	Mouse
Key lime	Colon	Human
Laurel leaf	Kidney, leukemia, skin	Human
Lavender	Mouth	Human
	Leukemia	Mouse
Lemon	Cervix, breast, lung, forestomach, general tumor	Mouse
	Cervical	Human

Lemongrass (East Indian)	Cervix, lung, colon, prostate, mouth, nerves	Human
Lemongrass (West Indian)	Mouth	Human
	Leukemia	Mouse
Mandarin	General tumor cell	Mouse
	Leukemia	Human
Mastic	Leukemia	Human
Melissa (lemon balm)	Brain, breast, colon, lung, leukemia	Human
	Skin	Mouse
Myrtle (bog)	Lung, colon	Human
Nut grass	Leukemia	Mouse
Onion	Skin	Mouse
	Leukemia	Human
Orange	Breast, cervix, liver	Rat
	Lung, forestomach	Mouse
Orange (bitter)	General tumor cell	Mouse
Oregano	Breast	Human
Rosemary	Breast, prostate	Human
Rosewood	Skin	Human
Sage	Breast, colon, kidney, prostate, skin	Human
East Mediterranean sage	Skin	Mouse
Sandalwood (East Indian)	Skin	Mouse
Spearmint	Mouth	Human
	Leukemia	Mouse
Sweet geranium	Leukemia	Human
Sweet marjoram	Lung	Human
Tangerine	Lung, forestomach	Mouse
Thyme	Breast, lung, mouth, prostate	Human
Tea tree	Skin	Human
Vetiver	Mouth	Human
	Leukemia	Mouse

CHEMOPROTECTIVE AND/OR
CHEMOTHERAPEUTIC ESSENTIAL OIL CONSTITUENTS

ESSENTIAL OIL CONSTITUENT	TYPE OF CANCER	CELLS TESTED
Alantolactone	Leukemia, stomach, uterus	Human
Allyl isothiocyanate	Various tissues	Rat
	Lung (melanoma cells)	Mouse
Ascaridole	Breast, colon, leukemia	Human
Benzaldehyde	Various	Human
Benzyl isothiocyanate	Breast, lung	Mouse
	Bladder	Rat
	Ovary	Human
Bergamottin	Breast	Human
Alpha-bisabolol	Brain, pancreas	Human
Alpha-cadinol	Colon	Human
Carvacrol	Breast, leukemia, lung	Human
	Skin	Mouse
Alpha-caryophyllene	Various cell lines	Human
(E)-cinnamaldehyde	Leukemia	Mouse
	Colon, melanoma	Human
Costunolide	Colon	Rat
Coumarin	Various	Human
Diallyl disulfide	Breast, colon, leukemia	Human
	Lung, forestomach	Rat
Diallyl sulfide	Breast, esophagus, liver	Rat
	Lung, skin	Mouse
Beta-elemene	Brain, lung, larynx, ovary	Human
Beta-eudesmol	Liver	Human
Eugenol	Liver, skin	Human
	Forestomach, skin	Human, mouse
Farnesol	Pancreas	Human, hamster
	Leukemia	Human
Geraniol	Colon	Human

	Skin, leukemia	Mouse
	Breast, liver	Rat
Beta-ionone	Breast	Rat
(Z)-Jasmone	Lung	Human
(+)-Limonene	Breast, liver, stomach	Rat
	Liver, lung, stomach	Human
	Lung (melanoma cells), stomach	Mouse
Linalool	Kidney, liver, leukemia, lymphoma, skin	Human
(-)-Menthol	Breast	Rat
Methoxsalen	Lung	Mouse
Methyl jasmonate	Breast, prostate, skin	Human
Myristicin	Lung	Mouse
Nerolidol	Colon	Rat
Perillyl alcohol	Lung, skin	Mouse
	Breast, colon, liver	Rat
	Pancreas	Hamster
Phenylethyl isothiocyanate	Colon, lung	Rat
	Lung	Mouse
Alpha-santalol	Skin	Mouse
Sclareol	Breast, colon, leukemia, lung, skin	Human
Terpinen-4-ol	Liver, leukemia, skin	Human
Thymoquinone	Connective tissue, forestomach, skin	Mouse
	Bone, colon, leukemia, prostate	Human
ar-Turmerone	Connective tissue	Mouse
Vanillin	Liver	Rat
Xanthorrhizol	Peritoneum	Mouse

STOP Before you start implementing these essential oils for cancer, be sure to review the known drug interaction chart in the Appendix B and consult with your physician if you're currently taking any medications. Also, don't forget that using essential oils while living a "fast food" lifestyle is like taking one step forward but two steps back! In other words, for essential oils to help you enjoy abundant health and wellness—free from chronic disease—it is vital to use them within the context of a healthy lifestyle. Go to Appendix A for our favorite "Disease-Busting Healthy Lifestyle Hacks" to learn more!

It's important to recognize that none of these studies evaluated human cancer patients under a clinical trial setting with a control group. All of these studies were human cell in vitro or animal evaluations. Thus, we cannot extrapolate dosing and other specific recommendations as we can with the other diseases discussed in this book.

Unfortunately, it is highly unlikely that we'll get to see the results of an actual clinical trial evaluating cancer patients, because researchers and ethics committees would deem it too dangerous to withhold medical treatment on a human volunteer to test how aromatherapy would fare against chemo or radiation.

Nonetheless, we are including a few considerations that you can discuss with your oncologist and a section below on how to use aromatherapy for cancer's side effects.

1. D-limonene

The most prominent and noteworthy component of citrus oils is d-limonene, confirmed to be a potent cancer-fighting agent. As described in the US National Library of Medicine's open chemistry database, PubChem: *"D-limonene is an oral dietary supplement containing a natural cyclic monoterpene and major component of the oil extracted from citrus peels with potential chemopreventive and antitumor activities."*

So basically, the limonene found in citrus and other essential oils can fight tumor growth by causing cancer cells to literally self-destruct. This suicide-triggering process is called apoptosis, also referred to as programmed cell death. For a full list of limonene-containing oils, see page 108 in chapter 6.

Application: In chapter 6, we shared several limonene-powered recipes to help with depression and substance abuse. Those same citrus-based remedies may also help with cancer. We recommend that you start there (page 101) to see how easy and pleasant it is to incorporate citrus oils into your daily cancer-fighting routine!

2. Sclareol

Sclareol, a constituent of clary sage essential oil, has promising anti-cancer effects. From studies dating back to 1999 and more recently, it can also trigger apoptosis like limonene can. Sclareol has also been shown to sensitize cervical cancer cells to chemotherapy drugs like bortezomib (Velcade), thus making chemotherapy more effective! And this isn't an anomaly. Just in 2019, sclareol was tested with the chemotherapy drug cisplatin, and similar results were found with cervical cancer cells—yet again, a perfect example of why "integrative oncology" is a valid approach to treating cancer in lieu of the completely conventional model.

As a stand-alone intervention, injecting sclareol into animals has been shown to decrease tumor size and enhance the effect of cancer therapy as an immunostimulant. While this does not tell us how much potential sclareol has to directly treat cancer, it's exciting to think about where that could go one day.

Application: Unless otherwise contraindicated by your oncologist, there should be no harm in applying a gentle 1 percent dilution of clary sage over the skin area covering a tumor or cancer of any kind. In fact, doing so may help your current treatments be more effective and reduce tumor size! (See our dilution chart on pages 26–28.)

ARE ESSENTIAL OILS ESTROGENIC?

This is one of the most consistent questions we receive regarding the use of essential oils for cancer, because of the myth that essential oils are "estrogenic" (having an estrogen-like effect on the body). This is particularly a concern for many women with estrogen-dominant breast cancer who are concerned about clary sage due to some scientists' claim that it contains a known estrogenic compound: sclareol.

Quick answer: There's nothing to worry about. Essential oils are not "estrogenic" in the way that should concern someone, nor are their individual compounds, but even if they were, the effects would be so minimal that they wouldn't cause any harm.

Essential oil safety expert Robert Tisserand puts it this way:

> On the basis of its structure, sclareol is unlikely to have any estrogenic action. Even if sclareol was estrogenic, at about 4 percent of clary sage oil, it would have to have a very high binding affinity for estrogen receptor sites for the essential oil to have any effect, and this is extremely unlikely.

Going back to our discussion in chapter 2 about essential oils being known as "harmonizers" and "adaptogens," the literature suggests that essential oils help the body facilitate either an increase or decrease of estrogen as needed. We see this with other phytoestrogens as well. Phytoestrogens are plant-based compounds that mimic estrogen in the body, meaning that they can interact with estrogen receptors in cells. These receptors mediate estrogen's functions within the body. However, the effects of phytoestrogens are much weaker than those of estrogen, and not all phytoestrogens work the same.

In some cases, they have been shown to have both estrogenic and antiestrogenic effects. This means that, while some phytoestrogens have estrogen-like effects and increase estrogen levels in your body, others block its effects and decrease estrogen levels. Like essential oils as a whole, phytoestrogens have the tendency to create homeostasis and overall healing in the body.

This is why we see sclareol having a profound effect on helping someone in their fight against cancer. Tisserand confirms this:

> *Sclareol does have an interesting anticancer activity, including in vitro action against human breast cancer MCF-7 cells (Dimas et al. 2006). An isomer, 13-epi-sclareol, which is also present in clary sage oil, inhibits the growth of breast and uterine cancers in vitro, and was slightly more potent than Tamoxifen, but was not toxic to normal cells (Sashidhara et al. 2007). This suggests the possibility that sclareol might actually inhibit estrogen, and might after all have some capacity to interact with estrogen receptor sites. What we do know is that sclareol will not give you breast cancer.*

The same is true with lavender, another oil that people are concerned is "estrogenic" and contraindicated in breast cancer treatment and even in children due to the ludicrous concern that it can cause gynecomastia (breast growth in boys).

USING ESSENTIAL OILS TO MANAGE CANCER SIDE EFFECTS

Cancer and its treatments can cause a plethora of side effects. Definitely speak up about any problems you have with your health-care team and ask for ways to reduce these so you feel better during your healing journey. We encourage you to consider the following ways aromatherapy can help.

Appetite and Weight Loss

Contrary to what we've learned about how citrus oils and peppermint oil can *suppress* appetite, lavender has been shown to *enhance* appetite and body weight. Similarly, other linalool-rich, calming oils help you enter that "rest and digest" state, which will help you better metabolize your food and enhance your ability to absorb the nutrients that you eat.

Application: If you're struggling to maintain a healthy weight because of cancer treatments or the disease itself, regularly diffuse lavender and the calming oils that we discussed in chapters 4 and 5 before and during meals.

Bruising and Edema (Swelling)

Arnica gel is our best friend as we treat the bumps and bruises our kids tend to get regularly. Fennel, geranium, helichrysum, lavender, rose, and Roman chamomile are our typical go-to oils here. We like making the following recipe. Though not used as commonly for bruises, these oils have been researched with success: black pepper, ginger, myrtle, marjoram, parsley, and violet.

Application: Make our Bruise Cream (page 206) and apply twice a day over the affected area.

BRUISE CREAM

10 drops fennel essential oil

10 drops geranium essential oil

10 drops helichrysum essential oil

10 drops lavender essential oil

10 drops Roman chamomile essential oil

10 drops rose essential oil (if you have some on hand)

2 ounces arnica gel

SUPPLIES

Small glass bowl

Small lidded glass jar

1. Drop the essential oils into a glass bowl.
2. Add the arnica gel and mix thoroughly.
3. Apply over bruises and swollen areas twice daily. A little bit goes a long way.
4. Store in a glass jar.

Constipation

Lack of bowel motility and constipation are regular concerns for cancer patients. A number of essential oils can help, including anise, caraway, coriander seed, fennel, ginger, peppermint, and tarragon. In a study conducted on elderly volunteers, a diluted blend of lemon, peppermint, and rosemary was massaged over the patients' abdomens every day for two weeks. Constipation quickly improved with increased bowel movement, and the benefits lasted nearly two weeks after therapy stopped!

Application: Make a 5 percent massage oil by mixing 20 drops each of lemon, peppermint, and rosemary essential oils with 2 ounces of Mama Z's Oil Base (page 25) and massage into the abdomen daily in a clockwise direction.

Diarrhea

As we'll discuss in chapter 16, enteric-coated capsules are the way to go if you're trying to treat inflammatory bowel disease. A 2019 study evaluated peppermint using these time-delayed capsules and observed that global symptoms of irritable bowel syndrome (IBS) were improved, including diarrhea. Another study published in 2019 evaluated what would happen if pig feed included a strong blend of cinnamaldehyde and thymol to help reduce diarrhea in lieu of using antibiotics. As expected, these essential oil compounds worked wonderfully!

Application: If you suffer from diarrhea, consider trying the capsule remedies we suggest in chapter 16. To make an adapted remedy based on the studies above, place 2 drops each of cinnamon bark, peppermint, and thyme essential oils in an enteric-coated capsule, fill with extra-virgin olive oil, and take once daily for two to four weeks until symptoms improve.

Fatigue

Lethargy, fatigue, and malaise (a general feeling of being unwell) are some of the most common complaints cancer patients experience. Thankfully, essential oils can help. Topical frankincense is particularly useful, according to some research. Be sure to try some (or all!) of the chronic fatigue recipes from chapter 7.

Application: Make a 2 percent frankincense-powered body oil simply by mixing 12 drops of your favorite frankincense essential oil with 2 ounces of Mama Z's Oil Base (page 25) and massage it into your neck, shoulders, and feet for an invigorating pick-me-up!

Flu-Like Symptoms

As we mentioned in chapter 2, the oils in our Immune-Boosting Blend were found to kill the flu virus when mixed together. Be sure to go back to page 49 to make this blend and Dr. Z's Immune-Boosting Snack (page 51); consult with your integrative oncologist to get the okay before taking them.

Other flu-like symptoms usually include malaise and achiness all over. This is where an evening aromatherapy bath can do wonders. It will help soothe achy muscles, provide for a gentle, relaxing detoxifying experience, and get you ready for a good night's sleep!

Application: Visit page 83 and make the Restful Evening Detox Bath recipe.

Alopecia (Hair Loss)

Yes, essential oils can help with hair loss, and we've guided many a chemo patient to regrowing their hair after treatment. Peppermint and rosemary oils are our go-to here. A 3 percent peppermint oil dilution was used with great success in one animal study. Compared to Rogaine, rosemary oil worked just as well, with significant hair growth in alopecia patients after six months!

Application: Make a 3 percent hair growth oil by mixing 18 drops each of peppermint and rosemary essential oils with 2 ounces of Mama Z's Oil Base (page 25); massage a small amount into your scalp after you shower every day.

Infection

Fighting infection can be a tough one, because many cancer treatments are immuno-suppressive. Be sure to check with your doctor before using essential oils to fight infection to make sure that you're not counteracting the therapies you're taking.

If you get the thumbs-up, then the sky's the limit. Virtually every essential oil is antimicrobial and can kill bacteria, fungi, and viruses. It's just a matter of choosing which oils for which infections.

Application: If your doctor okays fighting an infection with essential oils, follow our Triple-Threat Infection-Fighting Protocol (page 131).

Radiation Burn and Skin Sensitivity

The only study we found evaluating how essential oils could help women undergoing radiation treatment was conducted a few years ago, and it was discovered that the aromatherapy preparation had just as positive an effect as RadiaPlex Rx gel, a common topical application used by cancer patients. Products were applied topically three times a day until one month post-radiation.

The oils you'll want to use for radiation burns should be gentle and healing for the skin, including frankincense, geranium, helichrysum, lavender, Roman chamomile, rose, and sandalwood.

Also, we feel that using a base like a calendula-infused oil can make all the difference in the world. Widely known for its soothing properties, calendula is commonly added to body-care ointments. The beautiful flower is also used to create a CO_2 extract or absolute that is rich in healing compounds like *alpha-cadinol*, which is heralded for anti-cancer properties.

Application: Try the Radiation Burn Cream recipe (page 210), which is powered by a homemade calendula-infused oil.

CALENDULA-INFUSED OIL

This traditional recipe is simple to prepare and has a plethora of uses! It is perfect used alone or as the primary carrier in healing creams, massage oils, and salves.

Dried organic calendula flowers (enough to fill the jar)
Extra-virgin olive oil

SUPPLIES
Quart-size mason jar and lid
Pint-size jars and lids, for storage (optional)

1. Fill a mason jar two-thirds with calendula flowers.
2. Pour extra-virgin olive oil into the jar until roughly 80 percent of the jar is full.
3. Stir well with a wooden spoon and seal the jar with the lid.
4. Place the jar on your countertop or windowsill, being sure it's exposed to the sun, and shake at least once every day to mix the contents.
5. After 4 to 6 weeks, strain out and discard the calendula using a cheesecloth-lined sieve.
6. Pour the infused oil back into mason jar or, if desired, into smaller glass containers, screw on the lid(s), and store.
7. Use as a stand-alone therapy over radiation burns or in the recipe below.

To watch us make this recipe and learn more about infusing herbs, go to EOApothecary.com.

RADIATION BURN CREAM

20 drops helichrysum essential oil

20 drops lavender essential oil

20 drops Roman or German chamomile essential oil

1 to 2 ounces Calendula-Infused Oil (page 209; see Note)

1 ounce fresh aloe vera gel (optional; see Note)

SUPPLIES

Medium glass bowl

Lidded glass jar or lotion dispenser

1. Drop the essential oils into a glass bowl.
2. Add the infused oil and aloe gel and mix thoroughly.
3. Apply the oil over radiation burns and sensitive areas once or twice a day.
4. Store in a lidded glass jar or lotion dispenser.

NOTE: *If you can get your hands on an aloe plant, which is exceptionally healing, you can use fresh aloe in this recipe with great success. If you don't have fresh aloe, do not substitute a store-bought version made with alcohol or preservatives; just use 2 ounces of calendula-infused oil instead.*

Other common side effects of cancer and cancer treatments that we didn't mention include low libido, memory, pain, and sleep problems, all of which have been discussed in previous chapters of this book, along with suggestions to help you remedy each one naturally with essential oils.

Thousands of testimonials and case studies alone should awaken us to the realization that essential oils can be quite effective in helping cancer patients. And, as long as there are no dangerous adverse reactions, what's the risk in trying?

At this point, an increasing number of doctors support the use of natural therapies such as essential oils as an adjunct to their standard of care—not to mention if you're working with an integrative oncologist. With them, the sky's the limit!

Chapter 12

Cardiovascular Disease

ts death threat is currently bigger than that of cancer, and it's the world's number one killer: cardiovascular disease. A catchall term for the group of disorders that affect the heart and blood vessels, cardiovascular disease (CVD) includes the following:

- Cardiomyopathies (heart muscle disease)
- Cerebrovascular disease (stroke)
- Congenital heart disease (birth defects)
- Coronary heart disease (heart attack)
- Heart failure
- Hypertension (high blood pressure)
- Peripheral vascular disease
- Rheumatic heart disease (caused by rheumatic fever)

In the United States, more than eighteen million adults suffer from CVD. Coincidentally, eighteen million adults worldwide die annually from CVD. In fact, 30 percent of all global deaths are caused by CVD. Unless something changes, it is expected that the number will jump to twenty-four million by 2030, with heart disease and stroke topping the list.

Once again highlighting the interconnectedness of the chronic diseases discussed in this book, the primary reason why these numbers are expected to rise is because of metabolic syndrome, a serious health condition that affects about 23 percent of adults and places them at higher risk of cardiovascular disease, diabetes, stroke, and diseases related to fatty buildups in artery walls. Metabolic syndrome occurs when someone has three or more of the following:

1. Abdominal obesity
2. Elevated triglyceride levels
3. Low HDL cholesterol levels
4. Elevated blood pressure
5. Elevated blood glucose

But the good news is that CVD and its risk factors (including metabolic syndrome) are treatable and preventable, because its causes—namely obesity, high blood pressure, stress, and other factors—are largely under our control.

THE STATIN AND ASPIRIN PROBLEM

As you may have guessed, CVD medications top the list of the most prescribed drugs on the market today. Of the top ten most prescribed drugs on the market, CVD meds hold six slots, with the current ranking of numbers one, two, five, six, eight, and nine. More than five hundred million prescriptions are filled every year on CVD drugs in the United States alone!

Two of these top-ten drugs are statins. Statins are used to regulate dyslipidemia, or abnormal amounts of lipids (e.g., triglycerides, cholesterol, and/or fat phospholipids) in the blood.

Yet, statins do not work for half the people prescribed them, according to a 2019 study published in journal *Heart*. Of 165,411 primary-care patients in the United Kingdom who were prescribed statins, 84,609 (51.2 percent) had experienced a "sub-optimal low-density lipoprotein cholesterol (LDL-C) response" to statin therapy within twenty-four months of taking the drug. Moreover, of the 165,411 patients, there were 22,798 CVD events, which caused the authors of the study to conclude that "optimal lowering of LDL-C is not achieved within 2 years in over half of patients in the general population initiated on statin therapy, and these patients will experience significantly increased risk of future CVD."

Nonetheless, every time the blood cholesterol guidelines are updated, the number of people on statins skyrockets. The biggest shift occurred in 2013, when 50 percent of all adults over forty years old were on statins because the American College of Cardiology/American Heart Association guidelines recommended that anyone with the following four "risk" factors should be on the drug:

1. Primary treatment for current atherosclerotic cardiovascular disease
2. Primary treatment for LDL-C levels over 190 mg (aged twenty-one years and older)
3. Primary prevention for adults aged forty to seventy-five with diabetes and LDL-C between 70 and 189
4. Primary prevention for adults aged forty to seventy-five without diabetes, but LDL-C between 70 and 189 as long as they had a 7.5 percent chance or greater of developing atherosclerotic cardiovascular disease in the next ten years as determined by a series of risk factors including blood pressure, race, and gender

Then, three years later, it was announced that both heart disease and stroke death rates increased for the first time in decades. Obviously, getting more people on statins wasn't the answer.

The same is true for preventive aspirin use. If you've had a heart attack or stroke, your doctor will probably recommend you take aspirin daily, unless you have a history of bleeding or some serious allergy. She will also most likely recommend you take aspirin if it is determined that you are at high risk of having a first heart attack. This has contributed to far too many people taking aspirin prophylactically. A Harvard study published in 2019 suggested that about 29 million (nearly 25 percent)

American adults aged forty without cardiovascular disease are currently taking aspirin each day. Among those people, 6.6 million (roughly 23 percent) are taking it without a doctor's recommendation!

What's the danger in prophylactic aspirin use?

First, according to a recently completed clinical trial of more than 16,700 healthy older Americans and Australians with no history of heart problems or stroke, taking a low dose of aspirin every day does *not* help people live longer free of disability, dementia, nonfatal heart attacks, coronary heart disease, or nonfatal and fatal ischemic stroke. In other words, people who take aspirin daily had nearly identical health outcomes as those who didn't take aspirin. Second, the study, called the Aspirin in Reducing Events in the Elderly (ASPREE) experiment, uncovered something quite concerning: people taking aspirin every day for CVD prevention are at a higher risk of cancer-related deaths compared to people who aren't on aspirin!

Just thinking of the tens of millions of well-intentioned people currently on statins and daily aspirin regimens, who are innocently and faithfully following misguided advice, breaks our hearts. Especially when a vast majority of CVD could be prevented by disciplined lifestyle changes.

Truth be told, the most efficient way to prevent and manage CVD is to do the following: reach your ideal weight, balance your blood sugar, regularly exercise, successfully manage stress, and, with your doctor's help, get off as many prescription drugs as you can. And essential oils can help you every step of the way!

SHOULD YOU AVOID GRAPEFRUIT OIL?

If you're currently taking medication for CVD, chances are your doctor has told you to not eat grapefruit or drink grapefruit juice. This is because furanocoumarins (bergamottin and dihydroxybergamottin) can interact adversely with several medications, including statins, drugs for hypertension and abnormal heart rhythms, and antianxiety drugs and corticosteroids.

In many cases, consuming grapefruit increases the level of the medicine in your blood, thus increasing the risk of side effects because too much of the drug stays in your body. Many drugs are metabolized with the help of an enzyme known as

CYP3A in the small intestine. Furanocoumarins have the tendency to block the action of CYP3A, thereby preventing medications from being broken down properly.

The furanocoumarins in grapefruit juice that interact with CYP3A, however, are not found in great enough quantities, because it is extracted from the rind, not the fruit. There are no traces of dihydroxybergamottin whatsoever, and only a negligible amount of bergamottin in the oil. In fact, experts emphatically conclude you'd have to consume more than 10 milliliters (about 2 teaspoons) of grapefruit oil per day to contradict its use in CVD patients. This, of course, should never happen.

Of course, be sure to consult with your cardiologist, but enjoying grapefruit oil shouldn't be a problem at all!

BLACK SEED OIL

Not an essential oil, black seed oil (*Nigella sativa* L.) is a fatty oil like olive oil that is helpful in treating cardiovascular disease. It contains thymoquinone, which has been well-established to have several pharmacological activities, including acting as an anti-inflammatory and antitumor agent, a pain reliever, a vascular relaxant, and an oxidative stress reducer. Thymoquinone also helps improve endothelial function in aging animals after fourteen days of therapy.

The endothelium is a thin membrane that lines the heart and blood vessels. Endothelial dysfunction can be caused by several conditions, including diabetes or metabolic syndrome, hypertension, smoking, and physical inactivity.

Application: For your capsules and topical applications, consider using *Nigella sativa* L. for enhanced CVD benefits.

THE ESSENTIAL OILS APPROACH TO CARDIOVASCULAR DISEASE

With more research, we are seeing validation from the scientific community that essential oils can play a pivotal role in CVD prevention and management. Specifically, consider a review published a few years ago:

Research on EO has the potential to identify new bioactive compounds and formulate new functional products for the treatment of cardiovascular diseases such as arterial hypertension, angina pectoris, heart failure, and myocardial infarction.

The review indicated a few of the reasons why:

Some EO, and their active ingredients, have been reported to improve the cardiovascular system significantly by affecting vaso-relaxation (and thus lowering blood pressure, and decreasing the heart rate and exert a hypotension activity.

Below, we take a look at the CVD risks and contributing factors that essential oils have been shown to help prevent and manage.

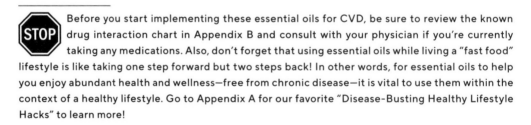

Before you start implementing these essential oils for CVD, be sure to review the known drug interaction chart in Appendix B and consult with your physician if you're currently taking any medications. Also, don't forget that using essential oils while living a "fast food" lifestyle is like taking one step forward but two steps back! In other words, for essential oils to help you enjoy abundant health and wellness—free from chronic disease—it is vital to use them within the context of a healthy lifestyle. Go to Appendix A for our favorite "Disease-Busting Healthy Lifestyle Hacks" to learn more!

GENERAL CARDIOPROTECTIVE ESSENTIAL OILS (HEART ATTACK AND STROKE)

If you're at risk of having a heart attack or stroke, consult with your cardiologist about taking two drops of the essential oils listed below (lavender, cinnamon bark, clove bud, or fennel seed) in a vegan gel capsule once or twice a day after eating. Be sure to fill up your capsule with a heart-healthy edible carrier oil like black seed or extra-virgin olive oil to help ensure safety and efficacy.

1. Lavender

Myocardial infarction (heart attack) is a common presentation of ischemic heart disease and a major cause of death worldwide. To help prevent heart attacks, having lavender on hand seems to be a good idea for a number of reasons. A study out of Iran induced heart attacks in lab rats and then injected lavender oil into the stomach of the animals affected. The essential oil profoundly amended ECG (electrocardiogram) pattern results, suggesting that lavender protects heart muscle myocardium against damage. The lavender injection also greatly reduced myeloperoxidase (MPO) and malondialdehyde (MDA).

- MPO is a toxic inflammatory enzyme that is elevated in people at risk for CVD (including heart attacks) and in patients with autoimmune disorders, such as multiple sclerosis and rheumatoid arthritis.
- MDA is one of the final products of polyunsaturated fatty acids peroxidation in the cells. An increase in free radicals causes overproduction of MDA. Malondialdehyde level is commonly known as a marker of oxidative stress and the antioxidant status in cancerous patients.

You may also find it helpful to know that bergamot is another oil that can help protect against endothelial dysfunction associated with cardiovascular disease.

2. Cinnamon Bark

If you're looking to improve your overall heart health, cinnamon bark may be able to help. It's well established in the literature that consuming 1, 3, or 6 grams of cinnamon every day reduces serum glucose, triglycerides, LDL cholesterol, and total cholesterol in people with type 2 diabetes, and preliminary research is also being conducted on the essential oil. For instance, a study on broiler chickens suggests that a daily supplement of cinnamon bark managed to help raise their HDL cholesterol (the good kind) and reduce LDL levels (the bad kind). It also supports the heart through increased antioxidant activity.

Another benefit of consuming cinnamon bark oil is cinnamaldehyde, its main component, which has been shown to inhibit blood clots in rat and mice studies. In a study from 2016, it was discovered that cinnamaldehyde inhibits neuron inflammation, making it a potential candidate for preventing stroke.

3. Clove Bud

This essential oil is known to help minimize "platelet aggregation." For perspective, platelets are a type of blood cell. They help form blood clots by sticking together (thus the term *aggregation*). A clot is what stops the bleeding when you have a wound. Without platelets, you could bleed to death. In cardiovascular disease, abnormal clotting occurs that can result in a heart attack or stroke. If plaque in a blood vessel ruptures, platelets sense the rupture but get confused. Thinking that an injury has taken place that will cause bleeding, they form a clot in the blood vessel, causing a blockage of blood flow.

Clove essential oil can help this situation by slightly thinning the blood to enhance circulation. It is also rich in eugenol, a component that was shown in a 2015 study to help prevent cardiac issues in rats induced with heart attacks. Treated rats showed improvement in cardiac injury, reduced inflammation of important proteins, and other preventive effects.

Because clove blends well with heart-healthy cinnamon bark and limonene-rich orange essential oils, consider taking one to two drops of each in your capsules

Note: If you're currently taking warfarin or other blood thinners, avoid ingesting clove bud oil because of its antiplatelet aggregation effects. It could cause internal bleeding.

4. Fennel Seed

When a blood clot completely obstructs a coronary artery supplying blood to the heart muscle, the heart muscle dies and someone experiences a heart attack and/or stroke. An interesting study suggests that ingesting fennel seed essential oil can reduce the risk of this happening.

Made from the crushed seeds of the plant, fennel essential oil is mostly associated with digestive health. But a 2007 study reported that the oil and its active ingredient, anethole, provided protection against stomach lesions as well as against blood clots in lab studies with animals. In fact, the researchers concluded that fennel oil and anethole have "a safe antithrombotic activity that seems due to their broad-spectrum antiplatelet activity, clot destabilizing effect and vasorelaxant action."

METABOLIC SYNDROME

If you're looking for the most efficient way to prevent and manage CVD, the biggest bang for your buck is to avoid metabolic syndrome in one fell swoop. From a natural living perspective, the lifestyle hacks we present in Appendix A are the way to go.

An aromatherapy approach is a fantastic complementary strategy, and you'll want to have these oils on hand to help address each of the factors associated with metabolic syndrome:

1. Abdominal obesity—lime, grapefruit, peppermint (see pages 245–252 for the entire list)
2. Elevated triglyceride levels—bergamot, lemon, lemongrass
3. Low HDL cholesterol levels—limonene-containing oil (citrus)
4. Elevated blood pressure—cinnamon bark, bergamot, lavender, ylang ylang
5. Elevated blood glucose—cinnamon bark, fenugreek, oregano (see chapter 14 for the entire list)

Be sure to follow the protocols starting on page 304 to help you reach your ideal weight and balance blood sugar. Additionally, see below for how to use limonene- and linalool-rich oils for hypertension and dyslipidemia.

5. Lemon

Limonene has long been known to help regulate cholesterol and blood glucose levels. In fact, it's been recommended as a dietary supplement to prevent and/or manage metabolic syndrome. It can also help with blood pressure and elevated heart rate.

In a recent study evaluating lemon, limonene, and a control, the famed citrus oil outperformed limonene by decreasing elevated triglyceride levels more efficiently. Yet, limonene outperformed lemon in increased HDL levels. This is one reason why we suggest using a citrus synergy blend to enhance the limonene interaction with other essential oils to enjoy complete heart health!

For a full list of limonene-containing oils, see page 108.

Application: Review chapter 6 and make our Citrus Delight Blend (page 102) and recipes to promote healthy cholesterol levels. A sample protocol you could follow would be the following: apply Citrus Delight Massage Oil (page 104) as a moisturizer or after you shower; take one Citrus Delight Capsule (page 106) twice daily with breakfast and dinner; and diffuse 6 drops of Citrus Delight Blend throughout the day. Try this for one month and monitor your cholesterol levels with your cardiologist.

6. Bergamot

Also containing linalool, limonene-rich bergamot oil is a must-have for all things heart health. Research from Korea suggests that it may have a protective effect on the inner lining of the small arteries in your body. In one lab study from 2009, it also provided protective effects against brain injury in rats caused by stroke.

Application: As with lemon above, review chapter 6 to make our Citrus Delight Blend (page 102) and corresponding remedies.

7. Ylang Ylang

With high blood pressure creating so many serious complications in the cardiovascular system, a study from Korea gives tremendous hope. The researchers studied the effect of ylang ylang aromatherapy on blood pressure and heart rate in twenty-nine healthy men who were divided in two groups: an ylang ylang group and a control group.

The researchers put three drops of ylang ylang oil into warm water and created incense. All of the subjects in the ylang ylang group smelled the fragrance for twenty minutes. The control group was not exposed to any aromatherapy.

At the end of the experimental period, those in the ylang ylang group showed significantly lower systolic and diastolic blood pressures and a lower heart rate than those in the control group. The researchers noted that their study "provides some evidences for the usage of ylang ylang as a medicinal agent."

Some people find the smell of linalool-rich ylang ylang too strong to tolerate as a stand-alone therapy, which is one reason why it's so frequently used in blends. As you may have guessed it, even when blended, ylang ylang doesn't lose its potent heart health properties. In fact, they are even enhanced!

To evaluate how an essential oil blend containing lavender, ylang ylang, marjoram, and neroli helps normalize blood pressure, eighty-three prehypertensive and hypertensive patients were advised to wear an aromatherapy necklace with two drops of a linalool-powered blend in the morning and at night. It was discovered that the inhalation of an essential oil had immediate and continuous effects on the home systolic blood pressure, daytime blood pressure, and salivary cortisol levels (stress reduction). The blend was lavender, ylang ylang, marjoram, and neroli (in a ratio of 20:15:10:2).

Another ylang ylang blend (lemon, lavender, and ylang ylang mixed 2:2:1) also produced a significant decrease in systolic blood pressure and normalized heart rate variability (a common CVD risk factor) in hypertension patients.

For a full list of linalool-containing oils, see page 86.

Application: Add 2 drops of lemon, 2 drops of lavender, and 1 drop of ylang ylang essential oil in your diffuser for a wonderfully soothing aroma throughout the day to promote balanced blood pressure. Alternatively, try the blend that worked so well in the research study above in your diffuser, aromatherapy inhaler, or necklace!

HYPERTENSION BLEND

30 drops lavender essential oil

22 drops ylang ylang essential oil

15 drops marjoram essential oil

3 drops neroli essential oil

SUPPLIES

5 ml bottle

1. Drop the essential oils in a 5 ml bottle. Cap the bottle and shake to combine.
2. Use as directed in the following recipes.

HYPERTENSION DIFFUSER BLEND

6 drops Hypertension Blend (recipe above)

SUPPLIES

Diffuser

1. Fill your diffuser with purified water as directed in the manufacturer's instructions.
2. Add the essential oil blend.
3. Turn on the diffuser and use throughout the day or at night to promote heart health. This recipe works well in an aromatherapy necklace.
4. Turn off the diffuser when done.

HYPERTENSION INHALER

20 drops Hypertension Blend (page 222)

SUPPLIES

Precut organic cotton pad

Aromatherapy inhaler

1. Place a cotton pad in the inhaler tube.

2. Drop the essential oils directly onto the cotton pad inside the tube. Alternatively, you can drop the blend into a glass bowl, roll the cotton pad in the oils to absorb them, and then insert it into the inhaler using tweezers.

3. Secure the cap and store the inhaler in a desk drawer, purse, or glove compartment so you have it handy.

4. When you're stressed, anxious, or simply want to enjoy a blood-pressure-supporting aromatic retreat, open the inhaler and take 10 deep breaths of the vapor from the tube.

5. Focus on your breathing as a stress-relieving meditation technique to help manage stress levels.

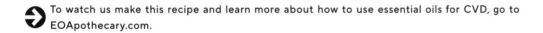 To watch us make this recipe and learn more about how to use essential oils for CVD, go to EOApothecary.com.

8. Bergamot

Bergamot really shines as a blend with other oils on this list of linalool-rich oils—and there is science to support the synergistic benefits of such a combination! Researchers had subjects inhale a blend of lavender, ylang ylang, and bergamot essentials oils for four weeks. Blood pressure, stress, anxiety, and levels of the stress hormone cortisol were all significantly reduced in the group treated with the blend compared to the control group.

Application: Enjoy the Hypertension Blend (page 222) recipes above by replacing neroli with bergamot essential oil.

9. Clary Sage

Clary sage is heart-protective because of its natural ability to relax the arteries. This action allows blood to better circulate throughout your body, reduces blood pressure, and improves the flow of oxygen to the muscles and organs.

A Korean study published in 2013 measured the effect of clary sage and lavender essential oils on blood pressure levels in female patients with incontinence and other urinary issues. The women inhaled either clary sage or lavender oil, and a control group was treated with sweet almond oil. Their blood pressure was then measured after inhaling the oils for an hour. Interestingly, those who inhaled clary sage oil experienced a significant reduction in blood pressure levels and breathing rate compared to both the lavender and control groups.

Application: In addition to enjoying clary sage by itself in your body oils, diffuser blends, and roll-ons, make our Healthy Heart Blend (page 225) and enjoy its recipes.

10. Lavender

The calming qualities of lavender help the heart by reducing blood pressure and easing the tension on blood vessels. This can prevent atherosclerosis and other cardiovascular problems, thus reducing your odds of stroke and heart attack. The *International Journal of Cardiology* reported that simply inhaling lavender improved coronary blood flow in thirty healthy adult men and reduced salivary cortisol levels (an indicator of stress). Animal lab studies also have shown that lavender oil lowered blood pressure and reduced stroke damage in rats.

Application: In addition to enjoying lavender by itself in your body oils, diffuser blends, and roll-ons, make our Healthy Heart Blend (page 225) and enjoy its recipes.

11. Rosewood

We see similar results in other oils rich in linalool. Take rosewood oil, for instance, which has been shown to help induce vagus nerve bradycardia (reduced heart rate) and the depressor reflex (rapid reduction in blood pressure and constricted blood vessel relaxation) when injected in rats. Note: Rosewood (also known as Brazilian rosewood) is an endangered species and is environmentally protected. There is still a lot of rosewood oil out there from previous distillations, so it's very possible to get your hands on some from companies that are committed to fair trade and sustainable practices.

Application: Add 1 drop of rosewood essential oil to the Healthy Heart Diffuser Blend (page 226) to promote proper cardiovascular function.

HEALTHY HEART BLEND

20 drops coriander seed essential oil

10 drops lavender essential oil

10 drops neroli essential oil

10 drops bergamot essential oil

10 drops clary sage essential oil

10 drops geranium essential oil

SUPPLIES

5 ml bottle

1. Drop the essential oils in a 5 ml bottle. Cap the bottle and shake to combine.

2. Use as directed in the following recipes.

HEALTHY HEART CAPSULE

Makes 1 dose

4 drops Healthy Heart Blend (recipe above)

Heart-healthy fatty oil like black seed oil or extra-virgin olive oil

SUPPLIES

Pipette

Size 00 vegan gel capsule

1. Using a pipette, drop the essential oil blend into the bottom half (the longer, narrower one) of the capsule. Fill this half to the brim with your heart-healthy oil.

continues

2. Fit the wider top half of the capsule over the bottom half and secure it snugly.

3. Immediately swallow the capsule with water after breakfast (see Note). Take daily and monitor results.

NOTE: *Do **not** make and store this capsule for future use. Also, this is not a long-term solution, and using it for more than four weeks at a time is not advisable. Be sure to switch up your protocol monthly and consult with your health-care provider first if you're currently taking medications. Discontinue if adverse reactions occur.*

HEALTHY HEART DIFFUSER BLEND

6 drops Healthy Heart Blend (page 225)

SUPPLIES
Diffuser

1. Fill your diffuser with purified water as directed in the manufacturer's instructions.

2. Add the essential oil blend.

3. Turn on the diffuser and use throughout the day or at night to promote heart health. This recipe works well in an aromatherapy necklace.

NOTE: *Add a drop of sustainably harvested rosewood essential oil if you can get your hands on some!*

HEALTHY HEART BODY OIL

16 drops Healthy Heart Blend (page 225)
2 ounces carrier oil or Mama Z's Oil Base (page 25)

SUPPLIES
Medium glass bowl
Lidded glass jar or lotion dispenser

1. Drop the essential oil blend into a glass bowl.

2. Add a carrier oil and mix thoroughly.

3. Apply after you shower or as a daily moisturizer to promote a systemic approach to heart health. Being sure to apply over your chest and abdomen. This recipe works well in an aromatherapy necklace.

4. Store in a glass jar or lotion dispenser.

NOTE: *Add 2 drops of sustainably harvested rosewood essential oil if you can get your hands on some!*

12. Citronella

Also containing linalool, citronella essential oil is used primarily to ward off bugs; however, science proves that it has far more benefits. Citronellol, its primary component, is actually used in folk medicine as an antihypertensive drug, and research in rat models confirms this. It's also known to be antibacterial, antifungal, antispasmodic, and anticonvulsant, thus making citronella quite the healer. Citronella oil is derived from the same family as lemongrass, and its clean, citrusy smell will bring summer to mind all year long!

Application: Citronella blends well with eucalyptus and lemongrass, so mix 2 drops each in your diffuser when you want to promote balanced blood pressure and heart health.

ROSEMARY FOR HYPOTENSION

For people with low blood pressure (hypotension), inhaling rosemary essential oil should be a consideration. Traditionally, rosemary has been inhaled to increase blood pressure, heart rate, and respiratory rate. But a seventy-two-month study evaluating thirty-two volunteers diagnosed with primary hypotension advised each patient to consume 1 milliliter (20 drops) of rosemary oil, and the results were even more profound.

As we discussed in chapter 2, the max daily oral dose of essential oils for adults ranges from 6 to 20 drops (in total) per day, and we caution anyone from ingesting

20 drops of rosemary essential oil unless otherwise directed by their health-care provider. Although you'll receive a lesser therapeutic effect, taking 3 or 4 drops in a vegan gel capsule once daily would be a much safer place to start. Nonetheless, the fact remains that rosemary should be a strong candidate when considering hypotension treatment.

Although cardiovascular disease comes in different types and stems from a variety of causes, employing a holistic approach to treat and prevent it shouldn't be a daunting task. Without doubt, that approach should definitely include diet, exercise, stress management, nutritional supplementation—and of course, essential oils!

Chapter 13

Chronic Respiratory Disease

W e must never underestimate the importance of our breath to life itself. It supplies our body and its various organs with oxygen, which is vital for our survival. Oxygen cannot be stored and must be replenished continuously. In fact, we can survive no longer than three minutes without air.

Sadly though, we are plagued in our society with chronic respiratory diseases that rob tens of millions of people across the world of precious oxygen and prevent them from experiencing abundant health. To make matters worse, if the situation progresses, and it often does, it can lead to death.

In fact, chronic respiratory diseases—asthma, pulmonary fibrosis, and chronic obstructive pulmonary disease (COPD), which includes both bronchitis and emphysema—are the fourth-leading cause of death in America. Globally, COPD is the third leading cause of death, which greatly contributes to the fourth leading cause of death: lower respiratory infections (bronchitis, pneumonia, and tuberculosis).

Because smoking is the leading cause of COPD and may cause up to 80 percent of cases, if this is an area that you struggle with, please review the addiction section in chapter 6 to get the aromatherapy support that you need to quit the habit.

And, because it is a well-established factor for developing COPD in adulthood, please take childhood asthma very seriously if your child is affected. In 2017, nearly

9 percent of children in the United States under the age of eighteen had asthma, and this epidemic is only getting worse.

The good news is that if you do have a respiratory disease, you can take actions that protect your health and boost your immunity. You can also start on preventive actions before you become ill! Learning how to protect yourself using essential oils for respiratory health can be the difference between getting sick and staying healthy.

QUICK NOTE ON INFLAMMATION

Asthma and COPD are both characterized by chronic inflammation in the airway and lungs. Thus, like most chronic diseases in this book, to successfully manage chronic respiratory conditions, you need to fix your inflammation problem.

The first step is to avoid contact with environmental exposures. Although it's impossible to avoid airborne toxins when you're outside or in public places, the best chance you have at preventing asthma and COPD is to breathe pure, fresh air in your home. Review chapter 3 for some tips on how to keep the air in your home pure and free of toxins.

The second step is to create an inflammation blend that suits your senses, and we know the main anti-inflammatory components to look for:

- **1,8-cineole**—found in eucalyptus (all types), galangal, niaouli, cajuput, cardamom, holy basil, laurel leaf, myrtle, rosemary, sage, spike lavender, and tea tree essential oils
- **Anethole**—found in anise, cedarwood, and fennel essential oils
- **Borneol**—found in lavender, rosemary, lavandin, spike lavender, and sage essential oils
- **Eugenol**—found in clove, black pepper, and basil essential oils
- **Menthol**—found in peppermint, corn mint, and lemon basil essential oils

In addition to the chemical components above, the following readily available essential oils have been shown to have very promising anti-inflammatory properties according to research studies:

- Caraway
- Clove
- Eucalyptus
- Ginger
- Lavender
- Marjoram
- Oregano
- Peppermint
- Roman chamomile
- Tea tree
- Thyme
- Turmeric

Safety Note: It's important to note that some essential oils experts claim that 1,8-cineole- and menthol-containing oils should not be used around the faces of children under three years old because of the potential to cause respiratory arrest and neurological problems.

Personally, we have not had any issues with using heavily diluted peppermint on or around our children, nor have our closest colleagues.

Still, not wanting to negate the advice of aromatherapists, use care with children under three years old and stick with the safe dilutions that we recommend for kids in chapter 2 if you use them topically.

THE ESSENTIAL OILS APPROACH TO RESPIRATORY SUPPORT

For people with chronic respiratory disease, viruses and bacteria can pose an especially harmful threat to your health and well-being. Extreme care should be taken with the flu, viruses, pneumonia, and other respiratory infections. Essential oils have been shown to help with all of these conditions, though they are not considered chronic diseases and are out of the purview of this book. Inhaling tea tree oil, for example, has been proven to have a strong anti-inflammatory influence on the immune system, which is one reason why we included it in our Easy Breathing Blend on page 232.

Focusing our attention specifically on chronic respiratory disease, we'll discuss asthma, pulmonary fibrosis, and COPD, which includes both bronchitis and emphysema. Symptoms shared by these illnesses are shortness of breath, coughing, wheezing, and a general inability to breathe normally.

You may be surprised to learn that using essential oils in *every* way, not just inhalation, can help solve the respiratory problems so many people have! Starting on page 236 is the list of essential oils that top the charts when it comes to managing chronic respiratory conditions, and here are some quick recipes that you can make using our favorite all-purpose respiratory support blend!

STOP Before you start implementing these essential oils for chronic respiratory disease, be sure to review the known drug interaction chart in Appendix B and consult with your physician if you're currently taking any medications. Also, don't forget that using essential oils while living a "fast food" lifestyle is like taking one step forward but two steps back! In other words, for essential oils to help you enjoy abundant health and wellness—free from chronic disease—it is vital to use them within the context of a healthy lifestyle. Go to Appendix A for our favorite "Disease-Busting Healthy Lifestyle Hacks" to learn more!

EASY BREATHING BLEND

20 drops eucalyptus essential oil (any species or a mixture)

15 drops orange essential oil

15 drops mandarin essential oil

10 drops cardamom essential oil

10 drops ginger essential oil

10 drops peppermint essential oil

5 drops tea tree essential oil

SUPPLIES

5 ml bottle

1. Drop the essential oils in a 5 ml bottle. Cap the bottle and shake to combine.

2. Use as directed in the following recipes.

EASY BREATHING DIFFUSER BLEND

5 or 6 drops Easy Breathing Blend (page 232)

SUPPLIES
Diffuser

1. Fill your diffuser with purified water as directed in the manufacturer's instructions.

2. Add the essential oil blend.

3. Turn on the diffuser when you want to promote easy breathing and respiratory support. It's great to run the diffuser during the day and night. This recipe works well in an aromatherapy necklace

EASY BREATHING INHALER

20 drops Easy Breathing Blend (page 232)

SUPPLIES
Precut organic cotton pad
Aromatherapy inhaler

1. Place a cotton pad in the inhaler tube.

2. Drop the essential oils directly onto the cotton pad inside the tube. Alternatively, you can drop the blend into a glass bowl, roll the cotton pad in the oils to absorb them, and then insert it into the inhaler using tweezers.

3. Secure the cap and store the inhaler in a desk drawer, purse, or glove compartment so you have it handy.

4. When you want instant respiratory support, open the inhaler and take 10 deep breaths of the vapor from the tube.

EASY BREATHING SPRITZER

10 drops organic 190-proof grain alcohol
10 drops Easy Breathing Blend (page 232)

continues

10 drops witch hazel

Distilled water, as needed

SUPPLIES

1-ounce spray bottle

1. Combine the grain alcohol, essential oil blend, and witch hazel in the bottle.

2. Fill with distilled water and shake gently to mix well.

3. Spray the air around you for an aromatic respiratory boost or on your sheets before you go to bed to promote better breathing at night.

NOTE: *This water-based formula will last for a couple of weeks. We've used it for as long as two months and have not noticed any bacterial overgrowth, which can happen with any water-based product. This may not be obvious at first, but the smell will become rancid and you will notice a change in color if it is contaminated.*

 To watch us make this recipe and learn more about our favorite ways to promote healthy, deep breathing, go to EOApothecary.com.

EASY BREATHING CAPSULE

Makes 1 dose

3 or 4 drops Easy Breathing Blend (page 232)

Organic virgin coconut oil, extra-virgin olive oil, or black seed oil (see Notes)

SUPPLIES

Pipette

Size 00 vegan gel capsule

1. Using a pipette, drop the essential oil blend into the bottom half (the longer, narrower one) of the capsule. Fill this half to the brim with the oil.

2. Fit the wider top half of the capsule over the bottom half and secure it snugly.

3. Immediately swallow the capsule with water after breakfast and/or dinner (see Notes). Take once or twice daily for inflammation and monitor respiratory symptoms.

NOTES: *Black seed oil has been shown to have powerful anti-inflammatory effects in COPD and emphysema. It can also help block lung damage and fibrosis. Using this fatty oil as the carrier in your Easy Breathing Capsule can help take your healing to the next level!*

*Do **not** make and store these capsules for future use. Also, this is not a long-term solution, and using it for more than four weeks at a time is not advisable. Be sure to switch up your protocol monthly and consult with your health-care provider first if you're currently taking medications. Discontinue if adverse reactions occur.*

EASY BREATHING ROLL-ON

12 drops Easy Breathing Blend (page 232)

Carrier oil of choice—jojoba and fractionated coconut oil absorb quickly—as needed

SUPPLIES

10 ml glass roller bottle

1. Drop the essential oil blend into the roller bottle.
2. Fill the roller bottle with your carrier oil of choice and shake well.
3. Apply over your chest and back of neck once daily or whenever you want to promote healthy respiratory function

EASY BREATHING BODY OIL

12 drops Easy Breathing Blend (page 232)

2 ounces carrier oil of choice or Mama Z's Oil Base (page 25)

SUPPLIES

Medium glass bowl

Lidded glass jar or lotion dispenser

1. Drop the essential oil blend into a bowl.
2. Add a carrier oil and mix thoroughly.
3. Use as a body oil after you shower and as a moisturizer throughout the day.

1. Eucalyptus

By far the most studied component in treating chronic respiratory disorders, the essential oils listed on page 230 that are rich in 1,8-cineole (or simply cineole) should definitely be in your medicine cabinet. Consider these your "all-purpose" respiratory support remedies. Here are some reasons why.

Caused by free radicals and oxidative stress, excess mucus secretion of your airways is a common feature of asthma and COPD. Research has shown that, because of its antioxidant and anti-inflammatory prowess, cineole has the uncanny ability to help resolve this condition, which can help promote true root-cause resolution for people suffering from chronic respiratory disorders.

Topping the charts with the most cineole content, eucalyptus oil has been the subject of much research focusing on respiratory diseases, including COPD and asthma. One study summed it up the best: "According to results, 1,8-cineole or eucalyptus EO can be effectively applied in the treatment of asthma, acute or chronic bronchitis, COPD, common cold and sinusitis."

Using eucalyptus via inhalation, topical application, and internally can all help. Several years ago, 242 COPD patients, all current or former smokers, were told to take their normally prescribed COPD medications as well as 200 milligrams (roughly six drops) of cineole or placebo three times daily for six months during wintertime. Those treated with cineole had improved airflow, reduced flare-ups and shortness of breath, and better overall health and quality of life.

Another study identified thirty-two airborne antituberculosis compounds in *Eucalyptus citriodora*, suggesting that simply diffusing the eucalyptus essential oil can help the spread of this horrible lung infection. Just imagine what it might do to the common cold or flu or coronavirus!

Application: Diffuse 5 or 6 drops of our Easy Breathing Blend (page 232) or equal parts of cardamom, eucalyptus, lemon, peppermint, rosemary, and tea tree essential oils for a synergistic respiratory blend!

2. Peppermint

Menthol is widely used as a flavoring agent in beverages, gum, and candy. Menthol is also used for burns and joint and muscle pain, as well as all things related to respiratory health: allergies, congestion, and deep breathing. It also so happens to be the primary component of peppermint essential oil.

An interesting study was conducted a couple years ago that evaluated how a blend of essential oils helped reduce lung and airway inflammation when exposed to microscopic air pollution (dangerous VOCs, heavy metals, endotoxins, pollen, fungal spores, viruses, and bacteria). This type of air pollution is well-known to be associated with the inflammation of many airway diseases, including allergic airway inflammation, asthma, and COPD. The oils tested were peppermint, frankincense, spruce, and eucalyptus. As expected, the blend performed superbly in reducing acute lung inflammation and systemic inflammation, which suggests these oils can help not only with COPD and asthma flare-ups but with total body support and a potential root-cause resolution!

Application: Diffuse 1 drop each of peppermint, frankincense, spruce, and eucalyptus essential oils throughout the day to support respiratory function, relieve inflammation, and reduce flare-ups. Alternatively, you can make a 2 percent topical body oil by mixing 3 drops of each oil with 1 ounce of Mama Z's Oil Base (page 25).

3. Ginger

Ginger oil's spicy and invigorating scent provides a comforting and warm aroma for any home. It also so happens to be a proven bronchodilator, meaning that it can help open the airways and help you breathe better. Researchers investigated ginger essential oil and its primary components citral and eucalyptol and uncovered that ginger oil in its whole form and isolated citral suppressed tracheal contraction, whereas isolated eucalyptol showed a relaxing effect on airways.

Interestingly, it was discovered that the use of propranolol reversed the beneficial bronchodilatory effects of both ginger oil and citral. Propranolol is a beta-blocker that is commonly prescribed for hypertension, atrial fibrillation, angina, migraines, tremors, and even medical conditions involving the thyroid and adrenal glands. So be sure to take this into consideration if you're on beta-blockers, because they may negate the effects of using essential oils to treat chronic respiratory conditions.

Application: In addition to trying the Easy Breathing recipes above, ginger blends wonderfully with respiratory supporting oils like fennel and citrus. Try diffusing equal parts of ginger, fennel, and orange essential oils, making a 2 percent body oil or ingesting 2 drops of each in a gel capsule filled with an edible carrier oil such as black seed or extra-virgin olive oil.

4. Lavender

Best known for relieving stress, headaches, and anxiety, lavender essential oil may also be beneficial for people suffering from asthma. In 2014, researchers in Japan discovered that nebulizing lavender oil for one month helped drastically decrease allergic inflammation and mucus cell formation, as well as reduced cytokine mRNA expression in lung tissue, which is a sign of lung disease. Chinese researchers found similar results with linalool (a main component of lavender).

Lavender is a flexible oil that blends well with many other oils. It has a long history in both traditional medicine and modern research, so the sky's the limit when using this ancient remedy!

Application: Use our Bye-Bye Allergy Blend in your diffuser, inhaler, gel capsule, or body oil for a synergistic approach to promoting healthy breathing and respiratory support.

BYE-BYE ALLERGY BLEND

20 drops lavender essential oil

20 drops lemon essential oil

20 drops peppermint essential oil

SUPPLIES

5 ml bottle

1. Drop the essential oils in a 5 ml bottle. Cap the bottle and shake to combine.
2. Use as directed in the following recipes.
3. Follow the Easy Breathing recipes on pages 232–235 for proper dilutions and use guides. Simply replace Easy Breathing Blend with Bye-Bye Allergy Blend for all remedies.

5. Mandarin

In 2012, researchers investigated the effects of oral doses of mandarin essential oil on a rat model of pulmonary fibrosis once per day for four weeks. Chronic pulmonary fibrosis is a condition where lung tissue becomes scarred over time, making proper lung function—and breathing—difficult and causing shortness of breath. Rats treated with mandarin oil had less lung inflammation and better fibrosis scores than those who were not.

Application: Enjoy a culinary dose of mandarin, an ingredient in our Easy Breathing recipes (pages 232–235), by using it as the citrus oil in Dr. Z's Citrus Soda Pop (page 267) and our Citrus Delight Cooler (page 106).

6. Orange

Orange essential oil is another excellent choice, thanks to its superior antioxidant abilities. And it's very versatile, easy to use, and affordable. It has proven anti-inflammatory benefits for the respiratory tract as a nasal spray when blended with soybean, aloe vera gel, coconut, and peppermint oils and vitamin E, according to a research study on healthy nonsmoking male volunteers. A key finding in this study was that "orange oil was demonstrated to have the ability to induce long-lasting gene expression of several antioxidant enzymes," which suggests that it can trigger the body's natural immune-fighting response to protect against airborne environmental exposure to toxins that can ultimately cause chronic respiratory disorders or flare-ups once the disease settles in!

In fact, many of the citrus oils have potent healing abilities because they contain limonene, shown in research to prevent bronchial obstruction and asthma in rats.

Application: Follow the recommendations above that we shared for mandarin. Both oils are very similar and can be used interchangeably.

Even with chronic conditions like asthma or COPD, there are ways you can control them and ease their symptoms. Essential oils have all the healing properties to minimize the severity of these respiratory diseases and more!

Chapter 14

Diabetes and Obesity

Currently, more than two billion people across the planet are overweight. That's roughly 25 percent of the entire global population (young and old), and every country is affected.

This number is three times what it was back in 1975 and a clear indication that an obesity pandemic is inevitable unless we do something drastic to stop it now. In fact, the most recent data suggests that by 2030, half of American adults and one-quarter of American children will be obese!

Let that sink in for a moment.

Arguably the most preventable and most dangerous chronic disease will be knocking on one out of every two doorsteps coming up in the next few years.

Not as prevalent but equally as alarming (and equally as preventable), just under five hundred million people across the globe are diabetic, and the number is projected to increase 25 percent by 2030 and 51 percent by 2045.

"DIABESITY"

Individually, type 2 diabetes and obesity are not only two of the most prevalent chronic diseases in the world but also the foremost preventable risk factors for other chronic diseases. To make matters worse, these two debilitating conditions—obesity and diabetes—are fueling a new one-plus-one-equals-three health crisis of what medical experts and medical researchers term *diabesity*. In other words, we've got three related epidemics going on in our country: obesity, type 2 diabetes, and diabesity.

What exactly is diabesity? Strictly speaking, diabesity is a medical term for the combination of obesity and diabetes—in other words, a condition in which obesity and diabetes coexist. It can develop at any stage of diabetes, from insulin resistance to full-blown diabetes.

Among the symptoms of diabesity are weight gain in the middle section of the body; hemoglobin A1c levels higher than 5.5 (a test used to diagnose diabetes); junk food cravings; indigestion; trouble losing weight; and fatigue, to name just a few.

However, the term *diabesity* is actually a bit misleading, because physically thin people can suffer from the entire spectrum of blood sugar disorders, all the way up to full-blown type 2 diabetes. The terms that describe this phenomenon are *skinny fat* and *metabolically obese*, in which someone appears to be thin but they actually have an abnormally high percentage of body fat and low amount of muscle mass. In short, their metabolisms behave as though they're obese (i.e., dyslipidemia, hyperglycemia, and insulin resistance) even when physically they're not.

Some may argue that diabesity is actually the leading cause of modern, chronic disease. The "diabese" have increased risks for the following:

- Alzheimer's disease and dementia
- Blindness
- Cancer
- Cardiovascular disease
- Digestive disorders
- Hypertension
- Kidney failure
- Respiratory disorders

The really good news is that diabesity—like obesity and type 2 diabetes—is completely preventable and largely reversible by simply following key lifestyle changes. Of these, nutrition is important, but we're not talking about fad diets or diets with "cheat meals" or "cheat days." None of these addressed the root of the problem regarding why someone needs to lose weight and what got them where they are.

Transformation, on the other hand, addresses these issues and much more. This is why our Essential Oils Diet protocol is a total, holistic transformation program that helps people in every area of life. You're only as strong as your weakest link, right? We help you fortify not only your physical health but your emotional, mental, and spiritual health as well. If you'd like to get plugged into our healthy transformation community and go deeper, visit EssentialOilsDiet.com.

MANAGING WEIGHT IS THE CRUX OF IT ALL

Being overweight is a major risk factor in developing type 2 diabetes. In fact, 30 percent of overweight people have the disease, and 85 percent of type 2 diabetics are overweight.

Because 85 percent of diabetics and 100 percent of people battling obesity are overweight, the obvious solution to these epidemics (and to stop diabesity) is to focus on healthy, sustainable weight loss strategies.

Not to mention, the effects of diabesity are endless. In fact, obesity alone is the leading cause of preventable death, second only to smoking. When combined with diabetes, we can expect diabesity to be number one by 2030.

It is truly a chronic condition, as no one wakes up one day overweight. It takes years to develop and generally requires several months to see a marked improvement and sometimes years to completely remedy. This prolonged healing process can take its toll on someone trying to lose weight.

There are umpteen reasons why someone may be overweight, and we cover the most prominent reasons and how to remedy them in our book *The Essential Oils Diet*. But none of this matters if you don't have a *why*.

THREE REASONS TO LOSE WEIGHT

First and foremost, if you want to lose weight (or need to shed some pounds to protect your health), it is absolutely critical to be firmly rooted in your *why*: the reason *why* motivates your behavior to reach your ideal weight. Once you do this, you'll be prepared to set up actionable steps that can help you overcome some struggles you may be having.

Having walked more than two thousand people through our Essential Oils Diet sixty-day weight-loss challenge, we have discovered that your *why* needs to be something other than "looking good" or trying to get healthy for the sake of preventing a serious sickness in the future. We have uncovered that most people require a significant, deeply rooted, life-transforming *why* to empower them to make the necessary changes to get healthy and enjoy the abundant life. Essentially, your *why* needs to focus on someone and/or something other than you. This brings an entirely new level of self-correction and accountability that no personal trainer or healthy-eating coach can create!

Here are three good reasons to lose weight:

1. For God. Our bodies are temples of the Holy Spirit, and the Bible says that we are to present them as living sacrifices to God. We are convinced that eating well and doing things that promote health and well-being are spiritual acts of worship. We choose to eat healthy foods for God, and we hold ourselves accountable to Him. To help you put this into perspective, think of the transient self-correction of millions of children trying to get on Santa's "good" list during Christmastime. What we're suggesting is infinitely more effective and life-altering than this.

2. For others. To be of utmost service to the world and to fulfill your full purpose in life, you cannot be weighed down by sickness and disease. We thus feel obligated to live our best for our friends, our family, and our entire online Natural Living Family. This gives our lives an eternal meaning and, again, holds us accountable to something other than getting into shape so we look good at the beach!

3. For yourself. It is your God-given inheritance to live an abundant life and feel confident in who you are and what you look like. You must love yourself without reservations. Going back to #2, have you ever wondered about the Golden Rule? How can you love others if you do not love yourself? You need to love yourself so that you can love others, and there's no better act of self-love than to be healthy and well-balanced physically, mentally, emotionally, and spiritually.

STOP Before you start implementing these essential oils for type 2 diabetes and obesity, be sure to review the known drug interaction chart in Appendix B and consult with your physician if you're currently taking any medications. Also, don't forget that using essential oils while living a "fast food" lifestyle is like taking one step forward but two steps back! In other words, for essential oils to help you enjoy abundant health and wellness—free from chronic disease—it is vital to use them within the context of a healthy lifestyle. Go to Appendix A for our favorite "Disease-Busting Healthy Lifestyle Hacks" to learn more!

THE ESSENTIAL OILS APPROACH TO WEIGHT LOSS

In addition to treating the root causes of weight gain, essential oils can directly curb hunger, treat food addiction, and trigger lipolysis (your body's natural fat-burning response). These recipes are a great place to start. Remember, you can customize them to your liking and according to the supplies that you have on hand.

WEIGHT LOSS BLEND

15 drops cinnamon bark essential oil

15 drops grapefruit essential oil

15 drops lime essential oil

15 drops peppermint essential oil

SUPPLIES

5 ml bottle

1. Drop the essential oils in a 5 ml bottle. Cap the bottle and shake to combine.
2. Use as directed in the following recipes.

WEIGHT LOSS CAPSULE

Makes 1 dose

2 or 3 drops Weight Loss Blend (recipe above)

Organic virgin coconut oil or extra-virgin olive oil

continues

SUPPLIES

Pipette

Size 00 vegan gel capsule

1. Using a pipette, drop the essential oil blend into the bottom half (the longer, narrower one) of the capsule. Fill this half to the brim with organic extra-virgin coconut or extra-virgin olive oil.

2. Fit the wider top half of the capsule over the bottom half and secure it snugly.

3. Immediately swallow the capsule with water after breakfast and/or dinner (see Note). Take once or twice daily and monitor your cravings, appetite, and weight loss.

NOTE: *Do not make and store these capsules for future use. Also, this is not a long-term solution, and using it for more than four weeks at a time is not advisable. Be sure to switch up your protocol monthly and consult with your health-care provider first if you're currently taking medications. Discontinue if adverse reactions occur.*

WEIGHT LOSS INHALER

20 drops Weight Loss Blend (page 245)

SUPPLIES

Precut organic cotton pad

Aromatherapy inhaler

1. Place a cotton pad in the inhaler tube.

2. Drop the essential oils directly onto the cotton pad inside the tube. Alternatively, you can drop the blend into a glass bowl, roll the cotton pad in the oils to absorb them, and then insert it into the inhaler using tweezers.

3. Secure the cap and store the inhaler in a desk drawer, purse, or glove compartment so you have it handy.

4. When you need appetite control or some help with unhealthy cravings or when you want to stimulate fat burning, open the inhaler and take 10 deep breaths of the vapor from the tube.

NOTE: *Alternatively, you can add 5 or 6 drops into a diffuser and use it throughout the day. This recipe works well in an aromatherapy necklace.*

WEIGHT LOSS BODY OIL

24 drops Weight Loss Blend (page 245)

2 ounces carrier oil of choice or Mama Z's Oil Base (page 25)

SUPPLIES

Medium glass bowl

Lidded glass jar or lotion dispenser

1. Drop the essential oil blend into a bowl.
2. Add a carrier oil and mix thoroughly.
3. Use as a body oil after you shower and as a moisturizer throughout the day.

For even more support in burning fat, try the following two recipes from The Healing Power of Essential Oils.

FAT-BURNING ROLL-ON

4 drops lime essential oil

3 drops peppermint essential oil

3 drops grapefruit essential oil

2 drops cypress essential oil

1 drop eucalyptus essential oil

1 drop cinnamon bark essential oil

Carrier oil of choice—jojoba and fractionated coconut oil absorb quickly—as needed

SUPPLIES

10 ml glass roller bottle

continues

1. Drop the essential oils into the bottle.
2. Fill the roller bottle with your carrier oil of choice and shake well.
3. Apply over problem areas, like the stomach, back of the thighs, and undersides of the upper arms, three or four times per week after showering.

NOTE: *Test a skin patch first on the back of your hand or bottoms of the feet to make sure your body responds well to the blend. Discontinue use immediately if irritation occurs.*

FAT-BURNING WRAP

Fat-Burning Roll-On (page 247)

SUPPLIES

1 yard muslin fabric, cut into strips wide enough to cover the body part you want to treat but small enough to be manageable
Plastic wrap

1. Right before bed, liberally apply the roll-on over any areas of concern.
2. Wrap each area of the body individually with muslin.
3. Wrap the fabric with two or three layers of plastic wrap.
4. When you wake up, unwrap each area and wipe yourself down with a towel before showering.

NOTE: *Wrapping the part of your body you're seeking to slim down after you've applied the Fat-Burning Roll-On will help increase absorption and prevent your sheets and clothes from absorbing the oils instead of your skin. This works great on the back of the legs to minimize cellulite!*

 To watch us make this recipe and learn more about reaching your ideal weight using essential oils, go to EOApothecary.com.

1. Lime

Lime essential oil might just turn out to be the fat-burning and weight-loss support that you've been looking for. Credited with naturally suppressing appetite, promoting weight loss, and preventing weight gain, lime oil can also, as suggested by a 2019 animal study, reduce cardiovascular disease risk factors such as elevated cholesterol, triglycerides, and LDL levels as well two key enzymes that indicate healing from liver damage (alanine aminotransferase and aspartate transaminase).

Application: In addition to trying the Fat-Burning Roll-On recipe (page 247), next time you get hungry between meals, make Dr. Z's Citrus Soda Pop (page 267) and enjoy a refreshing drink while burning fat! Lime also blends well with bergamot and frankincense, which makes for a wonderful diffuser remedy (below)!

HAPPY AND FOCUSED DIFFUSER BLEND

2 drops bergamot essential oil

2 drops frankincense essential oil

2 drops lime essential oil

SUPPLIES

Diffuser

1. Fill your diffuser with purified water as directed in the manufacturer's instructions.

2. Add the essential oils to the water.

3. Diffuse throughout the day to perk up your mood, help you focus, and support you in your weight loss goals.

2. Grapefruit

We've all heard of the "grapefruit diet," so it's not surprising that grapefruit essential oil is an effective weight-loss tool, but for different reasons than you may be familiar with.

In evaluating the effects of inhaled grapefruit and lavender essential oils, investigators found that nerve impulses were extensively affected, leading to fat-burning and appetite-reducing benefits.

Need to reduce your waistline? Grapefruit essential oil to the rescue. Grapefruit oil, as part of a topical blend, massaged onto the abdomen contributed to reduced waist circumferences and body composition changes in women who participated in a recent study.

Application: You can make a simple grapefruit body oil by mixing 15 drops of grapefruit essential oil with 1 ounce of Mama Z's Oil Base (page 25) and applying it after you shower. Just remember that grapefruit is a known photosensitizer, so be careful not to expose your skin to the sun after applying. Also, diffusing grapefruit with other citrus oils like lemon, orange, petitgrain, and neroli before and during meals makes a pleasant, refreshing aroma that promotes healthy eating habits.

3. Peppermint

Effective at relieving digestive symptoms like bloating, gas, and indigestion, inhaling peppermint can also reduce or eliminate food cravings and help you feel full faster, thus reducing caloric intake.

Application: Use peppermint essential oil with orange oil in your personal inhaler or diffuser for an instant mood boost or energy jolt, to reduce unhealthy food cravings, and to curb your appetite. If you get a hankering for something sweet, try this fast and easy recipe.

CITRUS MINT COCOA BITE

1 tablespoon organic virgin coconut oil

2 teaspoons raw cacao powder

1 dropperful vanilla-flavored liquid stevia

1 drop peppermint essential oil

1 drop orange essential oil

Small glass bowl

1. Mix all the ingredients in a glass bowl until smooth and blended.
2. Eat a spoonful when you want a quick burst of energy or when you're hungry between meals.
3. Cover and store in a small glass container.

4. Spearmint

Since spearmint is a cousin to peppermint, you'll find that the two oils have a lot of similarities. One study evaluated how inhaling a "fresh" blend of essential oils containing spearmint versus a "sweet" oil (vanilla) affected chocolate cravings in college-age females. The fresh blend included spearmint, grapefruit, tangerine, lemon, and ocotea essential oils. As expected, the fresh spearmint-powered blend reduced cravings, whereas the vanilla essential oil increased them.

Application: Follow the recipe for Citrus Mint Cocoa Bite (page 250), but substitute spearmint essential oil for the peppermint.

5. Fennel

Tasty, aromatic, and a global favorite, fennel will help manage anxiety, cramps, digestive upset, and a number of other health conditions. You may be surprised how useful it can be to your overall health!

Korean researchers in 2015 set out to discover whether or not fennel essential oil could decrease appetite in people with weight-management issues. In this small study of thirty-two obese female patients, they found that the group who inhaled fennel oil twice a week for a month had a significant decrease in appetite, compared to a nontreatment control group.

Fennel has also been shown to reduce intestinal spasms and increase motility of the small intestine, which is vital to properly digest and metabolize the foods that you eat.

Application: For our female readers, apply a 2 percent dilution of fennel over your abdomen in a clockwise direction twice a day during your next period to alleviate stomach cramps, enhance digestion, and decrease unhealthy food cravings.

For our male readers, follow the same instructions when you're feeling stressed or anxious.

THE ESSENTIAL OILS APPROACH TO BALANCING BLOOD SUGAR

Most of us are already familiar with substances that are beneficial for insulin sensitivity, with ground cinnamon topping the list of kitchen remedies to help deal with blood sugar and diabetes. Aromatherapy has even more to offer—with some oils appearing to benefit the insulin response and others working to ease the symptoms that diabetes can cause.

Essential oils for diabetes are best used as integrative components of our wellness routines. For the diabetic who now focuses their lifestyle on managing both the causes and symptoms of the disease, having such a versatile tool kit can be a lifeline.

Before we dive into specific oils and how they can help you naturally balance blood sugar, we'd like to highlight one particular study that evaluated powerful blends and share some recipes based on the findings.

Powerful Synergy Blends

One of the most intriguing things about essential oils is their ability to *synergize*—the phenomenon in which combinations of oils create even more potent healing properties than they possess individually. This is a fundamental concept behind creating blends.

In 2005, Georgetown University Medical Center researchers took note of the benefits of synergy when they studied using essential oils to lower elevated blood sugar. Instead of isolating a single oil for their research, they experimented with blends of multiple oils that have been suggested as beneficial for diabetes. We like this animal study for a couple reasons: it highlights the synergistic power of blending, and it provides the surprising benefits of using essential oils the right way.

The following three essential oil blends were tested:

1. Oregano, cinnamon, fenugreek, cumin, and fennel
2. Oregano, cinnamon, fenugreek, cumin, myrtle, allspice, and ginger
3. Oregano, cinnamon, fenugreek, cumin, and myrtle

Each blend was mixed with both pumpkinseed oil (an unusual carrier oil) and extra-virgin olive oil. A control group of rats received only water. The other three groups were given two or three drops orally of an essential oil blend in the carrier oil. (Smaller animals received two drops, and larger animals received three drops.) All three blends demonstrated significantly improved insulin sensitivity, systolic blood pressure, and reduced weight, with the third blend producing the most dramatic results.

Following are four blends and recipes from this research study that we featured as part of our *Essential Oils Diet* book protocol. The results we've heard from our readers have been astounding!

As a rule of thumb, you'll want to switch your protocol every three to four weeks for the best results. Use only one of these recipes at a time; in other words, don't take capsules at the same time you use a body oil or a roll-on.

BLOOD SUGAR–BALANCING BLEND (OPTION #1)

15 drops oregano essential oil

15 drops cinnamon bark essential oil

15 drops fenugreek essential oil

15 drops cumin essential oil

15 drops myrtle essential oil

BLOOD SUGAR-BALANCING BLEND (OPTION #2)

50 drops cinnamon bark essential oil

25 drops cumin essential oil

10 drops fenugreek essential oil

BLOOD SUGAR-BALANCING BLEND (OPTION #3)

50 drops Melissa (lemon balm) essential oil

25 drops French lavender essential oil

10 drops geranium essential oil

BLOOD SUGAR-BALANCING BLEND (OPTION #4)

50 drops bergamot essential oil

20 drops peppermint essential oil

10 drops French lavender essential oil

5 drops oregano essential oil

SUPPLIES

5 ml essential oil bottle

1. Drop the essential oils for each option in a 5 ml bottle. Cap the bottle and shake to combine.

2. Use as directed in the following recipes.

BLOOD SUGAR-BALANCING ROLL-ON

10 drops Blood Sugar-Balancing Blend of your choice (recipes above)

Carrier oil of choice—jojoba and fractionated coconut oil absorb quickly—as
  needed

SUPPLIES

10 ml glass roller bottle

1. Drop the essential oil blend into the roller bottle.
2. Fill the roller bottle with your carrier oil of choice and shake well.
3. Apply over your abdomen and lower back twice a day.

NOTE: *Test these blends first on the back of your hand or bottoms of your feet to ensure your body responds well to the blend. Immediately discontinue use if irritation occurs.*

BLOOD SUGAR–BALANCING BODY OIL

15 drops Blood Sugar–Balancing Blend of your choice (page 254)
1 ounce carrier oil of choice, such as Mama Z's Oil Base (page 25) or
    fractionated coconut, jojoba, or sweet almond oil

SUPPLIES
Small glass jar with a tight-fitting lid

1. Drop the essential oil blend into the glass jar.
2. Add the carrier oil and mix thoroughly.
3. Apply over your abdomen and lower back twice a day.

NOTE: *First test this on the back of your hand or bottoms of your feet to make sure your body responds well to the blend. Discontinue use immediately if irritation occurs.*

BLOOD SUGAR–BALANCING CAPSULE

Makes 1 dose

3 drops Blood Sugar–Balancing Blend of your choice (recipes above)
Organic virgin coconut oil or extra-virgin olive oil

SUPPLIES
Pipette
Size 00 vegan gel capsule

continues

1. Using a pipette, drop the essential oil blend into the bottom half (the longer, narrower one) of the capsule. Fill this half to the brim with organic extra-virgin coconut or extra-virgin olive oil.

2. Fit the wider top half of the capsule over the bottom half and secure it snugly.

3. Immediately swallow the capsule with water after breakfast and/or dinner (see Note). Take once or twice daily, and monitor your sugar cravings and blood sugar.

NOTE: *Do not make and store these capsules for future use. Also, this is not a long-term solution, and using it for more than four weeks at a time is not advisable. Be sure to switch up your protocol monthly and consult with your health-care provider first if you're currently taking medications. Discontinue if adverse reactions occur.*

ANTIDIABETIC ESSENTIAL OILS

1. Cinnamon Bark and Leaf

Cinnamon has been heavily researched in the treatment of diabetes, with a great deal of focus placed on it for pancreatic support, glucose lowering, weight loss, and general diabetes prevention and management.

Traditionally extracted from the *Cinnamomum zeylanicum* tree, cinnamon oil comes from either the inner bark or the leaves. Cinnamon bark essential oil is composed primarily of cinnamaldehyde and camphor, both potent antioxidants and antidiabetics.

Cinnamaldehyde has been shown to reduce blood glucose. Another compound, cinnamic acid, improves glucose tolerance and has the potential to stimulate insulin production. Both offer promise as natural remedies for prediabetes and type 2 diabetes.

Cinnamon leaf essential oil contains more eugenol, which is used to relieve pain and inflammation and fight bacteria. Although it is generally not prescribed as a diabetic remedy, evaluation found that "all tested doses of [cinnamon leaf essential oil] significantly lowered fasting blood glucose and fructosamine." The researchers pointed to pancreatic support as the likely mechanism leading to the blood sugar benefits.

We don't have an exact directive from studies and research to tell us how to maximize cinnamon's potential for diabetic wellness, but we can glean some helpful tidbits:

- Internal use seems to be the most effective.
- Cinnamon in all forms appears to lower blood sugar.
- A little dab'll do!

Application: Try one of the Blood Sugar–Balancing Blend options (pages 253–254) and remedies. Remember, cinnamon is a strong oil and can be an irritant if not used properly.

Be sure to monitor your blood sugar carefully when using cinnamon in any form, and consult with your doctor before adjusting medication. Your body might just respond a little *too* well to cinnamon's strengths.

2. Lemon Balm (Melissa)

Like cinnamon, some herbs and their essential oil are simply regarded as antidiabetic. Those are the words anyone with a diagnosis or pre-diagnosis of diabetes wants to hear! Let's fight this disease right at its core, where the body stops short of breaking down glucose into usable energy.

A few years ago, a fascinating study evaluated twenty-nine essential oils that were purchased from the Taiwan market and evaluated them to determine how they affected specific fat cells' consumption and accumulation of glucose over time. Essentially, this lab study was attempting to re-create how fat cells react to essential oils in someone's bloodstream. Beating out all the others in efficacy, lemon balm essential oil not only helped increase glucose consumption (similar to how the diabetes drug metformin performs), but it also significantly slowed fat accumulation. You may find it interesting to know that peppermint, lavender, bergamot, cypress, niaouli, rose geranium, and ravensara essential oils did not increase glucose consumption, but they did slow down fat-buildup activity.

These in vitro results have been confirmed elsewhere. Lemon balm essential oil's actions and potential benefits have been precisely tracked in animals. Of the mice that received a low-dose, heavily diluted amount of lemon balm essential oil, markers of diabetes were reduced in multiple facets. Ultimately, the researchers concluded that lemon balm "administered at low concentrations is an efficient hypoglycaemic agent, probably due to enhanced glucose uptake and metabolism."

Once more, we see that using minute amounts of these potent digestive-health essential oils can make a potentially substantial difference for those battling blood sugar imbalances.

Application: One drop is plenty in a gel capsule filled with extra-virgin olive oil. Also use the Blood Sugar–Balancing Blend Option #3 (page 254) in roll-on or body oil. As with all hypoglycemic/antidiabetic substances, be sure to monitor your levels carefully and work with your doctor closely.

3. Rosemary

Traditionally used by ancient cultures for mental clarity, digestive relief, and muscle pain, this essential oil is derived from the popular culinary herb. But don't restrict this powerful oil to the kitchen; it may help protect you from diabetes.

In a review of the scientific literature available on rosemary, researchers concluded that it has both antidiabetic and anti-obesity effects, making it a possibly powerful therapeutic against diabesity.

Application: Rosemary is a vital ingredient in our all-purpose Immune-Boosting Blend (page 49), which doubles up as a wonderful diabetes remedy. Use this blend in your diffuser, in your inhaler, and as a 2 percent body oil. Two or three drops of this blend can also be safely consumed in a vegan gel capsule filled with extra-virgin olive oil as well. Note that rosemary has the tendency to raise blood pressure, so be sure to consult with your physician before using rosemary if you've been diagnosed with hypertension.

4. Clove Bud

Some essential oils, such as clove bud, work on the enzymes involved in sugar metabolism. In 2015, researchers discovered that clove bud essential oil inhibited key enzymes and lipid processes that can lead to type 2 diabetes in mice. They concluded that the antioxidant properties of clove could be used to manage or prevent diabetes caused by oxidative stress.

Keep in mind that clove essential oil, while a beneficial antioxidant, is also quite powerful. Take caution when using this oil. If you are on a blood-thinning medication, check with your doctor before adding clove oil to your regimen.

Application: Like rosemary, clove is a staple in our all-purpose Immune-Boosting Blend (page 49). Use this blend in your diffuser, in your inhaler, and as a 2 percent body oil. Two or three drops of this blend can also safely be consumed in a vegan gel capsule filled with extra-virgin olive oil as well.

5. French Lavender

Lavender angustifolia (English lavender) is the lavender variety that most people buy. *Lavandula stoechas* (French lavender), on the other hand, is not sold as widely. Both are similar in that they contain soothing properties, but French lavender has been evaluated specifically in regard to diabetes, and researchers have found that it not only protects against diabetes and oxidative stress but also reverses toxin-induced damage done to liver and kidney enzymes.

Simply adding a few drops of French lavender essential oil to your diffuser and applying a lavender-infused body oil can do wonders to reduce stress and help you sleep at night. For a diabetes remedy, however, you'll most likely have to ingest it.

Application: Make the Blood Sugar–Balancing Blend Option #3 or #4 (page 254) and one of the remedies that follow. Alternatively, you can add 2 or 3 drops in a vegan gel capsule filled with extra-virgin olive oil for two weeks and monitor your blood sugar levels to determine the effectiveness.

With our discussion of essential oils for weight control, diabetes, and diabesity, we hope we have broadened your tools beyond cutting calories and working out. Both are important, but there is so much more you can do in order to maintain a trim, diabetes-free body, and essential oils can be a big part of your transformation.

Chapter 15

Fatty Liver

Most people we know aren't too concerned about liver disease. In fact, it's not even on their radar! This just may prove to be a grave oversight, as liver disease is skyrocketing and no one seems to be taking notice. Without a doubt, we have a global public health crisis on our hands, one that should be grabbing our attention.

SURPRISING STATS

Let's look at the prevalence of liver disease in the United Kingdom, for example:

- Liver disease is the third leading cause of premature death.
- Since 1970, deaths caused by liver disease have increased by 400 percent. This is in stark contrast to the other major causes of disease (e.g., heart disease and cancer), in which deaths have stabilized or decreased.
- 75 percent of people are diagnosed at an advanced stage when it is too late for lifestyle changes or effective intervention.
- 90 percent of liver disease is *preventable*.

This last point is key: with the *proper lifestyle changes*, liver disease would quickly become a nonissue.

Mention liver disease to most people and one word will spring to mind: cirrhosis, a scarring of the liver commonly caused by chronic alcoholism. Maybe that's why so many folks aren't taking their liver health seriously.

If you don't struggle with alcohol, then the liver is fine, right?

Wrong.

There is another, much more insidious and less obvious liver condition that is fast becoming an epidemic: nonalcoholic fatty liver disease, or NAFLD. That's a mouthful, and it doesn't have a high public profile like other chronic diseases, including heart disease, cancer, or diabetes. Few people—except perhaps those employed in the medical field—have even heard of it.

Yet, this hidden illness strikes more than 25 percent of all adults worldwide, and it is the most common liver disease in children and adolescents in developed countries. In the United States, NAFLD is the most common liver disease, and 30 to 40 percent of all American adults have it.

Let that sink in for a moment. . . .

When we first learned about NAFLD, we were shocked. Quickly approaching diagnosis in one of every two adults you meet on the streets of America, NAFLD, like obesity and type 2 diabetes, is one of the most easily preventable causes of death in the United States. In fact, NAFLD may overtake heart disease as the number one cause of premature death in the coming years.

In and of itself, NAFLD is obviously extremely dangerous, but if it advances to nonalcoholic steatohepatitis (NASH), it can lead to cirrhosis and liver cancer. Unfortunately, experts are not sure why some people with NAFLD have NASH while others do not, which adds complexity to an already confounding chronic disease.

More common in people who suffer from obesity, type 2 diabetes, and metabolic syndrome, NAFLD has been found in 40 to 80 percent of people who have type 2 diabetes and in 30 to 90 percent of people who are obese. This is why adopting a healthy, holistic lifestyle is key to enjoy a long, robust, abundant life. And, of course, essential oils can help!

WHAT CAUSES NAFLD?

This dangerous condition develops when there is a buildup of fat in liver cells that is *not* caused by alcohol. It is normal for the liver to have some fat, but a liver is considered fatty if more than 5 to 10 percent of the liver's weight is fat.

As you'll see with most of the chronic diseases addressed in this book, one chronic health condition can increase your risk of developing another. There is also growing evidence of links between NAFLD and depression. Moreover, the liver tends to develop more fat in those who are obese or who have diabetes, high cholesterol, or high triglycerides. Your risk increases with every pound of excess weight, for example. More than 70 percent of people with NAFLD are obese.

Oxidative stress is also a key risk factor. Causes include alcohol, drugs, viral infections, environmental pollutants, and dietary components. This is why curcumin (the primary chemical in turmeric) has been repeatedly touted as "a lead compound in the prevention and treatment of oxidative associated liver diseases."

NAFLD is often a symptomless chronic disorder. If symptoms do crop up, they are generally vague and nonspecific and may include fatigue, depression, malaise (feeling unwell), or a dull ache in your upper right abdomen, which might indicate an enlarged liver.

This poses a problem since NAFLD is frequently misdiagnosed, which can lead to a catastrophic problem because many physicians end up treating just the symptoms, leaving fatty liver to advance on its own without addressing the proper lifestyle modifications needed to stop progression.

At a more advanced stage, NAFLD may cause the following:

- Poor appetite
- Weight loss
- Nausea
- Weakness
- Yellowing of the skin and eyes and dark cola-colored urine
- Bleeding from engorged veins in your esophagus or intestines

- Fluid in your abdominal cavity (ascites)
- Itching
- Swelling of your legs and feet from retained fluid (edema)
- Mental confusion, such as forgetfulness or trouble concentrating
- Liver failure

If your doctor suspects NAFLD, you'll undergo any number of tests, including blood tests, liver enzyme and liver function tests, tests for chronic viral hepatitis (hepatitis A, hepatitis C, and others), and imaging procedures like an abdominal ultrasound, computerized tomography (CT) scanning, or magnetic resonance imaging (MRI) of the abdomen.

If other tests are inconclusive, your doctor may recommend a liver biopsy, in which a sample of tissue from your liver is removed. It will then be examined in a laboratory to look for signs of inflammation and scarring.

THE ESSENTIAL OILS APPROACH TO NAFLD

Keeping your liver healthy is vital to supporting all of your body's systems. An unhealthy liver can slow down the natural filtration process that your body uses to flush out harmful toxins.

Essential oils can help this process and assist in supporting your liver health. Another benefit is to use oils to create your own natural and nontoxic cleaning and personal care products so that you reduce your exposure to toxins in the home—and save money while doing so. Essential oils can also be used in place of over-the-counter remedies that could unnecessarily be harming your liver.

Also, don't forget to use your essential oils to manage the risk factors associated with fatty liver. Targeted aromatherapy strategies can be wonderfully effective at helping you lose weight, balance blood sugar, increase insulin sensitivity, and boost energy.

Before you jump in, however, keep in mind that there are some safety risks to using essential oils for liver disorders. If overly consumed, repeated high doses can lead to toxicity and exacerbate liver damage as essential oils constituents accumulate in your body, especially in adipose tissues. Stick to the recipes and applications below, and be sure to consult with your physician before starting a new protocol.

Essential oils have so much power to improve your health and well-being! Here is a rundown of the best essential oils for your liver and how to use them on a daily basis.

 Before you start implementing these essential oils for NAFLD, be sure to review the known drug interaction chart in Appendix B and consult with your physician if you're currently taking any medications. Also, don't forget that using essential oils while living a "fast food" lifestyle is like taking one step forward but two steps back! In other words, for essential oils to help you enjoy abundant health and wellness—free from chronic disease—it is vital to use them within the context of a healthy lifestyle. Go to Appendix A for our favorite "Disease-Busting Healthy Lifestyle Hacks" to learn more!

1. Anise

Let's start with anise, arguably one of the most underappreciated essential oils. Proven to have "beneficial effects in the treatment of NAFLD," anise oil taken internally can help lower cholesterol levels, reduce biomarkers of oxidative stress, and protect against liver damage in NAFLD-induced rats. With a strong licorice-like taste, this anethole-rich remedy is one of those love-it-or-hate-it type of oils, so start slowly and work your way up to using more of it.

Application: Start by taking 1 or 2 drops of anise in a vegan gel capsule once a day for one month. Be sure to fill up your capsule with an edible carrier oil to help ensure safety and efficacy.

2. Fennel

With a milder licorice flavor than its cousin anise, fennel is an aromatic herb that has been widely used as both a spice and a medicine all over the world. Along with anise and myrtle, fennel essential oil is rich in a chemical called anethole, which is well-known to reduce inflammation and fight cancer. It's also praised for its protection against toxin-induced liver damage.

Application: Make this Liver-Protecting Roll-On, which is powered by anethole-rich oils, and use it daily.

LIVER-PROTECTING ROLL-ON

8 drops fennel essential oil

6 drops anise essential oil

2 drops myrtle essential oil

Carrier oil of choice—jojoba and fractionated coconut oil absorb quickly—as needed

SUPPLIES

10 ml glass roller bottle

1. Drop the essential oils into the roller bottle.
2. Fill the roller bottle with your carrier oil of choice and shake well.
3. Apply over the liver (upper right-hand portion of the abdominal cavity) once daily for up to one month.

3. Ginger

One of the most-favored spices in the world, ginger has many proven health benefits, including some pertaining to liver health. Rich in antioxidants, ginger essential oil (and its component citral) has been shown to be highly proficient at protecting the liver from NAFLD caused by a high-fat diet. Specifically, research has shown that ginger oil and citral "effectively enhanced the antioxidant capacities and reduced inflammatory response," suggesting they can protect against steatohepatitis (a type of fatty liver characterized by inflammation).

Application: Try an ancient Indian culinary approach to taking ginger by adding it to our essential-oil-powered Easy Golden Milk (page 266).

EASY GOLDEN MILK

Serves 2

1½ cups unsweetened vanilla-flavored almond milk

1½ cups unsweetened vanilla-flavored coconut milk

1 tablespoon organic virgin coconut oil

1½ teaspoons organic ground turmeric

½ teaspoon organic pumpkin pie spice blend

2 drops cinnamon bark essential oil

1 drop black pepper essential oil

1 drop clove bud essential oil

1 drop ginger essential oil

Healthy sweetener to taste—coconut sugar, maple syrup, or stevia all work great

1. In a small saucepan set over low to medium heat, combine all ingredients.
2. Whisk frequently until the liquid is hot. Do not let it boil.
3. Serve immediately. This is perfect as a soothing, healing nighttime drink before bed.
4. Any leftovers can be refrigerated for up to 1 week. Reheat gently before serving.

4. Clove Bud

Like many essential oils, clove bud is exceptionally rich in antioxidants, which can help prevent liver disease due to its ability to fight disease-causing free radicals.

Research has shown that there are also beneficial compounds, such as eugenol, in clove oil that promote liver health. One animal study that fed rats a high fructose diet and induced fatty liver disease uncovered that daily oral administration of both clove essential oil and eugenol improved fatty liver and helped balance blood lipid levels.

We do know that the eugenol in clove oil can be contraindicated with certain medications like blood thinners and might increase the chances of bruising and bleeding. So check with your doctor before adding this spicy compound to your regimen.

Application: Enjoy a cup of the Easy Golden Milk recipe (page 266) every night before bed for a month and see how your symptoms improve.

5. Lime

There are about sixty active compounds in lime essential oil, several of which are considered to be liver-protective. Known for its purifying properties, lime oil is often used as an internal cleanser.

In a recent animal study, eight weeks of ingesting lime oil produced significant improvements in total cholesterol, triglycerides, and LDL levels, as well two key enzymes that indicate healing from liver damage (alanine aminotransferase and aspartate transaminase).

Application: Make Dr. Z's Citrus Soda Pop and enjoy a refreshing drink while protecting your liver!

DR. Z'S CITRUS SODA POP

Serves 4

4 dropperfuls vanilla-flavored liquid stevia

2 teaspoons fresh lime juice

2 teaspoons fresh lemon juice

3 drops lime essential oil

3 drops lemon essential oil

2 drops bergamot essential oil

32 ounces sparkling water

Lemon and/or lime wedges, for garnish

1. In a large glass container, mix together the stevia, citrus juices, and essential oils.
2. Add the sparkling water.
3. Serve over ice, garnished with a lime or lemon wedge.

To watch us make this recipe and learn more about how to harness the power of essential oils to promote liver health and banish unhealthy food cravings, go to EOApothecary.com.

6. Rosemary

This highly popular oil appears to stimulate the production and flow of bile, a fluid that aids digestion and is secreted by the liver and stored in the gallbladder. Rosemary thus has a healing effect on the liver, encouraging it to work more efficiently, and it is often used to treat liver problems, including cirrhosis and jaundice.

Research has shown that seven days of oral rosemary essential oil therapy helped defend rats from developing acute liver disease after they were exposed to a compound that causes NAFLD, presumably due to the oil's antioxidant capacity.

An interesting observation in this study confirmed what we've been saying for a long time: "less is more" when it comes to using essential oils. It was discovered that dosing the rosemary essential oil at 10 milligrams per kilogram of body weight (e.g., twenty drops for a 130-pound person) exacerbated bilirubin values, thus indicating impaired excretory function of the liver. On the contrary, a 5 milligram per kilogram body weight dose (e.g., ten drops for a 130-pound adult) did not exhibit that effect.

Note that the aromatherapy texts and safety manuals state that the max oral dose of rosemary is 2 milligrams (mg) per kilogram (kg) of body weight a day (roughly four drops for a 130-pound person), so be careful that you don't overdo it.

Application: Safely consume rosemary oil by adding Dr. Z's Immune-Boosting Snack (page 51) to your daily natural health regimen.

7. Oregano

Although there is no research specifically on oregano essential oil and fatty liver, multiple studies have evaluated carvacrol (its primary chemical constituent) as an emerging liver healer. It has been shown to reduce weight, lower cholesterol, and decrease triglycerides—all of which are elevated in NAFLD.

One fascinating study fed mice three different diets for ten weeks: normal, high-fat, and carvacrol-supplemented high-fat diets. Compared to mice fed the high-fat diet, those fed the carvacrol-supplemented diet had significantly lower levels of fat in their liver and more sufficient levels of alanine aminotransferase and aspartate transaminase in their bloodstream. It was also observed that carvacrol inhibited the expression of genes involved in inflammation.

The daily carvacrol intake of the mice in the study (100 mg/kg body weight) was equivalent to approximately 8 milligrams per kilogram human body weight (seventeen drops for a 130-pound person), though consuming this amount in oregano every day would be dangerous. The daily doses of carvacrol dietary supplements range from one to ten drops for a 130-pound person.

Application: In addition to enjoying a culinary approach to ingesting oregano oil (e.g., adding 2 or 3 drops in your pizza or pasta sauce), consider taking 3 or 4 drops in a vegan gel capsule daily for two to three weeks—keeping a keen eye on the signs and symptoms of fatty liver. Be sure to add an edible carrier oil to fill your capsule.

8. Eucalyptus

Of all the essential oils rich in 1,8-cineole, eucalyptus—all varieties—ranks the highest. This is important because 1,8-cineole has been discussed as a potential therapy candidate for NASH. It has been shown to improve steatosis (increased fat buildup in the liver) and fibrosis (scar tissue).

In addition to fat in your liver, NASH is categorized by hepatitis (inflammation of the liver) and liver cell damage, and experts estimate that upward of 20 percent of people with NAFLD have NASH.

Application: Safely consume rosemary oil by adding Dr. Z's Immune-Boosting Snack (page 51) to your daily natural health regimen.

9. Spearmint

Spearmint essential oil is rich in the chemical carvone, known to be protective against various health conditions, including liver issues.

After male mice were fed a high-fat diet and injected twice a week with carvone for eight weeks, researchers observed that it prevented weight gain, fat accumulation in the liver, and insulin resistance.

Application: As green tea is well-known to reduce the risk of liver disease, try this refreshing, minty iced matcha latte recipe for a morning pick-me-up.

SPEARMINTY ICED MATCHA LATTE

Serves 2

1 tablespoon matcha green tea powder

1 cup unsweetened vanilla-flavored almond milk, chilled

1 cup unsweetened vanilla-flavored coconut milk, chilled

4 dropperfuls vanilla-flavored liquid stevia

3 drops spearmint essential oil

1. Pour the matcha, almond and coconut milks, stevia, and essential oil into a blender.

2. Blend for 30 seconds, until frothy.

3. Pour the mixture into a 32-ounce glass bottle.

4. Fill to the top with ice. Serve immediately or refrigerate, shaking before use.

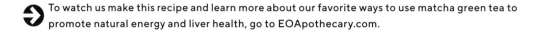 To watch us make this recipe and learn more about our favorite ways to use matcha green tea to promote natural energy and liver health, go to EOApothecary.com.

We think you'll be delighted at how just a few oils and various combinations of oils can have such a noticeable impact on your liver and help you feel vibrant enough to pursue abundant and radiant health in all areas of your life. Keep reading for more ways to deepen your experience of essential oils' power to heal.

Chapter 16

Inflammatory Bowel Diseases

nflammatory bowel disease, or IBD, is the name for a group of digestive disorders that cause chronic inflammation in the digestive tract. The two most common forms of IBD are Crohn's disease and ulcerative colitis (UC). Crohn's disease can affect the entire digestive tract, from the mouth to the anus, while UC affects the inner lining of the large intestine.

An estimated 1.3 percent of US adults (three million) report being diagnosed with IBD. It's like having Montezuma's revenge that never stops. Not making the headlines like the more prevalent chronic diseases such as cancer and obesity, IBD is the hidden risk factor no one is talking about. Compared to adults without IBD, those with IBD are more likely to have conditions that include the following:

- Arthritis
- Cardiovascular disease
- Cancer
- Kidney disease
- Respiratory disease
- Liver disease

Specifically, ulcerative colitis symptoms can vary, depending on the severity of inflammation and where it occurs and may include the following:

- Diarrhea, often with blood or pus
- Abdominal pain and cramping
- Rectal pain
- Rectal bleeding or passing small amount of blood with stool
- Urgency to defecate
- Inability to defecate despite urgency
- Weight loss
- Fatigue
- Fever
- Ulcers in large intestines
- Failure to grow in children

As for Crohn's, when the disease is active (it does go into remission), signs and symptoms may include these:

- Diarrhea
- Fever
- Fatigue
- Abdominal pain and cramping
- Blood in your stool
- Mouth sores
- Reduced appetite and weight loss
- Ulcers anywhere along the gastrointestinal tract
- Pain or drainage near or around the anus, due to inflammation from a tunnel into the skin (fistula)

The exact cause of both diseases remains unknown. Previously, diet and stress were suspected, but now doctors know that these factors may aggravate but don't cause IBD. Several factors, such as heredity and a malfunctioning immune system, likely play a role in their development.

Both conditions are typically treated with medications or surgery, but science is showing that essential oils may help relieve inflammation, inhibit ulcer formation, and alleviate other issues associated with these diseases.

BOWEL, GUT, AND ENTERIC-COATED CAPSULES

The word *bowel* is a popular term for the small and large intestines and should not be confused with the gut.

When you ask most people what the gut is, they'll likely think of their stomach. They may recall how they oftentimes get that "gut feeling" (or visceral response) when they have to make an important decision and their instincts kick in.

From a medical perspective, however, the gut is a bit more complicated. Technically referring to any part of your gastrointestinal tract from your mouth to your anus, the gut is split up into three sections: foregut (mouth to stomach), midgut (small intestines), hindgut (large intestines).

Thus, the bowel is synonymous with the midgut and hindgut.

Why is this important?

Because the only way to effectively treat inflammatory bowel diseases naturally is through time-release (or delayed-release) capsules. A simple gel capsule won't help work because the supplements or essential oils that you may take to treat IBD will be dissolved in your stomach.

Also known as enteric-coated, these capsules are unlike vegan capsules in that they contain an acid-resistant coating to bypass gastric juice (i.e., stomach acid) and reach the intestines. Composed of hydrochloric acid, potassium chloride, and sodium chloride, your stomach acid breaks down pretty much everything you consume, so a special delivery system is required if you want a therapeutic agent to reach your bowels. Enteric-coated capsules are activated only when they reach an alkaline environment, which usually happens in the small intestines and sometimes in the large intestines.

Up until lately, we've only seen polymer-based enteric-coated capsules, but the recent demand has motivated suppliers to offer vegan, nonplastic versions. Try searching online for "vegan, acid-resistant, enteric capsules" and you'll find some good options. Size 00 will meet all of your aromatherapy recipes. No need to go larger than that.

WILL ESSENTIAL OILS KILL YOUR MICROBIOME?

One of the most interesting aspects of health is the role played by your gut "microbiome." This newly discovered organ weighs 7 ounces and is composed of important fungi, bacteria, viruses, and other microorganisms. They number around one hundred trillion or so, literally outnumbering human cells by ten to one! But they're not just lodgers. Most important are the bacteria. Most bacteria are our allies, because without beneficial bacteria to balance the harmful strains, we are susceptible to intestinal damage, illness, mental and emotional stress, and much more.

The friendly bacteria play a vital role in keeping us healthy. They influence how every part of the body works, including how easily you lose (or gain) weight and even how your brain receives pain messages.

The gut actually has a nervous system dubbed "the second brain," and 80 percent of all neurotransmitters are produced there. In fact, your immune system lives here, helping to defend you against insults from unhealthy food particles, chemicals, pollutants, drugs, bacteria, and other invaders.

When we say, "You are what you eat," it's not just a quip or playful admonition. What enters your digestive system quite literally shapes your gut health. The digestive tract is a center of nutrition, of course, but also of immunity and even neural processes. If the gut is faltering, the whole body suffers.

A question we commonly receive is whether essential oils, because they are such potent antimicrobial agents, will kill both the good and bad bacteria in our body. These people are concerned about the health of their microbiome, and rightfully so!

From what we can tell in the medical literature, essential oils contain a property known as "cell selectivity." Innately, they respond favorably to probiotics ("good" bacteria) by leaving them alone, and target pathogenic microbes ("bad" bacteria). One study, for example, evaluated thymol and geraniol (components of thyme and rose oils, respectively) and discovered that they both were "effective in suppressing pathogens in the small intestine, with no concern for beneficial commensal colonic bacteria in the distal gut." Similar studies have found the same characteristics in bitter orange, caraway, and lavender essential oils.

We have no explanation for this fascinating phenomenon other than God, in His infinite wisdom, knew what He was doing when He created plants and humans. Time and time again, we see how the human body and nature work together in harmony for health and abundant life.

THE ESSENTIAL OILS APPROACH TO IBD

Essential oils for irritable bowel disorders and complete gut health are powerful and should be treated with the respect they deserve. Technically not under the chronic disease umbrella, several related conditions are primary risk factors for or symptoms of IBD: irritable bowel syndrome (IBS), intestinal permeability ("leaky gut" syndrome), dysbiosis and small intestine bacterial overgrowth (SIBO), nausea, and general indigestion. These also may be remedied using essential oils.

If you have or suspect a disease or chronic ailment, seek a doctor and professional for advice. Then consider essential oils and their gut-healing benefits with your physician, as backed by science.

STOP Before you start implementing these essential oils for IBD and gut health, be sure to review the known drug interaction chart in Appendix B and consult with your physician if you're currently taking any medications. Also, don't forget that using essential oils while living a "fast food" lifestyle is like taking one step forward but two steps back! In other words, for essential oils to help you enjoy abundant health and wellness—free from chronic disease—it is vital to use them within the context of a healthy lifestyle. Go to Appendix A for our favorite "Disease-Busting Healthy Lifestyle Hacks" to learn more!

IMPORTANT DIY CAPSULE REMINDER

It is *not* advisable to make and store the capsule remedies and recipes below ahead of time with enteric-coated capsules. They should be made "to order" before each use. The longer the essential oils sit in capsules, the more likely they are to erode and break down the capsules. And this defeats the purpose of the time-delayed, enteric-coated capsule. This is particularly true of the more caustic ("hot") essential oils like cinnamon, oregano, and thyme. Even if they are diluted properly, they may end up breaking down the capsule lining after a few days or weeks. It's just not worth the mess and headache (and cost!) of wasting your oils to make them ahead of time.

When taking essential oil capsules, always consume them after a meal; preferably after breakfast or dinner to provide daytime or nighttime benefits. And limit yourself to two doses a day, being sure to separate applications six to eight hours apart. Stick with the dilutions we provide, because they are all well within the safe maximum oral dose guidelines.

Taking DIY essential oil capsules is not a long-term solution, and using them for more than four weeks at a time is not advisable. The purpose of these remedies is to help you heal, and, hopefully, you can reduce or omit any medications you may be taking under the guidance of your medical provider.

If you experience relief, but the issue you're looking to resolve is still lingering, then be sure to switch up your protocol monthly to prevent any potential of bacterial resistance. And, as always, consult with your health-care provider first if you're currently taking medications. Discontinue if adverse reactions occur.

Synergy Blends

To understand whether essential oils can play a dominant role in successfully managing IBS, researchers evaluated the antibacterial activity of several different essential oils against active *E. coli*. Several key findings were uncovered:

- Coriander seed, fennel, mandarin, peppermint, sage, tea tree, and thyme essential oils all blocked the growth of *E. coli*.
- Lavender, lemon balm, lemongrass, pine, and rosemary oils exhibited strong antibacterial activity for more than six hours, the approximate length of time that would elapse between typical IBS medicine doses.
- According to the researchers conducting the study, "Any one of these

essential oils, or a mixture of them, would be a potential candidate for the reversal of SIBO and treatment of IBS."

- Researchers also suggested taking advantage of synergy blends instead of using single oils, because "the larger number of compounds would act on a wider range of bacteria, the oils might act synergistically to have a stronger effect on any given bacterium," and there would be a reduced chance of producing bacteria resistant to treatment.
- Finally, they concluded that, because of their GRAS (generally recognized as safe) status on the FDA list of food additives and overall effectiveness to not only kill but prevent the growth of bacteria, coriander seed, lemon balm, and peppermint essential oils "would be very good candidates for the treatment of IBS, either singly or in combination."

We like this blend for more than just IBS and suggest you consider it for IBD and its symptoms as well.

IBD SYNERGY CAPSULE

Makes 1 dose

2 drops coriander seed essential oil

2 drops lemon balm (Melissa) essential oil

2 drops peppermint essential oil

Organic virgin coconut oil or extra-virgin olive oil

SUPPLIES

Pipette

Size 00 vegan enteric-coated capsule

1. Using a pipette, drop the essential oils into the bottom half (the longer, narrower one) of the capsule. Fill this half to the brim with organic extra-virgin coconut or extra-virgin olive oil.

continues

2. Fit the wider top half of the capsule over the bottom half and secure it snugly.

3. Immediately swallow the capsule with water after breakfast and/or dinner. Take once or twice daily and monitor symptoms.

➲ To watch us make this recipe and learn more about our favorite ways to promote natural gut health, go to EOApothecary.com.

1. Peppermint

This essential oil is well-known for its digestive remedy capabilities, especially for IBS and SIBO. In the most comprehensive meta-analysis to date, peppermint oil was shown to be a safe and effective therapy for pain and total body symptoms in adults with IBS. Researchers have noted that peppermint oil improved symptoms through its antimicrobial activity in the small intestine.

Application: Make the IBD Synergy Capsule (page 277) or add 3 or 4 drops of peppermint essential oil to a vegan enteric-coated capsule and fill with extra-virgin olive oil. Take once or twice daily for one week and monitor your IBD symptoms.

2. Caraway

Compared to commonly prescribed drugs like prednisolone, Asacol (mesalamine), and hydrocortisone acetate, researchers suggest that caraway essential oil is a viable colitis therapy option, successfully reducing colon tissue lesions and colitis symptoms in animals after just five days of administration. The interesting thing about this particular study is that positive results were observed at all doses and administrative routes (oral and injection into the abdomen). This suggests that topical application over the abdomen could offer some colitis relief and may be used in addition to taking enteric-coated capsules.

Additionally, caraway has been tested with other essential oils to treat gut issues. One study, for instance, mixed caraway with peppermint and discovered that this blend treated functional dyspepsia (non-ulcer stomach pain) with great success.

Application: In addition to taking a Microflora-Friendly Capsule (page 280), make this refreshing ointment for invigorating, aromatic relief from IBD symptoms.

COLITIS-SOOTHING OINTMENT

15 drops orange essential oil

15 drops caraway essential oil

15 drops peppermint essential oil

2 ounces carrier oil of choice or Mama Z's Oil Base (page 25)

SUPPLIES

Medium glass bowl

Lidded glass jar or lotion dispenser

1. Drop the essential oils into a bowl.

2. Add a carrier oil and mix thoroughly. Store in glass container.

3. Massage the mixture into the abdomen in a clockwise direction after breakfast and dinner daily or when colitis symptoms flare up.

3. Bitter Orange

During an evaluation of how eight essential oils performed at treating intestinal dysbiosis specifically with the intent to determine the safety of the gastrointestinal tract microflora, bitter orange, caraway, and lavender topped the charts. Acknowledging the concern many people have about essential oils hurting the microbiome, the researchers concluded that "the herbs from which these oils are derived have long been used in the treatment of gastrointestinal symptoms, the in vitro results of this study suggest that their ingestion will have little detrimental impact on beneficial members of the [gastrointestinal tract] microflora."

Application: To support a healthy microbiome and soothe unpleasant gut symptoms, try taking a gentle Microflora-Friendly Capsule (page 280) daily after breakfast.

MICROFLORA-FRIENDLY CAPSULE

Makes 1 dose

2 drops bitter orange essential oil

2 drops caraway essential oil

2 drops lavender essential oil

Organic virgin coconut oil or extra-virgin olive oil

SUPPLIES

Pipette

Size 00 vegan enteric-coated capsule

1. Using a pipette, drop the essential oils into the bottom half (the longer, narrower one) of the capsule. Fill this half to the brim with organic extra-virgin coconut or extra-virgin olive oil.

2. Fit the wider top half of the capsule over the bottom half and secure it snugly.

3. Immediately swallow the capsule with water after breakfast and/or dinner. Take once or twice daily and monitor your symptoms.

4. Oregano

Oregano oil is another option for treating IBD supported by the medical literature. A recent study published in 2019 observed that a mixture of *Laetiporus sulphureus* mushrooms and oregano, cinnamon, and clove essential oils was found to decrease the activity of Crohn's disease in human volunteers.

Additionally, oregano essential oil has been shown to repair the gut lining and could be a viable solution for leaky gut.

Application: For IBD, leaky gut, and overall intestinal health, add 3 or 4 drops of oregano essential oil to a vegan enteric-coated capsule and fill with extra-virgin olive oil. Take once or twice daily for one week and monitor your IBD symptoms.

OREGANO: NATURE'S ANTIBIOTIC

Most people are unaware that antibiotics come in multiple forms. Beyond the indication of broad-spectrum antibiotics, there are more qualifications that determine how an antibiotic is most effectively used: gram-negative and gram-positive bacteria are affected in their own ways, and certain antibiotics will be more effective against one than the other.

Several years ago, an analysis of oregano oil's efficacy against three gram-negative bacteria (*E. coli, Salmonella typhimurium, Pseudomonas aeruginosa*) and two gram-positive (*Staphylococcus aureus, Bacillus subtilis*) bacteria. Oregano herb was harvested at three different growth stages (late vegetative, early vegetative, and flowering), distilled into three essential oils and evaluated, and all three were effective in vitro against all five bacterial strains.

With clear results against these common bacteria, particularly the food-safety-related *E. coli* and *S. typhimurium,* adding oregano essential oil in your culinary preparations (like pizza or pasta sauce) seems wise for gastrointestinal protection and disease prevention.

To avoid antibiotics for non-life-threatening infections, consider making the Triple-Threat Infection-Fighting Protocol (page 131), or try two or three drops of oregano essential oil in a vegan enteric-coated gel capsule filled with extra-virgin olive oil. Take once or twice daily for one week after meals and monitor your symptoms. It can do wonders for your health!

5. Thyme

Consuming thyme essential oil can also be a potent healing remedy. Evaluating a combination of oregano and thyme oils on mice with colitis, researchers observed that daily doses decreased mortality, accelerated weight gain, and reduced colon damage. Thymol and carvacrol (the primary components of thyme and oregano) are also fantastic for promoting intestinal integrity and immune responses.

Application: Place 2 drops each of thyme and oregano essential oils into a vegan enteric-coated capsule and fill with extra-virgin olive oil. Take once or twice daily for one week after meals and monitor your IBD symptoms.

5. Cumin

Several years ago, a study out of Iran directed fifty-seven IBS patients to stop taking all IBS medications for four weeks, and they were given a 2 percent prediluted oral dose of cumin essential oil instead: ten drops fifteen minutes after breakfast and fifteen minutes after dinner to mimic the manner in which most IBS patients take their prescriptions. The results were astounding: a decrease in abdominal pain, bloating, incomplete defecation, fecal urgency, and presence of mucus discharge in stool were statistically significant during and after cumin therapy. Improvements in stool consistency and defecation frequency were also both statistically significant in patients with constipation-dominant patterns of IBS.

Application: Make our Gentle Cumin Capsule to naturally manage IBS and IBD symptoms and gastrointestinal complaints.

GENTLE CUMIN CAPSULE

Makes 1 dose

2 to 3 drops cumin essential oil
Unrefined, organic coconut oil or extra-virgin olive oil

SUPPLIES
Pipette
Size 00 vegan gel capsule

1. Using a pipette, drop the essential oils into the bottom half (the longer, narrower one) of the capsule. Fill this half to the brim with coconut or extra-virgin olive oil.
2. Fit the wider top half of the capsule over the bottom half and secure it snugly.
3. Immediately swallow the capsule (see Note) with water after breakfast and/or dinner. Take once or twice daily and monitor symptoms.

6. Ginger

Ginger essential oil is a standout when it comes to easing nausea, and it presents itself as a potential solution for a nagging symptom that IBD patients suffer from: ulcers.

In 2015, researchers evaluated the anti-ulcer activity of turmeric and ginger essential oils in lab rats with stomach ulcers. Not only were internal hemorrhaging of the stomach wall and ulcer size greatly reduced after consuming both oils, but there was a marked increase in antioxidant levels as well. Culinary preparations would make sense here, providing a digestive system boost to your regular mealtime.

Application: Find creative ways of adding 1 drop each of ginger and turmeric essential oils to your favorite dishes a few times a week to enjoy a subtle culinary dose that promotes overall gut health throughout your upper gastrointestinal tract. For a more targeted approach to treat ulcers, take ginger and turmeric essential oils. For stomach ulcers: Mix 3 drops each of ginger and turmeric essential oils in a vegan gel capsule and fill with extra-virgin olive oil. For intestinal ulcers: Mix 3 drops each of ginger and turmeric essential oils in a vegan enteric-coated gel capsule and fill with extra-virgin olive oil. Take once or twice daily for one week after meals, and monitor your ulcer symptoms.

7. Turmeric

When combined with ginger, we've just seen that turmeric can do wonders for gut ulcers. When used alone, it can be just as powerful for gut inflammation caused by IBD. In fact, compared to stand-alone curcumin (a healing powerhouse in its own right), turmeric essential oil has been proven to provide "superior anti-inflammatory efficacy" in animals with colitis.

Application: Place 3 drops of turmeric essential oil or CO_2 in a vegan enteric-coated gel capsule and fill with extra-virgin olive oil. Take once or twice daily for one week after meals and monitor your IBD symptoms.

8. Patchouli

Rectal administration of medications is oftentimes the only thing that offers relief for people suffering from IBD flare-ups.

This is where patchouli oil suppositories can help. Patchouli is widely used to treat gastrointestinal diseases, including IBD, in Asian countries, including China. A recent study tested this ancient tradition and discovered that rectal administration of patchouli oil "significantly alleviated colonic damage and reduced disease activity indicators," including inflammation.

When applying essential oils around or in sensitive areas like the vagina and rectum, remember to never use more than a 1 percent dilution (6 drops of essential oils per 1 ounce of carrier oil).

Application: Use an enema to administer a 0.5 to 1 percent dilution of patchouli essential oil into the rectum three times per week, and monitor IBD symptoms.

SOOTHING IBD SUPPOSITORIES

16 to 24 drops patchouli essential oil (see Notes)

4 ounces organic virgin coconut oil, melted and cooled slightly, or Mama Z's Oil Base (page 25)

SUPPLIES

Silicone mini ice cube tray

Medium glass bowl

1. In a glass bowl, thoroughly mix together the essential oil and coconut oil.
2. Divide and fill the mini ice cube tray and put them in the freezer to harden. Each ice cube tray represents 1 application.
3. Take out 1 application upon waking and insert into rectum right before going into

shower. Alternatively, you can insert the suppository right before bed, but you'll need to use a pad or undergarment protector to soak up the excess oil as it melts to prevent damaging your clothes and sheets.

4. Store in freezer uncovered.

NOTES: *As long as you hover between a 0.5 and 1 percent dilution, you can use a variety of essential oils for rectal suppositories to offer IBD relief. Peppermint works great for soothing hemorrhoids, pain, and itching. Lavender, Roman chamomile, frankincense, and geranium are always safe go-to oils for all things healing and soothing. Just steer clear of the caustic ones like cinnamon, oregano, thyme, and clove. And be sure to consult with your physician to help you monitor results.*

Treat suppositories as you would internal-use essential oils. Start slowly and be very careful to observe for any adverse reactions. Discontinue use immediately if anything unpleasant occurs. Remember, using essential oils therapeutically should only help and should never hurt in any way.

8. Geranium

In Iran, geranium oil is regularly used to treat inflammatory disease, pain, anxiety, and sadness as well as gastrointestinal symptoms. Researchers recently tested this traditional approach in a lab setting on rats with acid-induced colitis and found that it had significant anti-inflammatory and anti-ulcer properties.

Application: Try the suppository recipe (page 284) using geranium essential oil for IBD pain and symptom relief.

9. Basil

Basil essential oil is also traditionally used in Middle Eastern countries to treat IBD. Investigators have discovered that basil oil inhibited acetic acid–induced colitis in rats. They recommend it as a possible supplementary remedy because it was observed not only to protect the colon from inflammation-induced colitis damage, but it also reduced ulcer severity and size.

Application: Place 3 drops basil essential oil in a vegan enteric-coated gel capsule and fill with extra-virgin olive oil. Take once or twice daily for one week after meals, and monitor your IBD symptoms.

10. Copaiba

The primary component of copaiba oil, beta-caryophyllene, is known to help protect the brain and improve symptoms related to Parkinson's disease. It has also been shown to successfully manage inflammatory bowel disease because of its antioxidative and/or anti-inflammatory properties. Other notable oils that are rich in beta-caryophyllene include black pepper, ylang ylang, lemon balm (Melissa), fenugreek, winter savory, clove bud, clove leaf, and black pine.

Application: Make the Beta-caryophyllene Capsule (page 291) or add 3 or 4 drops of copaiba essential oil into a vegan enteric-coated capsule and fill with extra-virgin olive oil. Take once or twice daily for one week, and monitor your IBD symptoms.

It never ceases to amaze us how one little itty-bitty drop of essential oils can do wonders for someone's health, and IBD is no exception! We have several friends and family members who have suffered greatly because of ulcerative colitis and Crohn's disease, and we know how debilitating IBD can be. We hope and pray that these remedies help you like they have our loved ones.

Chapter 17

Parkinson's Disease and Epilepsy

For most of us, taking a walk, picking up a mug of coffee, or signing a document are second-nature activities that come easily, and we do them every day without even thinking about them. But for millions of people with "movement disorders," such tasks are painstakingly difficult. They suffer from brain disorders that ruthlessly erode their ability to control their body movements.

Movement, such as reaching for something on a shelf, seems simple but is actually a complex process that requires activities from several different parts of the brain working in tandem with muscles and nerves.

When this process goes awry, a person is said to have a movement disorder—neurological syndromes in which there may be too much movement or very little. They are associated with pathological changes in the brain that lead to difficulty in walking, moving around, or maintaining posture and normal body balance. Movement disorders are quite prevalent, and many of them are hereditary.

The two most common movement disorders, Parkinson's disease and epilepsy, also fall under the chronic disease umbrella, and they will be the focus of this last chapter, as essential oils play a part in managing symptoms.

UNDERSTANDING PARKINSON'S DISEASE AND EPILEPSY

Nearly one million people in the United States are living with Parkinson's disease (PD), according to the Parkinson's Foundation. Most are over age fifty, although a version of the disease called young-onset Parkinson's can strike people under age forty—which is what happened to actor Michael J. Fox.

The second most common neurodegenerative disease after Alzheimer's, PD affects ten million adults globally, including 1 percent of all people over sixty years of age in industrialized countries. Its prevalence is expected to double by 2030. There is no known cure for the disease, but it is not known to be a cause of death. At the disease's worst, patients become bedridden.

In Parkinson's disease, there is a degeneration of nerve cells in the substantia nigra, a region of the brain that produces dopamine, a brain chemical that sends signals within the brain to allow smooth movement of the muscles. Dopamine is lost, causing nerve cells to become overactive. As a result, patients are unable to control their movement, and walking, arm movement, and facial expression become impaired. This loss of dopamine is a key factor as to why essential oils can help, as we'll see below.

Also, conditions known as essential tremors and restless legs syndrome (RLS) are both closely connected to PD, according to epidemiologic and genetic studies. In fact, RLS is characterized by low dopamine levels, and patients can benefit from similar treatments as for Parkinson's.

Another major movement disorder is epilepsy, a brain disorder that causes often-sudden, recurrent seizures. A seizure is a surge of electrical activity in the brain.

Epilepsy is a fairly common neurological disorder that affects sixty-five million people globally people around the world, and about three million in the United States. It is more common in young children and older adults and occurs in more men than women.

There's also no known cure for epilepsy, but it can be managed with medications and other strategies. Treatment plans are based on the severity of symptoms and how well someone responds to therapy. What is really exciting is the amount of research we now have regarding essential oils as a complementary therapy for epilepsy.

CBD FOR PARKINSON'S AND SEIZURES

In recent years, the scientific community has shown increased interest in CBD due to its good safety profile and neuroprotective properties. This neuroprotective action is due to its anti-inflammatory and antioxidant properties. CBD contains significant anti-inflammatory qualities in several experimental studies and has been shown to help manage the onset, severity, and symptoms associated with seizures and Parkinson's.

In fact, according to a recent literature review, "The results of scientific studies obtained so far [in] the use of CBD in clinical applications could represent hope for patients who are resistant to all conventional anti-epileptic drugs." This is true even for infants and children!

When making the following topical preparations and capsule remedies, consider adding in a dose of CBD to enhance the efficacy.

Consult with your medical team to determine if CBD is a good fit for you.

THE ESSENTIAL OILS APPROACH TO PARKINSON'S DISEASE

Because PD is characterized by the loss of dopamine-producing neurons, cancer drugs that raise dopamine levels have been studied, and it's been observed that they ease Parkinson's symptoms. It's logical to assume that aromatherapy can help as well, because inhaling essential oils triggers communication signals from the nose through the olfactory system to stimulate the brain to release the neurotransmitters dopamine as well as serotonin.

As we've seen in our discussions about depression and Alzheimer's disease, clary sage, galbanum, and lemon have all been shown to increase dopamine levels. Be sure to include these oils in your regular diffuser blends, spritzers, and aromatherapy inhalers.

Gamma-aminobutyric acid (GABA) also plays a role in Parkinson's. A major inhibitory neurotransmitter in the central nervous system, dysfunction or deficiency of the GABAergic system has been implicated in epilepsy. As we learned in our discussion about sleep, stress, and depression, valerian, lemon balm, and linalool-rich oils such as rosewood, coriander seed, magnolia, neroli, lavender, ylang ylang, petitgrain, clary sage, bergamot, and geranium are known to increase GABA levels. Be sure to include these oils in your regular diffuser blends, spritzers, and aromatherapy inhalers as well as in your topical applications. Because essential oils contain small, fat-soluble molecules, they can penetrate through the skin after topical application, enter into the blood, and cross the blood-brain barrier.

Note: As a general rule, all of the recipes in this section have the potential to help restless legs syndrome patients as well. For people with essential tremors, we'd recommend starting slow (inhalation) and working your way up to more concentrated doses (topical application, then ingestion under the guidance of a health professional).

1. Copaiba

As discussed in the previous chapter, the primary component of copaiba oil, betacaryophyllene, is known to help prevent and successfully manage inflammatory bowel disease because of its antioxidative and anti-inflammatory properties. In a recent study, however, it was also uncovered that oral dosing helps improve motor dysfunction, guards against loss of neurons, and protects important mechanisms that are damaged by Parkinson's in animals.

Other notable oils that are rich in beta-caryophyllene include black pepper, ylang ylang, lemon balm (Melissa), fenugreek, winter savory, clove bud, clove leaf, and black pine.

Application: Consult with your physician about trying the Beta-caryophyllene Blend and recipes below.

BETA-CARYOPHYLLENE BLEND

20 drops copaiba essential oil

20 drops fenugreek essential oil

15 drops black pepper essential oil

15 drops clove bud essential oil

5 drops lemon balm (Melissa) essential oil

SUPPLIES

5 ml bottle

1. Drop the essential oils in a 5 ml bottle. Cap the bottle and shake to combine.
2. Use as directed in the following recipes.

BETA-CARYOPHYLLENE CAPSULE

Makes 1 dose

3 or 4 drops Beta-caryophyllene Blend (page 290)

1 dose full-spectrum CBD (follow manufacturer's instructions for dosage)

Organic virgin coconut oil or extra-virgin olive oil

SUPPLIES

Pipette

Size 00 vegan gel capsule

1. Using a pipette, drop the essential oil blend and CBD into the bottom half (the longer, narrower one) of the capsule. Fill this half to the brim with organic extra-virgin coconut or extra-virgin olive oil.
2. Fit the wider top half of the capsule over the bottom half and secure it snugly.
3. Immediately swallow the capsule with water after breakfast and/or dinner (see Note). Take once or twice daily and monitor your symptoms.

NOTE: *Do not make and store these capsules for future use. Also, this is not a long-term solution, and using it for more than four weeks at a time is not advisable. Be sure to switch up your protocol monthly and consult with your health-care provider first if you're currently taking medications. Discontinue if adverse reactions occur.*

BETA-CARYOPHYLLENE DIFFUSER BLEND

5 or 6 drops Beta-caryophyllene Blend (page 290)

SUPPLIES

Diffuser

1. Fill your diffuser with purified water as directed in the manufacturer's instructions.
2. Add the essential oil blend.
3. Turn on the diffuser when you want to promote healthy motor and brain function. This works well running during the day and/or at night and can be used in an aromatherapy necklace.

BETA-CARYOPHYLLENE ROLL-ON

12 drops Beta-caryophyllene Blend (page 290)

Carrier oil of choice—jojoba and fractionated coconut oil absorb quickly—as needed

SUPPLIES

10 ml glass roller bottle

1. Drop the essential oil blend into the roller bottle.
2. Fill the roller bottle with your carrier oil of choice and shake well.
3. Apply over your chest and back of the neck once daily or whenever you want to promote healthy motor and brain function.

THE ENDOCANNABINOID SYSTEM

Discovered in the 1990s when researchers were studying tetrahydrocannabinol (THC—a known cannabinoid), the endocannabinoid system (ECS) is crucial for our survival as it plays a critical role in maintaining homeostasis of many processes in the human body, including pain, memory, mood, appetite, stress, sleep, metabolism, and immune and reproductive functions.

For the ECS to work properly, it requires cannabinoids, compounds made both by the body and in nature (e.g., cannabis), which bind with and trigger cannabinoid receptors that, in turn, produce a variety of physiological responses such as pain relief, insomnia relief, increased appetite, reduced stress, euphoria, and the feeling of being "high."

There are two receptors of primary interest to us:

- CB1 receptors found in the central nervous system (i.e., brain and spinal cord) can trigger the sensation of being high.
- CB2 receptors found in the peripheral nervous system, immune cells, muscles, skin, and vital organs that will not get you high when triggered.

THC is the famous cannabinoid in cannabis that causes people to get high, and it can bind with both CB1 and CB2 receptors.

What does this have anything to do with aromatherapy?

Well, because of beta-caryophyllene, the first known "dietary cannabinoid," has been approved by the FDA as GRAS (generally recognized as safe) to be used in food.

It also happens to be the primary sesquiterpene in black pepper, clove, hops, rosemary, copaiba, and cannabis, which binds with CB2 receptors.

Meaning, when you use copaiba, black pepper, or any essential oil that contains beta-caryophyllene, you activate the ECS without any psychotropic effects (i.e., you won't get high).

2. Palmarosa

Originating from a wild grass native to India, palmarosa offers support at your body's cellular level. It is known as an antiseptic, an antiviral, a bactericidal, a digestive aid, and a hydrating substance.

Palmarosa may also help the brain detox and protect against PD. A pesticide called rotenone has been implicated as a possible contributor to Parkinson's disease. In a 2018 study, mice with rotenone-induced Parkinson's disease were given geraniol, the primary component of palmarosa essential oil. The test uncovered that pretreating mice with geraniol not only protected brain cells from damage but improved oxidative stress, promoted proper mitochondrial function, and helped reduce cell death.

Palmarosa's citrusy, floral scent is uplifting and stimulating and provides critical protection for brain cells.

Application: Try mixing the essential oils of two members of the *Cymbopogon* genus, palmarosa and lemongrass, together in your diffuser for a unique, refreshing aroma. Also consult with your physician about taking these oils in a vegan gel capsule with CBD.

3. Lemongrass

A research design similar to the one described above was followed in India, but this study compared lemongrass essential oil with levodopa, a dopamine therapy commonly used to help PD patients. The brain-protecting efficacy of lemongrass was comparable with the drug, as well as the ability to reduce the presence of key enzymes such as glutamic pyruvic transaminase and lactate dehydrogenase, which are markers of the disease.

What's interesting here is that the author called out the limitations of modern Western medicine in alleviating PD, claiming that current treatments do little to address root issues and may even "accelerate further damage." His point that "herbal medicines are now in great demand among the population in developing countries not because they are inexpensive but also for better cultural acceptability, better compatibility with the human body and minimal side effects" is well received and should be heeded by all.

Application: For a topical remedy with inhalation benefits for brain health and to reduce PD symptoms, mix 15 drops each of lemongrass and palmarosa essential oils with 2 ounces of Mama Z's Oil Base (page 25) and add in 2 doses of CBD oil (per packaging instructions). Apply over the back of the neck twice daily.

4. Fennel

Estrogen, a female hormone, may reduce or slow the progression of Parkinson's disease, according to Mayo Clinic research. The studies showed that women on estrogen are 40 percent less likely to develop the disease, and women with Parkinson's who took estrogen showed improvements in memory, motor skills, and thinking. In addition, women are only half as likely to get the disease as men, more evidence that estrogen may be helpful in treating Parkinson's.

Which brings us to fennel essential oil, which contains a complex of compounds that have the tendency to bring estrogen balance to the body. An Iranian study observed that fennel oil protected female mice with Parkinson's and without ovaries from motor impairment, compared to the mice who did not receive the oil therapy. If you're a woman with Parkinson's, you might want to consider using fennel essential oil, especially if you are estrogen deficient. The oil might also be a powerful protective therapy against the disease, but of course, more research is needed.

Application: Inhaling fennel in a personal inhaler or ultrasonic diffuser is a great place to start. Also consult with your physician about taking 2 or 3 drops in a vegan gel capsule with CBD.

THE ESSENTIAL OILS APPROACH TO EPILEPSY

In 2019, the University of Texas in San Antonio published the most thorough paper on essential oils for the treatment of epilepsy to date. The review made the following key points:

- Approximately 20 to 30 percent of patients with epilepsy suffer from seizures that cannot be controlled using any antiepileptic drugs (AEDs) that are currently available.
- A large amount of evidence suggests that natural medicines may be one potential source of new antiepileptic drugs.
- EOs have been used as anticonvulsants in traditional medicine in many cultures worldwide, especially in the Middle East, India, China, and Brazil. It

is no surprise that much of the research on EOs and their antiepileptic effects has been produced by institutions in these regions.

- EOs have been documented for anxiolytic, sedative, neuroprotective, and anticonvulsive properties by academic research groups worldwide.
- Compounds found in EOs have been shown to interact with and exert pharmacological action on central nervous system targets involved in epilepsy.
- Basil, clove, dill, lavender, lemongrass, peppermint, spearmint, and other EOs containing the beneficial constituents discussed below are good candidates for evaluation as antiepileptic drugs.

Application: Start out by diluting one essential oil from the list above with Mama Z's Oil Base (page 25) to 2 percent for an invigorating body oil and massage it into your shoulders and back of your neck. Monitor results with your doctor. Alternatively, add a few drops to your diffuser or 20 drops in your inhaler for on-the-go support. Also, consult with your physician about taking 2 or 3 drops in a vegan gel capsule with CBD.

ESSENTIAL OILS CONSTITUENTS THAT MAY HELP WITH SEIZURES

The University of Texas at San Antonio review went on to discuss the most potent anti-seizure oils, noting that each contains at least one of the following therapeutic constituents:

- asarone—clinically used as medication for treating epilepsy
- carvone—a relaxant that has been used medicinally since ancient times
- citral—a detoxifier than aids in brain function
- eugenol—a potent antioxidant that increases the levels of dopamine and serotonin in the brain
- linalool—which can block certain receptors in the brain that can significantly lower the chance of seizures

According to review, the most potent essential-oil constituents that have helped prevent and manage seizures are carvone, citral, eugenol, and linalool. This is where your favorite essential oils fall in the mix.

Essential Oils Rich in Carvone

- Spearmint (57.2 to 71.6 percent)
- Caraway (47.3 to 59.5 percent)
- Dillseed (27.3 to 53.3 percent)
- Verbena (43.3 to 46.1 percent)
- Dill weed (31.6 to 42.4 percent)

Essential Oils Rich in Eugenol

- Clove bud (73.5 to 96.9 percent)
- Clove leaf (77.0 to 88.0 percent)
- Cinnamon leaf (68.6 to 87.0 percent)
- Basil, holy (31.9 to 50.4 percent)
- Basil, sweet (9.4 to 15.2 percent)
- Cinnamon bark (2.0 to 13.3 percent)
- Laurel leaf (1.2 to 3.0 percent)
- Jasmine absolute (1.1 to 3.0 percent)

Essential Oils Rich in Linalool

See page 86 from chapter 5.

CAN ESSENTIAL OILS CAUSE SEIZURES?

The 2019 study out of Texas referenced above made a point to note that some essential oils have convulsant effects and can trigger seizures in both epileptic and healthy people:

> *Internal use of EOs like sage, hyssop, rosemary, camphor, pennyroyal, eucalyptus, cedar, thuja, and fennel can cause epileptic seizures because they contain thujone, 1,8-cineole, camphor, or pinocamphone, which have been identified as convulsive agents.*

Note the implication of "*internal* use."

But what about *inhalation* and *topical* use?

In 2011, a report described a four-year old girl who experienced a seizure after being exposed *topically* to a head-lice preparation containing eucalyptus. And between 2015 and 2016, ten cases of eucalyptus *inhalation*-induced seizures were diagnosed in the literature.

Nonetheless, you'll definitely want to stay away from ingesting the oils claimed to cause seizures if this is something you or a loved one may be prone to. And use caution with inhalation and topical use. This is not to say that you have to completely avoid these oils, but just be careful. One of our aromatherapist friends has a child with epilepsy and tells us she regularly uses oils with 1,8 cineole (i.e., eucalyptus, rosemary, and sage) with no problem. Go figure.

Maybe there's more to the story than blanket thou-shall and thou-shall-not lists.

Take rosemary, for example. It's on the thou-shall-not list above, but it has been praised for modulating T-type calcium channels (or TTCCs), which play important roles in neuronal excitability, neuroprotection, sensory processes, and sleep. They also play important roles in epilepsy and pain. One study evaluating lavender and rosemary, as well as their major active compounds linalool and rosmarinic acid, discovered that they inhibit TTCCs, which contributes to the anxiolytic and the neuroprotective effects of these oils.

So, if one compound in rosemary can trigger a seizure but another compound reduces its effects, what do you do?

Like everything else we've discussed in this book, listen to your body, be sure to consult your doctor regarding the natural therapies you want to experiment with, and always use caution when self-treating a chronic illness.

So often we feel hopeless for seemingly hopeless conditions like the ones we have covered in this chapter. But there is a great deal of hope in these complex healing substances known as essential oils. They work holistically to balance the body and mind—and in doing so, help us achieve deeper healing.

Conclusion

"Is anyone among you sick? Let him call for the elders of the church, and let them pray over him, anointing him with oil in the name of the Lord. And the prayer of faith will save the one who is sick, and the Lord will raise him up."

—JAMES 5:14-15

When we read this Scripture, we are humbled by God's provision—that He gave us so many healing oils for our use and benefit. All through the Bible, there are references to how Jesus, His disciples, and many others anointed people with olive oil and essential oil extracts and healed them.

This powerful image, disregarded for centuries, now has been brought to light with growing scientific verification of how well plant-based medicine can help not only prevent but also treat so many chronic diseases today. Our hope is that through the words in this book you have been moved, touched, and, most of all, motivated to continue the journey, knowing that these highly concentrated plant compounds have extraordinary properties to treat, soothe, and support the body to heal the most serious illnesses of our time.

We hope, too, that you have a better understanding of how your body works, from shoring up its defenses to strengthening its self-healing powers. When you understand these innate, amazing forces, the better prepared you will be to enhance both the length and quality of your life. And the more you know, the better prepared you are to make healthy choices—from nutrition to exercise to better lifestyle habits.

Yes, chronic conditions make life more difficult, but we have more resources than ever—including essential oils—to join with medical assistance to greatly restore and optimize our health and give you and your family the abundant life you so deserve.

Your health, as well as the health of your family, is very, very precious. Take the necessary steps to restore it and preserve it.

You are in our prayers as you go forward, live fully, and create wonderful healing experiences for you and your loved ones.

Appendix A

Disease-Busting Healthy Lifestyle Hacks

Highlighting the interconnectedness of chronic disease, this brings up the recurring theme of our book, namely, that our society can reduce a significant number of deaths caused by chronic disease by simply adopting a few effective lifestyle changes, in addition to incorporating essential oils into our own personal health program.

Every disease discussed in this book shares many of the same risk factors, and the prevention strategies are nearly identical. That's why all of the major health agencies around the globe say the same thing: eat healthy, exercise regularly, avoid alcohol, stop smoking, get ample sleep, and reduce stress.

So, instead of repeating ourselves over and over again in each chapter, here is a quick rundown for your consideration.

ADOPT HEALTHY NUTRITIONAL PRACTICES

At the core of our being, we are what we eat. Proper nutrition prevents or helps people successfully manage every chronic disease discussed in this book.

Dr. Z's nutrition professor in chiropractic college said something that forever marked the way he views food: everything you eat will either turn into healthy flesh or diseased cells. This puts a more real-life spin on the famous Hippocrates quote "Let food be thy medicine," doesn't it?

The bottom line is that foods containing antioxidant-rich, bioactive ingredients promote healing and reduce inflammation, a primary factor that is the underlying cause of most chronic diseases. Nonfoods (i.e., processed, junk foods), white sugar, white flour, preservatives, chemical dyes, and the entire gamut of what makes most store-bought consumables dangerous produce the exact opposite effect.

We invite you to pick up our book *The Essential Oils Diet* to learn more about how bioactive compounds (including essential oils!) can help you live a long, healthy, and disease-free life.

REACH YOUR IDEAL WEIGHT

True, most people can benefit from shedding a few pounds, but note how we didn't simply say, "Lose weight." The key is to reach the weight that best fits your body type, and there is no one-size-fits-all approach.

Being overweight and clinically obese is more than how you look. It is not only a primary cause of premature death and a chronic disease in its own right but a serious medical condition associated with type 2 diabetes that increases your risk of other health problems.

The good news is that even if you lose a modest amount of weight, you can improve or prevent the health problems associated with chronic disease. Visit chapter 14 to see how you can use essential oils to reduce blood sugar and reach your ideal weight. Also, thousands of people have found our book *The Essential Oils Diet* to be a useful resource in reaching their ideal weight, and we invite you to learn more at EssentialOilsDiet.com.

GET MOVING

You were designed by God to move, not sit all day, which will only make your health worse by reducing blood flow, oxygen, metabolic function, digestion, and brain function—not to mention cause stiff, achy joints!

Get regular exercise, as much as you can. Taking a walk around the block can be a good start. Gradually progress with longer-duration and more frequent exercise, pursuing physical activities you enjoy. Watch a free screening of Mama Z's home fitness class to see how easy it is to incorporate daily exercise into your natural health regimen at MamaZExercise.com.

STOP SMOKING

Smoking hurts and constricts blood vessels to most of our major organs. We know from research that smoking increases chronic disease and is a primary cause of death worldwide.

Smoking cessation will definitely lower your risk and greatly improve your health. Read chapter 6 to learn how essential oils can help you quit the habit!

MANAGE STRESS

Chronic stress is a killer. Period. Unfortunately, many people today have trouble controlling it, and they resort to unhealthy habits like eating sugary foods, drinking alcohol, or using nicotine to cope; however, these behaviors simply cause more bodily damage.

Stress-relieving activities should include daily relaxation time, meditation, prayer, taking essential oils for stress, and deep breathing. You might also consider therapy with a qualified counselor. And explore other stress-relieving movement therapies such as yoga and tai chi.

When you successfully manage your stress levels, expect to see improvements throughout your entire body, mind, and spirit. Read chapter 5 for suggestions on how essential oils can help.

EASE BACK ON ALCOHOL

We once heard a pastor say that you're never going to hear someone tell you that alcohol saved their marriage. From drunk-driving to cirrhosis to saying things you'll later regret, there are definitely more risks associated with drinking booze than benefits.

Alcohol is linked to virtually every chronic condition, and it's important to keep in mind that alcohol is known as an anti-nutrient, because chronic consumption depletes your body of vital vitamins and minerals.

If you feel like you need to curb your drinking, there are many sources of help, including Alcoholics Anonymous (AA), hospital-run programs, and faith-based programs. Generally, these involve various types of support and behavior change.

After you stop drinking, or at least ease back on it, expect your abstinence to improve every aspect of your life. Read chapter 6 for some practical ways essential oils can help if this is an area you struggle with.

ENJOY A THERAPEUTIC MASSAGE

Not only exceptionally relaxing, therapeutic massage is also quite healing. Lymphatic drainage massage can help clear toxins that may be accumulating due to sluggishness, sports massage can help loosen joints and keep you limber, and deep tissue massage will work out the trigger points and can be quite stimulating if the right essential oils are used.

TRY ACUPUNCTURE

The practice of acupuncture is an ancient system that recognizes disease is due to imbalances in the flow of qi (pronounced "chee") or the "life energy" that moves through everyone. Qi is believed to be disrupted by stress, poor diet, fatigue, and excessive heat or cold.

REVISIT MEDICATIONS

Talk to your doctor about medications you're taking. Baby aspirin, antihistamines, cold medications, antidepressants, and some blood pressure drugs may make you groggy and fatigued and exacerbate the symptoms of many diseases. Others may contribute to weight gain.

There is also the issue of antibiotics. According to the Centers for Disease Control and Prevention, "Up to one-third to one-half of antibiotic use in humans is either unnecessary or inappropriate. Each year in the United States, 47 million unnecessary antibiotic prescriptions are written in doctor's offices, emergency rooms, and hospital-based clinics, which makes improving antibiotic prescribing and use a national priority."

Using essential oils can help reduce the dose that you need and can support getting you off these drugs, but only do this under the guidance of your physician, as the consequences can be detrimental if done improperly.

SUPPLEMENTS

In addition to essential oils, supplements such as magnesium, fish oil, vitamin D$_3$, and probiotics can help with total body health. Several pain-relieving supplements, for example, have been fairly well-researched, including devil's claw, curcumin/turmeric, capsaicin, white willow bark, and many *Boswellia* species. Discuss your situation with your natural health-care provider regarding any supplements or botanicals that might work best for you.

GET QUALITY SLEEP

Sleep is healing; without good, quality sleep, your body simply cannot repair its tissues, organs, and overall systems. Practice good sleep habits, and talk to your doctor if you snore loudly or have periods where you stop breathing or gasp during sleep (symptoms of sleep apnea). Remember that many essential oils can help you get a good night's sleep. Chapter 4 will help you learn how to use essential oils to get a better night's sleep.

LIMIT CHEMICAL EXPOSURE

Environmental pollutants inside and outside your home also contribute to chronic disease. As we have pointed out, filter your water, make your own cleaning products with essential oils, and avoid known toxins whenever you can. Check out chapter 3 for some easy-to-make home recipes to replace many of the store-bought products that aren't doing your body any favors.

Appendix B

Drug Interaction Chart

ESSENTIAL OIL LIST OF POTENTIAL DRUG INTERACTIONS (PRESCRIPTION DRUGS)

CATEGORY	GENERIC	BRAND NAME(S)	POTENTIAL INTERACTIONS (ORAL USE)	CONTRAINDICATION (ORAL USE)
Sleep and Anxiety	doxepin, zolpidem	Ambien, Edluar, Intermezzo, Silenor, Zolpimist	Blue Cypress, Blue Tansy,* German Chamomile,* Australian Sandalwood, Vitex, Yarrow*	n/a
Sleep and Anxiety	eszopiclone, triazolam, zaleplon	Lunesta, Halcion, Sonata	Blue Tansy, German Chamomile, Yarrow	n/a
Stress and Anxiety	alprazolam, buspirone, chlordiazepoxide, clonazepam, diazepam	BuSpar, BuSpar Dividose, Klonopin, Librium, Libritabs, Mitran, Poxi, Valium, Vanspar, Xanax	Blue Tansy, German Chamomile, Yarrow	n/a

CATEGORY	GENERIC	BRAND NAME(S)	POTENTIAL INTERACTIONS (ORAL USE)	CONTRAINDICATION (ORAL USE)
Depression and Substance Abuse	escitalopram, fluoxetine, paroxetine, sertraline	Brisdelle, Lexapro, Paxil, Paxil CR, Pexeva, Prozac, Rapiflux, Sarafem, Selfemra, Zoloft	Blue Cypress, Blue Tansy,* Cinnamon Leaf, Clove Bud, German Chamomile,* Australian Sandalwood, Vitex, Yarrow*	n/a
Depression and Substance Abuse	isocarboxazid, phenelzine	Marplan, Nardil	Cinnamon Leaf, Clove Bud	n/a
Chronic Fatigue and Fibromyalgia	armodafinil, modafinil, trazodone	Desyrel, Desyrel Dividose, Nuvigil, Oleptro, Provigil	Blue Tansy, German Chamomile, Yarrow	n/a
Chronic Fatigue and Fibromyalgia	cyclobenzaprine, dextroamphetamine and amphetamine tablets, duloxetine lisdexamfetamine, metaxalone, tramadol	Adderall, Amrix, Comfort Pac with Cyclobenzaprine, ConZip, Cymbalta, Fexmid, Flexeril, Irenka, Skelaxin, Ultram, Ultram ER, Vyvanse	Blue Cypress, Blue Tansy,* German Chamomile,* Australian Sandalwood, Vitex, Yarrow*	n/a
Libido and Erectile Dysfunction	sildenafil, tadalafil, vardenafil	Adcirca, Cialis, Levitra, Revatio, Staxyn, Viagra	Blue Tansy, German Chamomile, Yarrow	n/a
Alzheimer's and Dementia	donepezil, haloperidol	Aricept, Aricept ODT, Haldol	Blue Cypress, Blue Tansy,* German Chamomile,* Australian Sandalwood, Vitex, Yarrow*	n/a
Alzheimer's and Dementia	ergoloid mesylates	Hydergine, Hydergine LC	Blue Tansy, German Chamomile, Yarrow	n/a
Bone and Joint Disorders	meloxicam, methylprednisolone, prednisone	Anjeso, Deltasone, Medrol, Medrol Dosepak, Mobic, Qmiiz OD, Rayos, Sterapred, Vivlodex	Blue Tansy, German Chamomile, Yarrow	n/a
Bone and Joint Disorders	celecoxib, diclofenac, diclofenac and misoprostol	Arthrotec, Cambia, Cataflam, Celebrex, Dyloject, Voltaren-XR, Zipsor, Zorvolex,	German Chamomile	n/a

CATEGORY	GENERIC	BRAND NAME(S)	POTENTIAL INTERACTIONS (ORAL USE)	CONTRAINDICATION (ORAL USE)
Cancer	etoposide, ixabepilone, vinblastine, vincristine, vinorelbine	Ixempra, Navelbine, Oncovin, Velban, Vincasar PFS	Blue Tansy, German Chamomile, Yarrow	n/a
Cardiovascular Disease	amlodipine benazepril, atorvastatin, diltiazem, felodipine, nifedipine, simvastatin, vorapaxar	Adalat, Adalat CC, Afeditab CR, Cardizem (including Cardizem CD, LA, and ZR), Cartia XT, Dilacor XR, Dilt-CD, Diltia XT, Dilt-XR, Diltzac, Matzim LA, Lipitor, Lotrel, Nifediac CC, Nifedical XL, Plendil, Procardia, Procardia XL, Taztia XT, Tiazac, Zocor, Zontivity	Blue Tansy, German Chamomile, Yarrow	n/a
Cardiovascular Disease	azilsartan medoxomil, rosuvastatin	Crestor, Edarbi, Ezallor Sprinkle	German Chamomile	n/a
Cardiovascular Disease	metoprolol, propranolol	Hemangeol, Inderal LA, Inderal XL, InnoPran XL, Inderal, Kapspargo Sprinkle, Lopressor, Toprol-XL	Blue Cypress, Blue Tansy,* German Chamomile,* Australian Sandalwood, Vitex, Yarrow*	n/a
Cardiovascular Disease	warfarin	Coumadin, Jantoven	Blue Tansy, Cassia, Cinnamon Bark, Cinnamon Leaf, Clove Bud, German Chamomile, Lavandin Abrialis, Lavandin Grosso, Lavandin Super, Oregano, Patchouli, Savory, Star Anise, Sweet Fennel, Thyme, Yarrow	Birch,* Wintergreen*

CATEGORY	GENERIC	BRAND NAME(S)	POTENTIAL INTERACTIONS (ORAL USE)	CONTRAINDICATION (ORAL USE)
Chronic Respiratory Disease	budesonide, fluticasone inhalation, mometasone inhalation, salmeterol inhalation	ArmonAir RespiClick 55, ArmonAir RespiClick 113, ArmonAir RespiClick 232, Arnuity Ellipta, Asmanex HFA, Asmanex Twisthaler 120 Dose, Asmanex Twisthaler 14 Dose, Asmanex Twisthaler 30 Dose, Asmanex Twisthaler 60 Dose, Asmanex Twisthaler 7 Dose, Entocort EC, Flovent Diskus, Flovent HFA, Flovent, Flovent Rotadisk, Flovent Diskus (obsolete), Ortikos, Serevent, Serevent Diskus, Uceris	Blue Tansy, German Chamomile, Yarrow	n/a
Chronic Respiratory Disease	umeclidinium	Incruse Ellipta	Blue Cypress, Blue Tansy,* German Chamomile,* Australian Sandalwood, Vitex, Yarrow*	n/a
Diabetes and Obesity	metformin	Fortamet, Glucophage, Glucophage XR, Glumetza, Riomet	Cassia, Cinnamon Bark, Dill Weed, Geranium, Lemon Basil, Lemon Myrtle, Lemon Tea Tree, Lemongrass, Litsea/ May Chang, Melissa, Myrtle, Oregano, Rose Geranium, Star Anise, Sweet Fennel, Turmeric Rhizome	n/a

CATEGORY	GENERIC	BRAND NAME(S)	POTENTIAL INTERACTIONS (ORAL USE)	CONTRAINDICATION (ORAL USE)
Diabetes and Obesity	glimepiride, tolbutamide	Amaryl, Orinase, Orinase Diagnostic, Tol-Tab	Cassia, Cinnamon Bark, Dill Weed, Geranium, German Chamomile, Lemon Basil, Lemon Myrtle, Lemon Tea Tree, Lemongrass, Litsea/ May Chang, Melissa, Myrtle, Oregano, Rose Geranium, Star Anise, Sweet Fennel, Turmeric Rhizome	n/a
Diabetes and Obesity	pioglitazone, nateglinide, repaglinide	Actos, Prandin, Starlix	Blue Tansy, Cassia, Cinnamon Bark, Dill Weed, Geranium, German Chamomile, Lemon Basil, Lemon Myrtle, Lemon Tea Tree, Lemongrass, Litsea/ May Chang, Melissa, Myrtle, Oregano, Rose Geranium, Star Anise, Sweet Fennel, Turmeric Rhizome, Yarrow	
Fatty Liver	pioglitazone	Actos	Blue Tansy, Cassia, Cinnamon Bark, Dill Weed, Geranium, German Chamomile, Lemon Basil, Lemon Myrtle, Lemon Tea Tree, Lemongrass, Litsea/ May Chang, Melissa, Myrtle, Oregano, Rose Geranium, Star Anise, Sweet Fennel, Turmeric Rhizome, Yarrow	n/a

CATEGORY	GENERIC	BRAND NAME(S)	POTENTIAL INTERACTIONS (ORAL USE)	CONTRAINDICATION (ORAL USE)
Inflammatory Bowel Diseases	budesonide, cyclosporine, dexamethasone	Baycadron, Decadron, Dexamethasone Intensol, DexPak, Entocort EC, Neoral, Ortikos, SandIMMUNE, TaperDex, UcerisGengraf, Zema-Pak, ZoDex, Zonacort	Blue Tansy, German Chamomile, Yarrow	n/a
Parkinson's and Epilepsy	carbamazepine, clonazepam, rasagiline, ropinirole	Azilect, Carbatrol, Epitol, Equetro, Klonopin, Requip, Requip XL, ReQuip Follow on Pack, ReQuip Starter Pack, Repreve, Requip Starter Kit, Tegretol, Tegretol XR	Blue Tansy, German Chamomile, Yarrow	n/a
Parkinson's and Epilepsy	phenobarbital, phenytoin	Dilantin, Luminal, Phenytek, Solfoton	German Chamomile	n/a
Parkinson's and Epilepsy	selegiline	Eldepryl, Zelapar	Blue Tansy, Citronella, Geranium, German Chamomile, Lemon Basil, Lemon Myrtle,* Lemon Tea Tree,* Lemongrass,* Litsea/ May Chang,* Melissa, Palmarosa, Rose Geranium, Yarrow	

Caution for all routes (inhalation, oral, topical)

This table covers prescription medications and potential essential oil interactions and contraindications.

Contraindicated essential oils should be avoided without question, whereas potential interactions include essential oils that might pose an issue for the noted method of use, but the evidence doesn't allow for firm conclusions to be drawn. Think of potential interactions as you would a yellow traffic light with the recommendation to proceed with caution, and contraindications as a red light telling you to stop and do not proceed.

*By default, most caution for potential interactions and contraindications center on oral use; however, there are exceptions and such exceptions are noted with an * where appropriate. If you are taking prescription medications, it is best to check with your health-care provider about whether essential oils used in the manners discussed in this book are in your best interest.*

Finally, this information is based on the most recent research and most respected aromatherapy texts available today. It is a highly curated compilation of the most reliable findings from aromatherapists, essential oil safety experts, and scientists. By design, we cover only the most commonly used essential oils on the market, and not esoteric oils not easily found. Thus, this list is not exhaustive, and not all combination drugs are noted. Other essential oils not listed on this chart may have potential interactions with your medications.

ESSENTIAL OIL LIST OF POTENTIAL DRUG INTERACTIONS (OTC)

CATEGORY	GENERIC	BRAND NAME(S)	POTENTIAL INTERACTIONS (ORAL USE)	CONTRAINDICATION (ORAL USE)
Pain Relief Medication	acetaminophen	Actamin, Anacin AF, Apra, Bromo Seltzer, Children's Tylenol, Elixsure Fever/Pain, Mapap, Medi-Tabs, Q-Pap, Silapap Childrens, Tactinal, Tempra Quicklets, Tycolene, Tylenol, Vitapap	Blue Tansy, German, Chamomile, Yarrow	n/a
Pain Relief Medication	aspirin	Arthritis Pain, Aspi-Cor, Aspir 81, Aspir-Low, Bayer Plus, Bufferin, Durlaza, Ecotrin, Ecpirin, Miniprin	Cassia, Cinnamon Bark, Cinnamon Leaf, Clove Bud, Sweet Fennel, Lavandin, Savory, Oregano, Patchouli, Star Anise, Thyme	Birch,* Wintergreen*
Pain Relief Medication	ibuprofen	Advil, Midol, Motrin, Motrin IB, Motrin Migraine Pain, Proprinal, Smart Sense Children's Ibuprofen, PediaCare Children's Pain Reliever/Fever Reducer, PediaCare Infant's Pain Reliever/Fever Reducer	German Chamomile	n/a
Pain Relief Medication	naproxen	Aleve, EC-Naprosyn, Flanax Pain Reliever, Midol Extended Relief, Naprelan, Naprosyn, Anaprox, Anaprox-DS, Naproxen Sodium, Aleve Caplet, Aleve Gelcap, Aleve Easy Open Arthritis	Blue Tansy, German, Chamomile, Yarrow	n/a

CATEGORY	GENERIC	BRAND NAME(S)	POTENTIAL INTERACTIONS (ORAL USE)	CONTRAINDICATION (ORAL USE)
Cough and Cold	dextromethorphan	Babee Cof, Benylin DM Pediatric, Buckleys Mixture, Creomulsion, Creo-Terpin, DayQuil Cough, Delsym, Delsym 12 Hour Cough Relief, Elixsure Cough, Robafen Cough Liquidgels, Robitussin CoughGels, Scot-Tussin Diabetic, Silphen DM, St. Joseph Cough Suppressant, Sucrets DM Cough, Theraflu Thin Strips Cough, Triaminic Long Acting Cough	Blue Cypress, Blue Tansy,* German Chamomile,* Australian Sandalwood, Vitex, Yarrow*	n/a
Antihistamine	diphenhydramine	Allergy Relief, Allermax, Banophen, Benadryl, Compoz Nighttime Sleep Aid, Diphedryl, Diphenhist, Dytuss, Nytol QuickCaps, PediaCare Children's Allergy, Q-Dryl, QlearQuil Nighttime Allergy Relief, Quenalin, Scot-Tussin Allergy Relief Formula, Siladryl Allergy, Silphen Cough, Simply Sleep, Sleepinal, Sominex, Tranquil, Twilite, Unisom Sleepgels Maximum Strength, Valu-Dryl, Vanamine PD, Z-Sleep, ZzzQuil	Blue Cypress, Blue Tansy,* German Chamomile,* Australian Sandalwood, Vitex, Yarrow*	n/a

* Caution for all routes (inhalation, oral, topical).

Sources: Drugs.com (http://www.drugs.com), and R. Tisserand and R. Young, *Essential Oil Safety: A Guide for Health Care Professionals,* 2nd ed., London: Churchill Livingstone, 2013, pp. 585 and 588.

Notes and References

Preface

Centers for Disease Control and Prevention. "About Chronic Diseases." National Center for Chronic Disease Prevention and Health Promotion. Last reviewed November 17, 2020. https://www.cdc.gov/chronicdisease/about/index.htm.

Introduction

Pearson, A. C. S., S. M. Cutshall, W. M. Hooten, et al. "Perspectives on the Use of Aromatherapy from Clinicians Attending an Integrative Medicine Continuing Education Event." *BMC Complementary and Alternative Medicine* 19, no. 1 (2019): 174.

PWC Global. "Chronic Diseases and Conditions Are on the Rise." Accessed December 15, 2020. https://www.pwc.com/gx/en/industries/healthcare/emerging-trends-pwc-healthcare/chronic-diseases.html.

Urbanet. "The World Urban Population: Infographics." August 25, 2016. https://www.urbanet.info/world-urban-population.

Chapter 1: A CLOSER LOOK AT CHRONIC DISEASE

Centers for Disease Control and Prevention. "Preventing Chronic Diseases and Reducing Health Risk Factors." Last reviewed October 25, 2013. https://www.cdc.gov/nccdphp/dch/programs/healthy communitiesprogram/overview/diseasesandrisks.htm.

Reger, M. A., I. H. Stanley, and T. E. Joiner. "Suicide Mortality and Coronavirus Disease 2019—A Perfect Storm?" *JAMA Psychiatry* 77, no. 11 (2020): 1093–94.

World Health Organization. "Overview." In *Preventing Chronic Diseases: A Vital Investment*, 1–32.

Geneva: World Health Organization, 2005. https://www.who.int/chp/chronic_disease_report/contents/en/.

Chapter 2: ALL YOU NEED TO KNOW TO START USING ESSENTIAL OILS

Bonn-Miller, M.O., M. J. E. Loflin, and B. F. Thomas. "Labeling Accuracy of Cannabidiol Extracts Sold Online." *JAMA* 318, no. 7 (2017): 1708–9.

Gill, L. L. "CBD May Be Legal, But Is It Safe?" *Consumer Reports*, April 15, 2019. https://www.consumerreports.org/cbd/cbd-may-be-legal-but-is-it-safe.

Chapter 3: PREVENTING CHRONIC DISEASE BY CREATING A HEALTHIER HOME

Agatonavic-Kustin, S., E. Kustrin, and D. W. Morton. "Essential Oils and Functional Herbs for Healthy Aging." *Neural Regeneration Research* 14, no. 3 (March 2019): 441–45.

Budson, A. E. "Does Air Pollution Cause Alzheimer's Disease?" *Harvard Health Blog*, July 23, 2020. https://www.health.harvard.edu/blog/does-air-pollution-cause-alzheimers-disease-2020072320627.

Choi, S. Y., and K. Park. "Effect of Inhalation of Aromatherapy Oil on Patients with Perennial Allergic Rhinitis: A Randomized Controlled Trial." *Evidence-Based Complementary and Alternative Medicine* 2016, no. 4 (March 13, 2016): 1–7.

Encyclopedia Britannica, s.v. "essential oil." Accessed December 15, 2020. https://www.britannica.com/topic/essential-oil.

Glassey, D. "The Vitalistic Healing Model." Pathways to Family Wellness, February 25, 2015. https://pathwaystofamilywellness.org/Holistic-Healthcare/the-vitalistic-healing-model/All-Pages.html.

Hongratanaworakit, T., and G. Buchbauer. "Evaluation of the Harmonizing Effect of Ylang Ylang Oil on Humans after Inhalation." *Planta Medica* 70, no. 7 (July 2004): 632–36.

Mahfoudhi, N., R. Ksouri, and S. Hamdi. "Nanoemulsions as Potential Delivery Systems for Bioactive Compounds in Food Systems: Preparation, Characterization, and Applications in Food Industry." In *Emulsions: Nanotechnology in the Agri-Food Industry*, vol. 3, 365–403. Boston: Academic Press, 2016.

Merriam-Webster, s.v. "adaptogen (*n.*)." Accessed December 15, 2020, https://www.merriam-webster.com/dictionary/adaptogen.

National Association for Holistic Aromatherapy. "What Is Aromatherapy?" Accessed December 15, 2020. https://naha.org/explore-aromatherapy/about-aromatherapy/what-is-aromatherapy.

Plant, J. "Effects of Essential Oils on Telomere Length in Human Cells." *Medicinal and Aromatic Plants* 5, no. 2 (January 2016).

Wu, S., K. B. Patel, L. J. Booth, et al. "Protective Essential Oil Attenuates Influenza Virus Infection: An In Vitro Study in MDCK Cells." *BMC Complementary and Alternative Medicine* 10, no. 1 (November 15, 2010): 69.

Zhao, C., Z. Xu, G.-C. Wu, et al. "Emerging Role of Air Pollution in Autoimmune Diseases." *Autoimmunity Reviews* 18, no. 6 (June 2019): 607–14.

Chapter 4: SLEEP DISORDERS AND INSOMNIA

American Sleep Association. "Sleep and Sleep Disorder Statistics." Accessed December 15, 2010. https://www.sleepassociation.org/about-sleep/sleep-statistics/.

Ariani, N. W. N. "Effect of Sandalwood Aromatherapy in Sleep Quality of Adolescents at Dharma Jati Orphanage II in the Year 2012." *Coping: Community of Publishing in Nursing* 1, no. 1 (2013).

Arzi, A., A. Green, and G. Givaty. "The Influence of Odorants on Respiratory Patterns in Sleep." *Chemical Senses* 35, no. 1 (November 2009): 31–40.

Atlantic Institute of Aromatherapy. "Blending with Rose." Accessed December 15, 2020. https://atlanticinstitute.com/blending-with-rose-2/.

Babar, A., N. A. Al-Wabel, S. Shams, et al. "Essential Oils Used in Aromatherapy: A Systemic Review." *Asian Pacific Journal of Tropical Biomedicine* 5, no. 8 (August 2015): 601–11.

Breus, M. J. "Understanding Valerian and Hops." The Sleep Doctor. June 17, 2019. https://thesleep doctor.com/2017/06/19/understanding-valerian-hops-how-valerian-and-hops-can-help-you-de -stress-relax-and-sleep-better/?cn-reloaded=1.

Centers for Disease Control and Prevention. "1 in 3 Adults Don't Get Enough Sleep." Last reviewed February 16, 2016. https://www.cdc.gov/media/releases/2016/p0215-enough-sleep.html.

Centers for Disease Control and Prevention. "Data and Statistics: Short Sleep Duration Among US Adults." Sleep and Sleep Disorders. Last reviewed May 2, 2017. https://www.cdc.gov/sleep/data _statistics.html.

Chang, Y. Y., C.-L. Lin, and L.-Y. Chang. "The Effects of Aromatherapy Massage on Sleep Quality of Nurses on Monthly Rotating Night Shifts." *Evidence-Based Complementary and Alternative Medicine* 2017, no. 1 (July 6, 2017).

Chattu, V. K., M. D. Manzar, S. Kumary, et al. "The Global Problem of Insufficient Sleep and Its Serious Public Health Implications." *Healthcare* 7, no. 1 (2019): 1.

Hafner, M., M. Stepanek, J. Taylor, et al. "Why Sleep Matters—The Economic Costs of Insufficient Sleep: A Cross-Country Comparative Analysis." *Rand Health Quarterly* 6, no. 4 (January 1, 2017): 11.

Hardy, M., M. D. Kirk-Smith, and D. D. Stretch. "Replacement of Drug Treatment for Insomnia by Ambient Odour." *The Lancet* 346, no. 8976 (September 9, 1995): 701.

Institute of Medicine (US) Committee on Sleep Medicine and Research. *Sleep Disorders and Sleep Deprivation: An Unmet Public Health Problem.* Edited by H. R. Colten and B. M. Altevogt. Washington, DC: National Academies Press, 2006.

Jager, W., G. Buchbauer, L. Jirovetz, et al. "Percutaneous Absorption of Lavender Oil from a Massage Oil." *Journal of the Society of Cosmetic Chemists* 43, no. 1 (1992): 49–54.

Keyhanmehr, A. S., M. Movahhed, S. Sahranavard, et al. "The Effect of Aromatherapy with *Rosa damascena* Essential Oil on Sleep Quality in Children." *Research Journal of Pharmacognosy* 5, no. 1 (2018): 41–46.

Kim, H.-B., S.-K. Myung, Y. C. Park, et al. "Use of Benzodiazepine and Risk of Cancer: A Meta-analysis of Observational Studies." *International Journal of Cancer* 140, no. 3 (September 2016): 513–25.

Kripke, D. F., R. D. Langer, and L. E. Kline. "Hypnotics' Association with Mortality or Cancer: A Matched Cohort Study." *British Medical Journal* 2, no. 1 (February 27, 2012): e000850.

Lally, P., C. H. M. van Jaarsveld, H. W. W. Potts, et al. "How Are Habits Formed: Modelling Habit Formation in the Real World." *European Journal of Social Psychology* 40, no. 6 (October 2010): 998–1009.

Lee, I. S., and G. J. Lee. "Effects of Lavender Aromatherapy on Insomnia and Depression in Women College Students." *Taehan Kanho Hakhoe Chi* 36, no. 1 (February 2006): 136–43.

Lillehei, A. S., and L. L. Halcon. "A Systematic Review of the Effect of Inhaled Essential Oils on Sleep." *Journal of Alternative and Complementary Medicine* 20, no. 6 (June 2014): 441–51.

Mantua, J., and R. M. C. Spencer. "Exploring the Nap Paradox: Are Mid-Day Sleep Bouts a Friend or Foe?" *Sleep Medicine* 37 (September 2017): 88–97.

Moss, M., L. Moss, K. A. Wesnes, et al. "Expectancy and the Aroma of Roman Chamomile Influence Mood and Cognition in Healthy Volunteers." *International Journal of Aromatherapy* 16, no. 2 (December 2006): 63–73.

Moss, M., S. Hewitt, L. Moss, et al. "Modulation of Cognitive Performance and Mood by Aromas of Peppermint and Ylang Ylang." *International Journal of Neuroscience* 118, no. 1 (January 2008): 59–77.

National Sleep Foundation. "National Sleep Foundation Recommends New Sleep Times." February 2, 2015. https://www.sleepfoundation.org/press-release/national-sleep-foundation-recommends-new-sleep-times.

Ohmori, A., K. Shinomiya, Y. Utsu, et al. "Effect of Santalol on the Sleep-Wake Cycle in Sleep-Disturbed Rats." *Japanese Journal of Psychopharmacology* 27, no. 4 (August 2007): 167–71.

Repasky, D. "How to Safely Put Essential Oils in Your CPAP for Aromatherapy!" CPAP.com. June 27, 2019. https://www.cpap.com/blog/essential-oils-cpap-aromatherapy/.

Suni, E. "Circadian Rhythm." Sleepfoundation.org. Last updated September 25, 2020. https://www.sleepfoundation.org/circadian-rhythm.

Taavoni, S., N. Ekabatani, M. Kashaniyan, et al. "Effect of Valerian on Sleep Quality in Postmenopausal Women: A Randomized Placebo-Controlled Clinical Trial." *Menopause* 18, no. 9 (September 2011): 951–55.

Takeda, A., W. Watanuki, and S. Koyama. "Effects of Inhalation Aromatherapy on Symptoms of Sleep Disturbance in the Elderly with Dementia." *Evidence-Based Complementary and Alternative Medicine* 2017, no. 7 (March 2017): 1–7.

Weil, A. 2010. "Can Inhaled Scents Be Harmful?" Drweil.com. October 22, 2010. https://www.drweil.com/health-wellness/balanced-living/healthy-living/can-inhaled-scents-be-harmful/.

Chapter 5: STRESS AND ANXIETY

American Psychological Association. *Stress in America: The State of Our Nation.* November 1, 2017. https://www.apa.org/news/press/releases/stress/2017/state-nation.pdf.

Bradley, B. F., S. L. Brown, S. Chu, et al. "Effects of Orally Administered Lavender Essential Oil on

Responses to Anxiety-Provoking Film Clips." *Human Psychopharmacology* 24, no. 4 (June 2009): 319–30.

Cho, M.-Y., E. S. Min, M.-H. Hur, et al. "Effects of Aromatherapy on the Anxiety, Vital Signs, and Sleep Quality of Percutaneous Coronary Intervention Patients in Intensive Care Units. *Evidence-Based Complementary and Alternative Medicine* 2013 (2013): 381381.

Choi, S. Y., P. Kang, H. S. Lee, et al. "Effects of Inhalation of Essential Oil of *Citrus aurantium* L. var. *amara* on Menopausal Symptoms, Stress, and Estrogen in Postmenopausal Women: A Randomized Controlled Trial." *Evidence-Based Complementary and Alternative Medicine* 2014, no. 2 (June 2014): 796518.

Goes, T.C., F. R. V. Ursulino, T. H. Almeida-Souza, et al. "Effect of Lemongrass Aroma on Experimental Anxiety in Humans." *Journal of Alternative and Complementary Medicine* 21, no. 12 (December 2015): 766–73.

Jafarzadeh, M., S. Arman, and F. F. Pour. "Effect of Aromatherapy with Orange Essential Oil on Salivary Cortisol and Pulse Rate in Children during Dental Treatment: A Randomized Controlled Clinical Trial." *Advanced Biomedical Research* 2, no. 1 (March 6, 2013): 10.

Kamkaen, N., N. Ruangrungsi, N. N. Patalung, et al. "Physiological and Psychological Effects of Lemongrass and Sweet Almond Massage Oil." *Journal of Health Research* 29, no. 2 (March–April 2015): 85–91.

Kheirkhah, M., N. S. V. Pour, L. Nisani, et al. "Comparing the Effects of Aromatherapy with Rose Oils and Warm Foot Bath on Anxiety in the First Stage of Labor in Nulliparous Women." *Iranian Red Crescent Medical Journal* 16, no. 9 (September 2014): e14455.

Komori, T., M. Kageyama, Y. Tamura, et al. "Anti-stress Effects of Simplified Aroma Hand Massage." *Mental Illness* 10, no. 1 (May 15, 2018): 7619.

Mohebitabar, S., M. Shirazi, S. Bioos, et al. "Therapeutic Efficacy of Rose Oil: A Comprehensive Review of Clinical Evidence." *Avicenna Journal of Phytomedicine* 7, no. 2 (May–June 2017): 206–13.

National Institute of Mental Health. "5 Things You Should Know About Stress." Accessed December 15, 2020. https://www.nimh.nih.gov/health/publications/stress/index.shtml.

Navarra, M., C. Mannucci, M. Delbò, et al. "*Citrus bergamia* Essential Oil: From Basic Research to Clinical Application." *Frontiers in Pharmacology* 6 (2015): 36.

Rashidi-Fakari, F., M. Tabatabaeichehr, and H. Mortazavi. "The Effect of Aromatherapy by Essential Oil of Orange on Anxiety during Labor: A Randomized Clinical Trial." *Iranian Journal of Nursing and Midwifery Research* 20, no. 6 (November–December 205): 661–64.

Salleh, M. R. "Life Event, Stress and Illness." *Malaysian Journal of Medical Sciences* 15, no. 4 (October 2008): 9–18.

Scholey, A., A. Gibbs, C. Neale, et al. "Anti-stress Effects of Lemon Balm–Containing Foods." *Nutrients* 6, no. 11 (November 2014): 4805–21.

Shirzadegan, R., M. Gholami, S. Hasanvand, et al. "Effects of Geranium Aroma on Anxiety among Patients with Acute Myocardial Infarction: A Triple-Blind Randomized Clinical Trial." *Complementary Therapy in Clinical Practice* 29 (November 2017): 201–6.

Swamy, M. K., and U. R. Sinniah. "A Comprehensive Review on the Phytochemical Constituents and Pharmacological Activities of *Pogostemon cablin* Benth.: An Aromatic Medicinal Plant of Industrial Importance." *Molecules* 20, no. 5 (May 2015): 8521–47.

Tisserand, R., and R. Young. *Essential Oil Safety: A Guide for Health Care Professionals.* 2nd ed., 585 and 588. London: Churchill Livingstone, 2013.

Chapter 6: DEPRESSION AND SUBSTANCE ABUSE

Abouhosseini Tabari, M., M. A. Hajizadeh, F. Maggi, et al. "Anxiolytic and Antidepressant Activities of *Pelargonium roseum* Essential Oil on Swiss Albino Mice: Possible Involvement of Serotonergic Transmission." *Phytotherapy Research* 32, no. 1 (February 2918): 1014–22.

Addiction Center. "Depression." Accessed December 15, 2020. https://www.addictioncenter.com/addiction/depression-and-addiction/.

Agatonovic-Kustrin, S., E. Kustrin, V. Gegechkori, et al. "Anxiolytic Terpenoids and Aromatherapy for Anxiety and Depression." *Advances in Experimental Medicine and Biology* 1260 (April 2020): 283–96.

American Addiction Centers. "Alcohol and Drug Abuse Statistics." Accessed October 5, 2020. https://americanaddictioncenters.org/rehab-guide/addiction-statistics.

Arpornchayanon, W., S. Chansakaow, T. Wongpakaran, et al. "Acute Effects of Essential Oil Blend Containing Phlai Oil on Mood among Healthy Male Volunteers: Randomized Controlled Trial." *Journal of Complementary and Integrative Medicine* 17, no. 2 (October 16, 2019): 20190097.

Bratskeir, K. "Can You Ever Go Off Antidepressants?" *Huffington Post.* Last updated March 5, 2019. https://www.huffpost.com/entry/going-off-antidepressants_l_5c7804cae4b0d3a48b578b9a.

Centers for Disease Control and Prevention. "Learn about Mental Health." Last reviewed January 26, 2018. https://www.cdc.gov/mentalhealth/learn/.

Chang, S. Y. "Effects of Aroma Hand Massage on Pain, State Anxiety and Depression in Hospice Patients with Terminal Cancer." *Journal of Korean Academic Medicine* 38, no. 4 (August 2008): 493–502.

Cioanca, O., L. Hritcu, M. Mihasan, et al. "Inhalation of Coriander Volatile Oil Increased Anxiolytic-Antidepressant-Like Behaviors and Decreased Oxidative Status in Beta-amyloid (1-42) Rat Model of Alzheimer's Disease." *Physiology & Behavior* 131 (May 28, 2014): 68–74.

Deng, X.-Y., H.-Y. Li, J.-J. Chen, et al. "Thymol Produces an Antidepressant-Like Effect in a Chronic Unpredictable Mild Stress Model of Depression in Mice." *Behavioural Brain Research* 291 (September 15, 2015): 12–19.

Greenfield, B. "In Recovery—from Antidepressants. How Patients Are Helping Each Other Withdraw." Yahoo Life. January 3, 2019. https://www.yahoo.com/lifestyle/recovery-antidepressants-patients-helping-withdraw-130646526.html.

Gu, S. M., S. Y. Kim, S. Lamichhane, et al. "Limonene Inhibits Methamphetamine-Induced Sensitizations via the Regulation of Dopamine Receptor Supersensitivity." *Biomolecules & Therapeutics* 27, no. 4 (July 1, 2019): 357–62.

Guzmán-Gutiérrez, S. L., H. Bonilla-Jaime, R. Gómez-Cansino, et al. "Linalool and β-Pinene Exert Their Antidepressant-Like Activity through the Monoaminergic Pathway." *Life Sciences* 128 (May 1, 2015): 24–29.

Harvard Health Publishing, Harvard Medical School. "Going Off Antidepressants." Harvard Women's Health Watch. Last updated March 25, 2020. https://www.health.harvard.edu/diseases-and-conditions/going-off-antidepressants.

Harvard Health Publishing, Harvard Medical School. "What Are the Real Risks of Antidepressants?" Last updated March 19, 2019. https://www.health.harvard.edu/mind-and-mood/what-are-the-real-risks-of-antidepressants.

Hoenen, M., K. Müller, B. Pause, et al. "Fancy Citrus, Feel Good: Positive Judgment of Citrus Odor, but Not the Odor Itself, Is Associated with Elevated Mood during Experienced Helplessness." *Frontiers in Psychology* 7 (February 2, 2016): 74.

Hongratanaworakit, T. "Relaxing Effect of Rose Oil on Humans." *National Product Communications* 4, no. 2 (February 2009): 291–96.

Kessler, R. C., M. Angermeyer, J. C. Anthony, et al. "Lifetime Prevalence and Age-of-Onset Distributions of Mental Disorders in the World Health Organization's World Mental Health Survey Initiative." *World Psychiatry* 6, no. 3 (October 2007): 168–76.

Matsumoto, T., H. Asakura, and T. Hayashi. "Effects of Olfactory Stimulation from the Fragrance of the Japanese Citrus Fruit Yuzu (*Citrus junos* Sieb. ex Tanaka) on Mood States and Salivary Chromogranin A as an Endocrinologic Stress Marker." *Journal of Alternative and Complementary Medicine* 20, no. 6 (June 1, 2014): 500–6.

Matsumoto, T., T. Kimura, and T. Hayashi. "Aromatic Effects of a Japanese Citrus Fruit—Yuzu (*Citrus junos* Sieb. ex Tanaka)—on Psychoemotional States and Autonomic Nervous System Activity during the Menstrual Cycle: A Single-Blind Randomized Controlled Crossover Study." *BioPsychoSocial Medicine* 10 (April 21, 2016): 11.

National Alliance on Mental Illness. "Substance Use Disorders." Reviewed May 2020. https://www.nami.org/About-Mental-Illness/Common-with-Mental-Illness/Substance-Use-Disorders.

National Health Service. "Side Effects: Antidepressants." Last reviewed August 16, 2018. https://www.nhs.uk/conditions/antidepressants/side-effects.

National Institute on Drug Abuse. "Comorbidity: Addiction and Other Mental Illnesses." US Department of Health and Human Services, National Institutes of Health. Last revised September 2010. https://www.drugabuse.gov/sites/default/files/rrcomorbidity.pdf.

National Institute on Drug Abuse. "Drug Abuse and Addiction: One of America's Most Challenging Public Health Problems." Accessed December 15, 2020. https://archives.drugabuse.gov/publications/drug-abuse-addiction-one-americas-most-challenging-public-health-problems/addiction-chronic-disease.

National Institute of Mental Health. "Suicide." Last updated September 2020. https://www.nimh.nih.gov/health/statistics/suicide.shtml.

Nazıroğlu, M., S. Kozlu, E. Yorgancıgil, et al. "Rose Oil (from *Rosa × damascena* Mill.) Vapor Attenuates Depression-Induced Oxidative Toxicity in Rat Brain." *Journal of Natural Medicines* 67, no. 1 (January 2013): 152–58.

Nikfar, S., and A. F. Behboudi. "Limonene." In *Encyclopedia of Toxicology*, 3rd ed., 78–82. Cambridge, MA: Academic Press, 2014.

Nutt, D., and L. Nestor. *Addiction.* 2nd ed. Oxford, UK: Oxford University Press, 2018.

Piccinelli, A. C., J. A. Santos, E. C. Konkiewitz, et al. "Antihyperalgesic and Antidepressive Actions of (R)-(+)-Limonene, α-phellandrene, and Essential Oil from *Schinus terebinthifolius* Fruits in a Neuropathic Pain Model." *Nutritional Neuroscience* 18, no. 5 (July 2015): 217–24.

Ritchie, H., and M. Roser. "Drug Use." Our World in Data. December 2019. https://ourworldindata.org/drug-use.

Rose, J. E., and F. M. Behm. "Inhalation of Vapor from Black Pepper Extract Reduces Smoking Withdrawal Symptoms." *Drug and Alcohol Dependence* 34, no. 3 (February 1994): 225–29.

Sasaki, K., A. El Omri, S. Konjo, et al. "*Rosmarinus officinalis* Polyphenols Produce Anti-depressant Like Effect through Monoaminergic and Cholinergic Functions Modulation." *Behavioural Brain Research* 238 (February 2013): 86–94.

Seol, G. H., H. S. Shim, P.-J. Kim, et al. "Antidepressant-Like Effect of *Salvia sclarea* Is Explained by Modulation of Dopamine Activities in Rats." *Journal of Ethnopharmacology* 130, no. 1 (July 6, 2010): 187–90.

Setzer, W. N. "Essential Oils and Anxiolytic Aromatherapy." *National Product Communications* 4, no. 9 (September 2009): 1305–16.

Sun, J. "D-Limonene: Safety and Clinical Applications." *Alternative Medicine Review* 12, no. 3 (September 2007): 259–64.

Tan, L. T. H., L. H. Lee, W. F. Yin, et al. "Traditional Uses, Phytochemistry, and Bioactivities of *Cananga odorata* (Ylang Ylang)." *Evidence Based Complementary and Alternative Medicine* 2015, no. 4 (August 2015): 896314.

US National Library of Medicine. "Living with a Chronic Illness—Reaching Out to Others." Medline Plus. Reviewed August 4, 2018. https://medlineplus.gov/ency/patientinstructions/000602.htm.

Villareal, M. O., A. Ikeya, K. Sasaki, et al. "Anti-stress and Neuronal Cell Differentiation Induction Effects of *Rosmarinus officinalis* L. Essential Oil." *BMC Complementary Medicine and Therapies* 17, no. 1 (December 22, 2017): 549.

Voinov, B., W. D. Richie, and R. K. Bailey. "Depression and Chronic Diseases: It Is Time for a Synergistic Mental Health and Primary Care Approach." *Primary Care Companion for CNS Disorders* 15, no. 2 (2013): PCC. 12r01468.

World Health Organization. "Depression." January 30, 2020. https://www.who.int/news-room/fact-sheets/detail/depression.

Zhang, L.-L., Z.-Y. Yang, G. Fan, et al. "Antidepressant-Like Effect of *Citrus sinensis* (L.) Osbeck Essential Oil and Its Main Component Limonene on Mice." *Journal of Agricultural and Food Chemistry* 67, no. 50 (March 24, 2019): 13817–28.

Chapter 7: CHRONIC FATIGUE SYNDROME AND FIBROMYALGIA

Ahmadifard M., S. Yarahmadi, A. Ardalan, et al. "The Efficacy of Topical Basil Essential Oil on Relieving Migraine Headaches: A Randomized Triple-Blind Study." *Complementary Medicine Research* 27, no. 5 (2020): 310–18.

Batista, P.A., M. F. Werner, E. C. Oliviera, et al. "The Antinociceptive Effect of (-)-Linalool in Models of Chronic Inflammatory and Neuropathic Hypersensitivity in Mice." *Journal of Pain* 11, no. 11 (November 2010):1222–29.

Felman, A. "Everything You Need to Know about Fibromyalgia." Medical News Today. January 5, 2018. https://www.medicalnewstoday.com/articles/147083.

Friedberg, F., N. Tintle, J. Clark, et al. "Prolonged Fatigue in Ukraine and the United States: Prevalence and Risk Factors." *Fatigue: Biomedicine, Health & Behavior* 3, no. 1 (2015): 33–46.

Fries, E., J. Hesse, J. Hellhammer, et al. "A New View on Hypocortisolism." *Psychoneuroendocrinology* 30, no. 10 (November 2005): 1010–16.

Han, C., F. Li, S. Tian, et al. "Beneficial Effect of Compound Essential Oil Inhalation on Central Fatigue." *BMC Complementary and Alternative Medicine* 18, no. 1 (November 26, 2018): 309.

Healthy Women. "Chronic Fatigue Syndrome." Accessed December 15, 2020. https://www.healthy women.org/condition/chronic-fatigue-syndrome/overview.

John Hopkins Medicine. "Forgiveness: Your Health Depends on It." Accessed December 15, 2020. https://www.hopkinsmedicine.org/health/wellness-and-prevention/forgiveness-your-health -depends-on-it.

Ko, G. D., A. Hum, G. Traitses, et al. "Effects of Topical O24 Essential Oils on Patients with Fibromyalgia Syndrome: A Randomized, Placebo Controlled Pilot Study." *Journal of Musculoskeletal Pain* 15, no. 1 (2007): 1, 11–19.

Marchese, A., I. E. Orhan, M. Daglia, et al. "Antibacterial and Antifungal Activities of Thymol: A Brief Review of the Literature." *Food Chemistry* 210 (November 2016): 402–14.

Mayo Clinic. "Fibromyalgia." Accessed December 15, 2020. https://www.mayoclinic.org/diseases -conditions/fibromyalgia/symptoms-causes/syc-20354780.

Meamarbashi A. "Instant Effects of Peppermint Essential Oil on the Physiological Parameters and Exercise Performance." *Avicenna Journal of Phytomedicine* 4, no. 1 (January–February 2014): 72–78.

Miller, L., and L. Sperry. "A Forgiveness Intervention for Women with Fibromyalgia Who Were Abused in Childhood: A Pilot Study." *Spirituality in Clinical Practice* 1, no. 3 (September 2014): 203–17.

Nascimento, S. S., A. S. A. Araújo, R. G. Brito, et al. "Cyclodextrin-Complexed *Ocimum basilicum* Leaves Essential Oil Increases Fos Protein Expression in the Central Nervous System and Produce an Antihyperalgesic Effect in Animal Models for Fibromyalgia." *International Journal of Molecular Science* 16, no. 1 (December 2019): 547–63.

Nascimento, S. S., E. A. Camargo, J. M. DeSantana, et al. "Linalool and Linalool Complexed in β-Cyclodextrin Produce Anti-hyperalgesic Activity and Increase Fos Protein Expression in Animal Model for Fibromyalgia." *Naunyn Schmiedeberg's Archives of Pharmacology* 387, no. 10 (June 2014): 935–42.

Price, S., and L. Price. *Aromatherapy for Health Professionals*. 4th ed., 102. London: Churchill Livingstone, 2012.

Riva, R., P. J. Mork, R. H. Westgaard, et al. "Fibromyalgia Syndrome Is Associated with Hypocortisolism." *International Journal of Behavioral Medicine* 17 (2010): 223–33.

Saiyudthong, S., and C. Marsden. "Acute Effects of Bergamot Oil on Anxiety-Related Behaviour and Corticosterone Level in Rats. *Phytotherapy Research* 25, no. 6 (June 2011): 858–62.

Sayorwan, W., N. Ruangrungsi. T. Piriyapunyporn, et al. "Effects of Inhaled Rosemary Oil on Subjective Feelings and Activities of the Nervous System." *Science Pharmaceutica* 81, no. 2 (April–June 2013): 531–42.

Toussaint, L., M. Overvold-Ronningen, A. Vincent, et al. "Implications of Forgiveness Enhancement in Patients with Fibromyalgia and Chronic Fatigue Syndrome." *Journal of Health Care Chaplaincy* 16, nos. 3–4 (2010): 123–39.

Tsubanova, N., T. Sevastyanova, E. Tsubanova, et al. "Aromatherapy with Essential Oils Treating Chronic Fatigue Syndrome." *Cyberlininka*. https://cyberleninka.ru/article/n/aromatherapy-with-essential-oils-treating-chronic-fatigue-syndrome.

US Department of Health and Human Services. "Autoimmune Diseases." Office on Women's Health. Last updated April 1, 2019. https://www.womenshealth.gov/a-z-topics/autoimmune-diseases.

Varney, E., and J. Buckle. "Effect of Inhaled Essential Oils on Mental Exhaustion and Moderate Burnout: A Small Pilot Study." *Journal of Alternative and Complementary Medicine* 19, no. 1 (January 2013): 69–71.

Watanabe, E., K. Kuchta, M. Kimura, et al. "Effects of Bergamot (*Citrus bergamia* (Risso) Wright & Arn.) Essential Oil Aromatherapy on Mood States, Parasympathetic Nervous System Activity, and Salivary Cortisol Levels in 41 Healthy Females." *Forsch Komplementmed* 22, no. 1 (February 2015): 43–49.

Wilson, J. L. "Adrenal Function in Chronic Fatigue Syndrome and Fibromyalgia." Presented at American College of Apothecaries, Wellness and Nutrition Solution Conference, Chicago, IL, May 4–6, 2017.

Chapter 8: LIBIDO AND ERECTILE DYSFUNCTION

Aleissa, M. "Effect of Ginger Supplements on Some Reproductive Parameters and Spermatogenesis of Mice." *Indian Journal of Fundamental and Applied Life Sciences* 4, no. 1 (January–March 2014): 271–77.

Bailey, E. "The Smell of Pumpkin Pie May Be Good for Your Sex Life." Health Central. November 14, 2012. https://www.healthcentral25:.com/article/the-smell-of-pumpkin-pie-may-be-good-for-your-sex-life.

Chen, L.-R., N.-Y. Ko, and K.-H. Chen. "Medical Treatment for Osteoporosis: From Molecular to Clinical Opinions." *International Journal of Molecular Sciences* 20, no. 9 (May 6, 2019): 2213.

Choi, S. Y., P. Kang, H. S. Lee, et al. "Effects of Inhalation of Essential Oil of *Citrus aurantium* L. var. *amara* on Menopausal Symptoms, Stress, and Estrogen in Postmenopausal Women: A Randomized Controlled Trial." *Evidence-Based Complementary and Alternative Medicine* 2014, no. 2 (June 2014): 796518.

De Pietro, MaryAnn. "What Happens When Estrogen Levels Are Low?" Medical News Today. February 27, 2018. https://www.medicalnewstoday.com/articles/321064#causes.

Farnia, V., M. Shirzadir, J. Shakeri, et al. "*Rosa damascena* Oil Improves SSRI-Induced Sexual Dysfunction in Male Patients Suffering from Major Depressive Disorders: Results from a Double-Blind, Randomized, and Placebo-Controlled Clinical Trial." *Neuropsychiatric Disease and Treatment* 11 (March 9, 2015): 625–35.

Ghannadi, A., F. Jaffary, and H. Najafzadeh. "Evaluation of the Prophylactic Effect of Fennel Essential Oil on Experimental Osteoporosis Model in Rat." *International Journal of Pharmacology* 2, no. 5 (2006): 588–92.

Gilhooly, P. E., J. E. Ottenweller, G. Lange, et al. "Chronic Fatigue and Sexual Dysfunction in Female Gulf War Veterans." *Journal of Sex and Marital Therapy* 27, no. 5 (2001): 483–87.

Holt, S. "Natural Approaches to Promote Sexual Function, Part 2: Stimulants and Dietary Supplements." *Alternative and Complementary Therapies* 5, no. 5 (August 2009): 279–85.

Hongratanaworakit, T. "Stimulating Effect of Aromatherapy Massage with Jasmine Oil." *National Product Communications* 5, no. 1 (January 2010): 157–62.

Khadivzadeh, T., M. N. Najafi, M. Ghazanfarpour, et al. "Aromatherapy for Sexual Problems in Menopausal Women: A Systematic Review and Meta-analysis." *Journal of Menopausal Medicine* 24, no. 1 (April 2018): 56–61.

Lee, K.-B., Y.-S. Kang, and E. Cho. "Changes in 5-Hydroxytryptamine and Cortisol Plasma Levels in Menopausal Women after Inhalation of Clary Sage Oil." *Phytotherapy Research* 28, no. 11 (November 2014): 1599–605.

Roozbeh, N., M. Ghazanfarpour, T. Khadivzadeh, et al. "Effect of Lavender on Sleep, Sexual Desire, Vasomotor, Psychological and Physical Symptom among Menopausal and Elderly Women: A Systematic Review." *Journal of Menopausal Medicine* 25, no. 2 (August 2019): 88–93.

Shiri, R., J. Koskimämi, M. Hakama, et al. "Effect of Chronic Diseases on Incidence of Erectile Dysfunction." *Urology* 62, no. 6 (December 1, 2003): 1097–102.

Slashdot. "Pumpkin Pie Increases Male Sex Drive." Accessed December 15, 2020. https://science.slashdot.org/story/10/11/23/1523245/pumpkin-pie-increases-male-sex-drive.

Tajuddin, A. S., S. Ahmad, A. Latif, et al. "Aphrodisiac Activity of 50% Ethanolic Extracts of *Myristica fragrans* Houtt. (Nutmeg) and *Syzygium aromaticum* (L) Merr. & Perry. (Clove) in Male Mice: A Comparative Study." *BMC Complementary and Alternative Medicine* 3, no. 1 (October 2003): 6.

WebMD. "Fibromyalgia and Sex." Last reviewed June 16, 2020. https://www.webmd.com/fibromyalgia/guide/fibromyalgia-and-sex#1.

Chapter 9: ALZHEIMER'S AND DEMENTIA

Agatonovic-Kustrin, S., E. Kustrin, and D. W. Morton. "Essential Oils and Functional Herbs for Healthy Aging." *Neural Regeneration Research* 14, no. 3 (March 2019): 441–45.

Ali, T. B., T. R. Schleret, B. M. Reilly, et al. "Adverse Effects of Cholinesterase Inhibitors in Dementia, According to the Pharmacovigilance Databases of the United-States and Canada." *PloS One* 10, no. 12 (December 2015): e0144337.

Alzheimer's Association (US). "What Is Dementia?" Accessed December 16, 2020. https://www.alz .org/alzheimers-dementia/what-is-dementia.

Alzheimer's Society (UK). "How Do Drugs for Alzheimer's Disease Work?" Accessed December 16, 2020. https://www.alzheimers.org.uk/about-dementia/treatments/drugs/how-do-drugs-alzheimers -disease-work.

Amiresmaeili, A., S. Roohollahi, A. Mostafavi, et al. "Effects of Oregano Essential Oil on Brain TLR4 and TLR2 Gene Expression and Depressive-Like Behavior in a Rat Model." *Research in Pharmaceutical Sciences* 13, no. 2 (April 2018): 130–41.

Asadbegi, M., P. Yaghmaei, I. Salehi, et al. "Investigation of Thymol Effect on Learning and Memory Impairment Induced by Intrahippocampal Injection of Amyloid Beta Peptide in High Fat Diet–Fed Rats." *Metabolic Brain Disease* 32, no. 3 (June 2017): 827–39.

Ayaz, M., A. Sadiq, M, Junaid, et al. "Neuroprotective and Anti-Aging Potentials of Essential Oils from Aromatic and Medicinal Plants." *Frontiers in Aging Neuroscience* 9 (May 2017): 168. https:// www.frontiersin.org/articles/10.3389/fnagi.2017.00168/full.

Ballard, C. G., J. T. O'Brien, K. Reichelt, et al. "Aromatherapy as a Safe and Effective Treatment for the Management of Agitation in Severe Dementia: The Results of a Double-Blind, Placebo-Controlled Trial with Melissa." *Journal of Clinical Psychiatry* 63, no. 7 (July 2002): 553–58.

Bonesi, M., F. Menichini, R. Tundis, et al. "Acetylcholinesterase and Butyrylcholinesterase Inhibitory Activity of *Pinus* Species Essential Oils and Their Constituents." *Journal of Enzyme and Inhibition Medicinal Chemistry* 25, no. 5 (July 2009): 622–28.

Chaiyana, W., and S. Okonogi. "Inhibition of Cholinesterase by Essential Oil from Food Plant." *Phytomedicine* 19, nos. 8–9 (April 2012): 836–39.

Chen, M., Y.-Y. Chang, S. Huang, et al. "Aromatic-Turmerone Attenuates LPS-Induced Neuroinflammation and Consequent Memory Impairment by Targeting TLR4-Dependent Signaling Pathway." *Molecular Nutrition & Food Research* 62, no. 2 (January 2018). https://doi/abs/10.1002/ mnfr.201700281.

Cioanca, O., M. Hăncianu, C. Mircea, et al. "Essential Oils from Apiaceae as Valuable Resources in Neurological Disorders: *Foeniculi vulgare aetheroleum*." *Industrial Crops and Products* 88 (October 2016): 51–57.

Cioanca, O., L. Hritcu, M. Mihasan, et al. "Inhalation of Coriander Volatile Oil Increased Anxiolytic–Antidepressant-Like Behaviors and Decreased Oxidative Status in Beta-Amyloid (1-42) Rat Model of Alzheimer's Disease." *Physiology & Behavior* 131 (May 2014): 68–74.

Encyclopedia.com. "Cholinesterase Inhibitors: Definition." Last updated December 2, 2020. https://www.encyclopedia.com/science-and-technology/biochemistry/biochemistry/cholinesterase.

Eriksson, P. S., E. Perfilieva, T. Björk-Eriksson, et al. "Neurogenesis in the Adult Human Hippocampus." *Nature Medicine* 4 (November 1998): 1313–17.

Fox, M., L. A. Knapp, P. W. Andrews, et al. "Hygiene and the World Distribution of Alzheimer's Disease: Epidemiological Evidence for a Relationship between Microbial Environment and Age-Adjusted Disease Burden." *Evolution, Medicine, and Public Health* 2013, no. 1 (January 2013): 173–86.

Haze, S., K. Seiko, and Y. Gozu. "Effects of Fragrance Inhalation on Sympathetic Activity in Normal Adults." *Japanese Journal of Pharmacology* 90, no. 3 (November 2002): 247–53.

Hucklenbroich, J., R. Klein, B. Neumaier, et al. "Aromatic-Turmerone Induces Neural Stem Cell Proliferation *In Vitro* and *In Vivo*." *Stem Cell Research & Therapy* 5, no. 4 (September 2014): 100.

Jimbo, D., Y. Kimura, M. Taniguchi, et al. "Effect of Aromatherapy on Patients with Alzheimer's Disease." *Psychogeriatrics* 9, no. 4 (December 2009): 173–79.

Jukic, M., O. Politeo, M. Maksimovic, et al. "*In Vitro* Acetylcholinesterase Inhibitory Properties of Thymol, Carvacrol and Their Derivatives Thymoquinone and Thymohydroquinone." *Phytotherapy Research* 21, no. 3 (March 2007): 259–61.

Kennedy, D., E. Okello, P. Chazot, et al. "Volatile Terpenes and Brain Function: Investigation of the Cognitive and Mood Effects of *Mentha × piperita* L. Essential Oil with In Vitro Properties Relevant to Central Nervous System Function." *Nutrients* 10, no. 8 (August 2018): 1029.

Kiendrebeogo, M., A. Y. Coulibaly, R. C. H. Nebie, et al. "Antiacetylcholinesterase and Antioxidant Activity of Essential Oils from Six Medicinal Plants from Burkina Faso." *Revista Brasileira de Farmacognosia* 21, no. 1 (January–February 2011): 63–69.

Lee, C., G. H. Park, C. Y. Kim, et al. "[6]-Gingerol Attenuates β-Amyloid-Induced Oxidative Cell Death via Fortifying Cellular Antioxidant Defense System." *Food and Chemical Toxicology* 49, no. 6 (March 2011): 1261–69.

Lee, S. Y. "The Effect of Lavender Aromatherapy on Cognitive Function, Emotion, and Aggressive Behavior of Elderly with Dementia." *Taehan Kanho Hakhoe Chi* 35, no. 2 (April 2005): 303–12.

Loizzo, M. R., F. Menichini, R. Tundis, et al. "In Vitro Biological Activity of *Salvia leriifolia* Benth Essential Oil Relevant to the Treatment of Alzheimer's Disease." *Journal of Oleo Science* 58, no. 8 (2009): 443–46.

Moss, M., L. Moss, K. A. Wesnes, et al. "Modulation of Cognitive Performance and Mood by Aromas and Peppermint and Ylang Ylang." *International Journal of Neuroscience* 118, no. 1 (February 2008): 59–77.

Moss, M., and L. Oliver. "Plasma 1,8-Cineole Correlates with Cognitive Performance Following Exposure to Rosemary Essential Oil Aroma." *Therapeutic Advances in Psychopharmacology* 2, no. 3 (June 2012): 103–13.

Perry, N., G. Court, N. Bidet, et al. "European Herbs with Cholinergic Activities: Potential in Dementia Therapy." *Geriatric Psychiatry* 11, no. 12 (December 1996): 1063–69.

Perry, N. S. L., J. Sampson, P. Houghton, et al. 2001. "In-Vitro Activity of *S. lavandulaefolia* (Spanish Sage) Relevant to Treatment of Alzheimer's Disease." *Journal of Pharmacy and Pharmacology* 53, no. 10 (October 2001): 1347–56.

Peters, J. M., T. Kratzsch, T. Hummel, et al. "Olfactory Function in Mild Cognitive Impairment and Alzheimer's Disease: An Investigation Using Psychophysical and Electrophysiological Techniques." *American Journal of Psychiatry* 60, no. 11 (December 2003): 1995–2002.

Price, S., and L. Price. *Aromatherapy for Health Professionals.* 4th ed., 265–68, 292. London: Churchill Livingstone, 2012.

Sabogal-Guáqueta, A. M., E. Osaorio, and G. P. Cardona-Gómez. "Linalool Reverses Neuropathological and Behavioral Impairments in Old Triple Transgenic Alzheimer's Mice." *Neuropharmacology* 102 (March 2016): 111–20.

Science Daily. "Meditation May Help Slow Progression of Alzheimer's Disease." November 18, 2013. https://www.sciencedaily.com/releases/2013/11/131118141817.htm.

Scuteri, D., L. A. Morrone, L. Rombolà, et al. "Aromatherapy and Aromatic Plants for the Treatment of Behavioural and Psychological Symptoms of Dementia in Patients with Alzheimer's Disease: Clinical Evidence and Possible Mechanisms." *Evidence-Based Complementary and Alternative Medicine* 2017, no. 6 (March 2017): 1–8.

Shytle, R. D., P. C. Bickford, K. Rezai-zedeh, et al. "Optimized Turmeric Extracts Have Potent Anti-amyloidogenic Effects." *Current Alzheimer Research* 6, no. 6 (December 2009): 564–71.

Snow, L. A., L. Hovanec, and J. Brandt. "A Controlled Trial of Aromatherapy for Agitation in Nursing Home Patients with Dementia." *Journal of Alternative and Complementary Medicine* 10, no. 3 (June 2004): 431–37.

Solomon, H. "The Therapeutic Potential of Rosemary (*Rosmarinus officinalis*) Diterpenes for Alzheimer's Disease." *Evidence-Based Complementary and Alternative Medicine* 2016, no. 6 (January 28, 2016): 1–14.

Tepe, A. S., and M. Ozaslan. "Anti-Alzheimer, Anti-diabetic, Skin-whitening, and Antioxidant Activities of the Essential Oil of *Cinnamomum zeylanicum*." *Industrial Crops and Products* 145 (March 2020): 112069.

Tisserand, R., and R. Young. *Essential Oil Safety: A Guide for Health Care Professionals.* 2nd ed., 517. London: Churchill Livingstone, 2013.

Tundis, R., M. R. Loizzo, M. Bonesi, et al. "Comparative Study on the Antioxidant Capacity and Cholinesterase Inhibitory Activity of *Citrus aurantifolia* Swingle, *C. aurantium* L., and *C. bergamia* Risso and Poit. Peel Essential Oils." *Journal of Food Science* 77, no. 1 (January 2012): H40–46.

Wang, P., Q. Luo, H. Qiao, et al. "The Neuroprotective Effects of Carvacrol on Ethanol-Induced Hippocampal Neurons Impairment via the Antioxidative and Antiapoptotic Pathways." *Oxidative Medicine and Cellular Longevity* 2017, no. 5 (January 2017): 1–17.

Yegambaram, M., B. Manivannan, T. G. Beach, et al. "Role of Environmental Contaminants in the Etiology of Alzheimer's Disease: A Review." *Current Alzheimer Research* 12, no. 2 (February 2015): 116–46.

Yu, H., Z.-L. Zhang, J. Chen, et al. "Carvacrol, a Food-Additive, Provides Neuroprotection on Focal Cerebral Ischemia/Reperfusion Injury in Mice." *PloS One* 7, no. 3 (March 2012): e33584.

Zhou, W., S. Fukumoto, and H. Yokogoshi. "Components of Lemon Essential Oil Attenuate Dementia Induced by Scopolamine." *Nutritional Neuroscience* 12, no. 2 (April 2009): 57–64.

Zotti, M., M. Colaianna, M. G. Morgese, et al. "Carvacrol: From Ancient Flavoring to Neuromodulatory Agent." *Molecules* 18, no. 6 (May 2013): 6161–72.

Chapter 10: BONE AND JOINT DISORDERS

Adam, B., J. Best, L. Bechmann, et al. "A Combination of Peppermint Oil and Caraway Oil Attenuates the Post-Inflammatory Visceral Hyperalgesia in a Rat Model." *Scandinavian Journal of Gastroenterology* 41, no. 2 (March 2006): 155–60.

American College of Rheumatology. "Fractures Can Lead to Premature Death in Older People." *Science Daily*. November 8, 2015. https://www.sciencedaily.com/releases/2015/11/151108084919.htm.

Ames-Sibin, A. P., C. L. Barizão, C. V. Castro-Ghizoni, et al. "β-Caryophyllene, the Major Constituent of Copaiba Oil, Reduces Systemic Inflammation and Oxidative Stress in Arthritic Rats." *Journal of Cellular Biochemistry* 119, no. 12 (December 2012): 10262–77.

Burns, E., and R. Kakara. "Deaths from Falls Among Persons Aged ≥65 Years—United States, 2007–2016." *Morbidity and Mortality Weekly Report* 67, no. 18 (May 2018): 509–14.

Cardia, G. F. E., S. E. Silva-Filho, E. L. Silva, et al. "Effect of Lavender (*Lavandula angustifolia*) Essential Oil on Acute Inflammatory Response." *Evidence-Based Complementary and Alternative Medicine* 2018, no. 2 (March 2018): 1–10.

Castro Ghizoni, C. V., A. P. A. Ames, O. A. Lameira, et al. "Anti-inflammatory and Antioxidant Actions of Copaiba Oil Are Related to Liver Cell Modifications in Arthritic Rats." *Journal of Cellular Biochemistry* 118, no. 10 (October 2017): 3409–23.

Centers for Disease Control and Prevention. "Deaths from Older Adult Falls." Home and Recreational Safety. Last reviewed July 9, 2020. https://www.cdc.gov/homeandrecreationalsafety/falls/data/deaths-from-falls.html.

Dolder, S., W. Hofstetter, A. Wetterwald, et al. "Effect of Monoterpenes on the Formation and Activation of Osteoclasts In Vitro." *Journal of Bone and Mineral Research* 21, no. 4 (April 2006): 647–55.

Elbahnasawy, A. S., E. R. Valleeva, E. M. El-Sayed, et al. "The Impact of Thyme and Rosemary on Prevention of Osteoporosis in Rats." *Journal of Nutrition and Metabolism* 2019, no. 11 (March 31, 2019): 1–10.

Filho, L. S. F., G. K. M. de Almeida, I. Couto, et al. "Therapeutic Ultrasound Associated with Copaiba Oil Reduces Pain and Improves Range of Motion in Patients with Knee Osteoarthritis." *Fisioterapia em Movimento* 30, no. 3 (September 2017): 443–51.

Han, X., D. Rodriguez, and T. L. Parker. "Biological Activities of Frankincense Essential Oil in Human Dermal Fibroblasts." *Biochimie Open* 4 (June 2017): 31–35.

Harvard Health Publishing, Harvard Medical School. "Osteopenia: When You Have Weak Bones, but

Not Osteoporosis." Last updated July 6, 2020. https://www.health.harvard.edu/womens-health/osteopenia-when-you-have-weak-bones-but-not-osteoporosis.

Hebert, P. R., E. J. Barice, and C. H. Hennekens. "Treatment of Low Back Pain: The Potential Clinical and Public Health Benefits of Topical Herbal Remedies." *Journal of Alternative and Complementary Medicine* 20, no. 4 (April 2014): 219–20.

Hibler, E. A., J. Kauderer, M. H. Greene, et al. "Bone Loss after Oophorectomy among High-Risk Women: An NRG Oncology/Gynecologic Oncology Group Study." *Menopause* 23, no. 11 (November 2016): 1228–32.

Jaffary, F., A. Ghannadi, and H. Najafzadeh. "Evaluation of the Prophylactic Effect of Fennel Essential Oil on Experimental Osteoporosis Model in Rats." *International Journal of Pharmacology* 2, no. 5 (2006): 588–92.

Kheirouri, S., V. Hadi, and M. Alizadeh. "Immunomodulatory Effect of *Nigella sativa* Oil on T Lymphocytes in Patients with Rheumatoid Arthritis." *Immunological Investigations* 45, no. 4 (May 2016): 271–83.

Kim, M.-J., E.-S. Nam, and S.-I. Paik. "The Effects of Aromatherapy on Pain, Depression, and Life Satisfaction of Arthritis Patients." *Journal of the Korean Academy of Nursing* 35, no. 1 (February 2005): 18694.

Li, X.-J., Y.-S. Li, W. K. Zhang, et al. "α-Pinene, Linalool, and 1-Octanol Contribute to the Topical Anti-Inflammatory and Analgesic Activities of Frankincense by Inhibiting COX-2." *Journal of Ethnopharmacology* 179 (February 2016): 22–26.

Li, X.-J., Z. Zue, S.-L. Han, et al. "Bergapten Exerts Inhibitory Effects on Diabetes-Related Osteoporosis via the Regulation of the PI3K/AKT, JNK/MAPK and NF-$\varkappa$B Signaling Pathways in Osteoprotegerin Knockout Mice." *International Journal of Molecular Medicine* 38, no. 6 (December 2016): 1661–72.

Mahboubi, M., L. M. T. Kashani, and M. Mahboubi. "*Nigella sativa* Fixed Oil as Alternative Treatment in Management of Pain in Arthritis Rheumatoid." *Phytomedicine* 46 (July 2018): 69–77.

Mühlbauer, R.C., A. Lozano, S. Palacio, et al. "Common Herbs, Essential Oils, and Monoterpenes Potently Modulate Bone Metabolism." *Bone* 32, no. 4 (April 2003): 372–80.

Nasiri, A., M. A. Mahmodi, and Z. Nobakht. "Effect of Aromatherapy Massage with Lavender Essential Oil on Pain in Patients with Osteoarthritis of the Knee: A Randomized Controlled Clinical Trial." *Complementary Therapies in Clinical Practice* 25 (November 2016): 75–80.

National Council on Aging. "Fall Prevention Facts." Accessed December 16, 2020. https://www.ncoa.org/news/resources-for-reporters/get-the-facts/falls-prevention-facts.

NIH Osteoporosis and Related Bone Diseases National Resource Center. "What People with Rheumatoid Arthritis Need to Know About Osteoporosis." Last reviewed November 2018. https://www.bones.nih.gov/health-info/bone/osteoporosis/conditions-behaviors/osteoporosis-ra.

Perna, S., D. Spadaccini, L. Botteri, et al. "Efficacy of Bergamot: From Anti-inflammatory and Anti-oxidative Mechanisms to Clinical Applications as Preventive Agent for Cardiovascular Morbidity, Skin Diseases, and Mood Alterations." *Food Science & Nutrition* 7, no. 2 (January 2019): 369–84.

Putnam, S. E., A. M. Scutt, K. Bicknell, et al. "Natural Products as Alternative Treatments for Metabolic Bone Disorders and for Maintenance of Bone Health." *Phytotherapy Research* 21, no. 2 (February 2007): 99–112.

Shoara, R., M. H. Hashempur, A. Ashraf, et al. "Efficacy and Safety of Topical *Matricaria chamomilla* L. (Chamomile) Oil for Knee Osteoarthritis: A Randomized Controlled Clinical Trial." *Complementary Therapies in Clinical Practice* 21, no. 3 (August 2015): 181–87.

Stanmore, E. K., J. Oldham, D. A. Skelton, et al. "Risk Factors for Falls in Adults with Rheumatoid Arthritis: A Prospective Study." *Arthritis Care & Research* 65, no. 8 (August 2013): 1251–58.

Tisserand, R., and R. Young. *Essential Oil Safety: A Guide for Health Care Professionals.* 2nd ed., 469. London: Churchill Livingstone, 2013.

US Food and Drug Administration. "FDA Drug Safety Communication: FDA Strengthens Warning that Non-aspirin Nonsteroidal Anti-Inflammatory Drugs (NSAIDs) Can Cause Heart Attacks or Strokes." Last updated February 26, 2018. https://www.fda.gov/drugs/drug-safety-and-availability/fda-drug-safety-communication-fda-strengthens-warning-non-aspirin-nonsteroidal-anti-inflammatory.

UW Health. "Rheumatoid Arthritis: Systemic Symptoms." Accessed December 16, 2020. https://patient.uwhealth.org/healthwise/article/aa19294.

Weaver, C. M., D. L. Alekel, W. E. Ward, et al. "Flavonoid Intake and Bone Health." *Journal of Nutrition in Gerontology and Geriatrics* 31, no. 3 (2012): 239–53.

World Health Organization. "Chronic Rheumatic Conditions." Accessed December 16, 2020. https://www.who.int/chp/topics/rheumatic/en.

World Health Organization. "Falls." January 16, 2018. https://www.who.int/news-room/fact-sheets/detail/falls.

Chapter 11: CANCER SUPPORT

Alammar, N., L. Wang, B. Saberi, et al. "The Impact of Peppermint Oil on the Irritable Bowel Syndrome: A Meta-analysis of the Pooled Clinical Data." *BMC Complementary and Alternative Medicine* 19, no. 1 (January 2019): 21.

Blowman, K., M. F. L. Lemos, M. Magalhäes, et al. "Anticancer Properties of Essential Oils and Other Natural Products." *Evidence-Based Complementary and Alternative Medicine* 2018, no. 7 (March 2018): 1–12.

Cancer Research UK. "1 in 2 People in the UK Will Get Cancer." February 4, 2015. https://www.cancerresearchuk.org/about-us/cancer-news/press-release/2015-02-04-1-in-2-people-in-the-uk-will-get-cancer.

Dimas, K., D. Kokkinopoulos, C. Demetzos, et al. "The Effect of Sclareol on Growth and Cell Cycle Progression of Human Leukemic Cell Lines." *Leukemia Research* 23, no. 3 (March 1999): 217–34.

Dimas, K., S. Hatziantoniou, S. Tseleni, et al. "Sclareol Induces Apoptosis in Human HCT116 Colon Cancer Cells in Vitro and Suppression of HCT116 Tumor Growth in Immunodeficient Mice." *Apoptosis* 12, no. 4 (April 2007): 685–94.

Gautam, N., A. K. Mantha, and S. Mittal. "Essential Oils and Their Constituents as Anticancer Agents: A Mechanistic View." *BioMed Research International* 2014, no. 4 (June 2014): 1–23.

Halm, M. A., C. Baker, and V. Harshe. "Effect of an Essential Oil Mixture on Skin Reactions in Women Undergoing Radiotherapy for Breast Cancer: A Pilot Study. *Journal of Holistic Nursing* 32, no. 4 (December 2014): 290–303.

Kim, M.-A., J.-K. Sakong, E.-J. Kim, et al. "Effect of Aromatherapy Massage for the Relief of Constipation in the Elderly." *Taehan Kanho Hakhoe Chi* 35, no. 1 (February 2005): 56–64.

Li, W., Z. Ping, G. Xuemei, et al. "Naturally Occurring Sclareol Diterpene Augments the Chemosensitivity of Human Hela Cervical Cancer Cells by Inducing Mitochondrial Mediated Programmed Cell Death, S-Phase Cell Cycle Arrest and Targeting Mitogen-Activated Protein Kinase (MAPK)/Extracellular-Signal-Regulated Kinase (ERK) Signaling Pathway." *Medical Science Monitor* 26 (January 2020): e920248.

McGinley, L. "The Disturbing Links between Too Much Weight and Several Types of Cancer." *Washington Post*, April 14, 2019.

National Center for Biotechnology Information. "PubChem Compound Summary for CID 440917, D-Limonene." Accessed December 16, 2020. https://pubchem.ncbi.nlm.nih.gov/compound/D-Limonene.

Noori, S., Z. M. Hassan, and O. Salehian. "Sclareol Reduces CD4+ CD25+ FoxP3+ Treg Cells in a Breast Cancer Model In Vivo." *Iranian Journal of Immunology* 10, no. 1 (March 2013): 1021.

Oh, J. Y., M. A. Park, and Y. C. Kim. "Peppermint Oil Promotes Hair Growth without Toxic Signs." *Toxicological Research* 30, no. 4 (December 2014): 297–304.

Orchard, A., and S. van Vuuren. "Commercial Essential Oils as Potential Antimicrobials to Treat Skin Diseases." *Evidence-Based Complementary and Alternative Medicine* 2017, no. 1 (January 2017): 1–92.

Panahi, Y., M. Taghizadeh, E. T. Marzony, et al. "Rosemary Oil vs Minoxidil 2% for the Treatment of Androgenetic Alopecia: A Randomized Comparative Trial." *Skinmed* 13, no. 1 (January–February 2015): 15–21.

Shen, J., A. Niijima, M. Tanida, et al. "Olfactory Stimulation with Scent of Lavender Oil Affects Autonomic Nerves, Lipolysis and Appetite in Rats." *Neuroscience Letter* 383, nos. 1–2 (July 2005): 188–93.

Siegel, R. L., K. D. Miller, and A. Jemal. "Cancer Statistics, 2020." *CA: A Cancer Journal for Clinicians* 70, no. 1 (January–February 2020): 7–30.

Tian, Q. Y., and X. S. Piao. "Essential Oil Blend Could Decrease Diarrhea Prevalence by Improving Antioxidative Capability for Weaned Pigs." *Animals* 9, no. 10 (October 2019): 847.

Tisserand, R. "Is Clary Sage Oil Estrogenic?" April 25, 2010. https://roberttisserand.com/2010/04/is-clary-sage-oil-estrogenic.

Tisserand, R., and Young, R. *Essential Oil Safety: A Guide for Health Care Professionals*. 2nd ed., 179–83. London: Churchill Livingstone, 2013.

Witt, C. M., L. G. Balneaves, M. J. Cardosa, et al. "A Comprehensive Definition for Integrative Oncology." *JNCI Monographs* 2017, no. 52 (November 2017).

World Health Organization. "Cancer." September 12, 2018. https://www.who.int/en/news-room/fact-sheets/detail/cancer.

Wu, S., J. L. Booth, K. B. Patel, et al. "Protective Essential Oil Attenuates Influenza Virus Infection: An In Vitro Study in MDCK Cells." *BMC Complementary and Alternative Medicine* 10, no. 1 (November 2010): 69.

Zhang, T., T. Wang, and P. Cai. "Sclareol Inhibits Cell Proliferation and Sensitizes Cells to the Antiproliferative Effect of Bortezomib via Upregulating the Tumor Suppressor Caveolin-1 in Cervical Cancer Cells." *Molecular Medicine Reports* 15, no. 6 (June 2017): 3566–74.

Chapter 12: CARDIOVASCULAR DISEASE

Akyea, R. K., J. Kai, N. Qureshi, et al. "Sub-optimal Cholesterol Response to Initiation of Statins and Future Risk of Cardiovascular Disease." *Heart* 105, no. 13 (July 2019): 975–81.

American Heart Association. "About Metabolic Syndrome." Last reviewed July 31, 2016. https://www.heart.org/en/health-topics/metabolic-syndrome/about-metabolic-syndrome.

American Heart Association News. "Heart Disease, Stroke Death Rates Increase Following Decades of Progress." American Heart Association. December 8, 2016.

Bastos, J. F. A., I. J. A. Moreira, T. P. Ribeiro, et al. "Hypotensive and Vasorelaxant Effects of Citronellol, a Monoterpene Alcohol, in Rats." *Basic and Clinical Pharmacology and Toxicology* 106, no. 4 (April 2010): 331–37.

Centers for Disease Control and Prevention. "Heart Disease in the United States." Last reviewed September 8, 2020. https://www.cdc.gov/heartdisease/facts.htm.

Cha, J. H., S. H. Lee, and Y. S. Yoo. "Effects of Aromatherapy on Changes in the Autonomic Nervous System, Aortic Pulse Wave Velocity and Aortic Augmentation Index in Patients with Essential Hypertension." *Journal the Korean Academy of Nursing* 40, no. 5 (October 2010): 705–13.

Chen, Y.-F., Y.-W. Wang, W.-S. Huang, et al. "Trans-Cinnamaldehyde, An Essential Oil in Cinnamon Powder, Ameliorates Cerebral Ischemia-Induced Brain Injury via Inhibition of Neuroinflammation Through Attenuation of iNOS, COX-2 Expression and NFκ-B Signaling Pathway." *NeuroMolecular Medicine* 18, no. 3 (September 2016): 322–33.

Ciftci, M., U. G. Simsek, A. Yuce, et al. "Effects of Dietary Antibiotic and Cinnamon Oil Supplementation on Antioxidant Enzyme Activities, Cholesterol Levels and Fatty Acid Compositions of Serum and Meat in Broiler Chickens." *Acta Veterinaria Brno* 79, no. 1 (March 2010): 33–40.

Costa, C. A. R. A., L. T. Bidinotto, R. K. Takahira, et al. "Cholesterol Reduction and Lack of Genotoxic or Toxic Effects in Mice after Repeated 21-Day Oral Intake of Lemongrass (*Cymbopogon citratus*) Essential Oil." *Food and Chemical Toxicology* 49, no. 9 (September 2011): 2268–72.

de Andrade, T. U., G. A. Brasil, D. C. Endringer, et al. "Cardiovascular Activity of the Chemical Constituents of Essential Oils." *Molecules* 22, no. 9 (September 2017): 1539.

de Siqueira, R. J., K. M. S. Rodrigues, M. T. B. da Silva, et al. "Linalool-Rich Rosewood Oil Induces Vago-Vagal Bradycardic and Depressor Reflex in Rats." *Phytotherapy Research* 28, no. 1 (January 2014): 42–48.

Drug Report. "The 50 Most Commonly Prescribed Drugs in America and Their Average Price." March 23, 2020. https://www.drugreport.com/50-commonly-prescribed-drugs-in-america/.

Fernandez, L. F., O. M. Palomino, and G. Fruots. "Effectiveness of *Rosmarinus officinalis* Essential Oil as Antihypotensive Agent in Primary Hypotensive Patients and Its Influence on Health-Related Quality of Life." *Journal of Ethnopharmacology* 151, no. 1 (2014): 509–16.

Harvard Health Publishing, Harvard Medical School. "A Major Change for Daily Aspirin Therapy." Harvard Health Letter. November 2019. https://www.health.harvard.edu/staying-healthy/a-major-change-for-daily-aspirin-therapy.

Hung, W.-L., J. H. Suh, and Y. Wang. "Chemistry and Health Effects of Furanocoumarins in Grapefruit." *Journal of Food and Drug Analysis* 25, no. 1 (January 2017): 71–83.

Hwang, J.-H. "The Effects of the Inhalation Method Using Essential Oils on Blood Pressure and Stress Responses of Clients with Essential Hypertension." *Taehan Kanho Hakhoe Chi* 36, no. 7 (December 2006): 1123–34.

Jing, L., Y. Zhang, S. Fan, et al. "Preventive and Ameliorating Effects of Citrus D-Limonene on Dyslipidemia and Hyperglycemia in Mice with High-Fat Diet-Induced Obesity." *European Journal Pharmacology* 715, nos. 1–3 (September 2013): 46–55.

Jung, D.-J., J.-Y. Cha, S.-E. Kim, "Effects of Ylang Ylang Aroma on Blood Pressure and Heart Rate in Healthy Men." *Journal of Exercise Rehabilitation* 9, no. 2 (April 2013): 250–55.

Khan, A., M. Safdar, M. M. A. Khan, et al. "Cinnamon Improves Glucose and Lipids of People with Type 2 Diabetes." *Diabetes Care* 26, no. 12 (December 2003): 3215–18.

Lee, H., M. Woo, M. Kim, et al. "Antioxidative and Cholesterol-Lowering Effects of Lemon Essential Oil in Hypercholesterolemia-Induced Rabbits." *Preventive Nutrition and Food Science* 23, no. 1 (March 2018): 8–14.

Mnafgui, K., R. Hajji, F. Derbali, et al. "Anti-inflammatory, Antithrombotic and Cardiac Remodeling Preventive Effects of Eugenol in Isoproterenol-Induced Myocardial Infarction in Wistar Rat." *Cardiovascular Toxicology* 16, no. 4 (October 2016): 336–44.

Paddock, C. "Daily Aspirin Does Not Make for a Longer, 'Disability-Free' Life." Medical News Today. September 19, 2018.

Saljoughian, S., S. Roohinejad, A. E. A. Bekhit, et al. "The Effects of Food Essential Oils on Cardiovascular Diseases: A Review." *Critical Reviews in Food Science and Nutrition* 58, no. 10 (July 2018): 1688–705.

Sayorwan, W., N. Ruangrungsi, T. Poroyapunyporn, et al. "Effects of Inhaled Rosemary Oil on Subjective Feelings and Activities of the Nervous System." *Scientia Pharmaceutica* 81, no. 2 (April–June 2013): 531–42.

Seol, G. H., Y. H. Lee, P. Kang, et al. "Randomized Controlled Trial for *Salvia sclarea* or *Lavandula angustifolia*: Differential Effects on Blood Pressure in Female Patients with Urinary Incontinence Undergoing Urodynamic Examination." *Journal of Alternative and Complementary Medicine* 19, no. 7 (July 2013): 664–70.

Shiina, Y., N. Funabashi, K. Lee, et al. "Relaxation Effects of Lavender Aromatherapy Improve Coronary Flow Velocity Reserve in Healthy Men Evaluated by Transthoracic Doppler Echocardiography." *International Journal of Cardiology* 129, no. 2 (September 2008): 193–97.

Tisserand, Hana. "Grapefruit Oil and Medication." Tisserand Institute. Accessed December 16, 2020. https://tisserandinstitute.org/learn-more/grapefruit-oil-and-medication.

Tognolini, M., V. Ballabeni, S. Bertoni, et al. "Protective Effect of *Foeniculum vulgare* Essential Oil and Anethole in an Experimental Model of Thrombosis." *Pharmacological Research* 56, no. 3 (September 2007): 254–60.

US Food and Drug Administration. "Grapefruit Juice and Some Drugs Don't Mix." Last updated July 18, 2017. https://www.fda.gov/consumers/consumer-updates/grapefruit-juice-and-some-drugs-dont-mix.

US National Library of Medicine. "Aspirin in Reducing Events in the Elderly (ASPREE)." Clinical-Trials.gov. Last updated May 30, 2019. https://clinicaltrials.gov/ct2/show/NCT01038583.

Vakili, A., S. Sharifat, M. M. Akhavan, et al. "Effect of Lavender Oil (*Lavandula angustifolia*) on Cerebral Edema and Its Possible Mechanisms in an Experimental Model of Stroke." *Brain Research* 1548 (February 2014): 56–62.

World Health Organization. "About Cardiovascular Diseases." Accessed December 16, 2020. https://www.who.int/cardiovascular_diseases/about_cvd/en.

You, J. H., P. Kang, S. S. Min, et al. "Bergamot Essential Oil Differentially Modulates Intracellular Ca2+ Levels in Vascular Endothelial and Smooth Muscle Cells: A New Finding Seen with Fura-2." *Journal of Cardiovascular Pharmacology* 61, no. 4 (April 2013): 324–28.

Ziaee, M., A. Khorrami, M. Ebrahimi, et al. "Cardioprotective Effects of Essential Oil of *Lavandula angustifolia* on Isoproterenol-Induced Acute Myocardial Infarction in Rat." *Iranian Journal of Pharmaceutical Research* 14, no. 1 (Winter 2015): 279–89.

Chapter 13: CHRONIC RESPIRATORY DISEASE

Ács, K., V. L. Balázs, B. Kocsis, et al. "Antibacterial Activity Evaluation of Selected Essential Oils in Liquid and Vapor Phase on Respiratory Tract Pathogens." *BMC Complementary and Alternative Medicine* 18, no. 1 (July 27, 2018): 227.

Adam, B., T. Liebregts, J. Best, et al. "A Combination of Peppermint Oil and Caraway Oil Attenuates the Post-inflammatory Visceral Hyperalgesia in a Rat Model." *Scandinavian Journal of Gastroenterology* 41, no. 2 (February 2006): 155–60.

Centers for Disease Control and Prevention. "Leading Causes of Death." Last reviewed October 30, 2020. https://www.cdc.gov/nchs/fastats/leading-causes-of-death.htm.

Centers for Disease Control and Prevention. "Most Recent National Asthma Data." Last reviewed October 26, 2020. https://www.cdc.gov/asthma/most_recent_national_asthma_data.htm.

El-Khouly, D., W. M. El-Bakly, A. S. Awad, et al. "Thymoquinone Blocks Lung Injury and Fibrosis by Attenuating Bleomycin-Induced Oxidative Stress and Activation of Nuclear Factor Kappa-B in Rats." *Toxicology* 302, nos. 2–3 (December 16, 2012): 106–13.

Gao, M., A. Singh, K. Macri, et al. "Antioxidant Components of Naturally-Occurring Oils Exhibit

Marked Anti-inflammatory Activity in Epithelial Cells of the Human Upper Respiratory System." *Respiratory Research* 12, no. 1 (July 13, 2011): 92.

Golab, M., and K. Skwarlo-Sonta. "Mechanisms Involved in the Anti-inflammatory Action of Inhaled Tea Tree Oil in Mice." *Experimental Biology and Medicine* 232, no. 3 (March 2007): 420–26.

Horváth, G., and K. Ács. "Essential Oils in the Treatment of Respiratory Tract Diseases Highlighting Their Role in Bacterial Infections and Their Anti-inflammatory Action: A Review." *Flavour and Fragrance Journal* 30, no. 5 (September 2015): 331–41.

Huo, M., X. Cui, J. Xue, et al. "Anti-inflammatory Effects of Linalool in RAW 264.7 Macrophages and Lipopolysaccharide-Induced Lung Injury Model." *Journal of Surgical Research* 180, no. 1 (December 2012): e47–54.

Jeena, K., V. B. Liju, and R. Kuttan. "Antioxidant, Anti-inflammatory and Antinociceptive Activities of Essential Oil from Ginger." *Indian Journal of Physiology and Pharmacology* 57, no. 1 (December 31, 2012): 51–62.

Jeurgens, L. J., I. Tuleta, M. Stoeber, et al. "Regulation of Monocyte Redox Balance by 1,8-Cineole (Eucalyptol) Controls Oxidative Stress and Pro-inflammatory Responses In Vitro: A New Option to Increase the Antioxidant Effects of Combined Respiratory Therapy with Budesonide and Formoterol?" *Synergy* 7 (December 2018): 1–9.

Kacem, R. "Neutrophils Involvements in COPD: Effects of Essential Oil Extracted from *Nigella sativa* (L.) Seeds on Human Neutrophil Functions and Elastase Activity." Doctoral thesis, Ferhat Abbas University of Setif, 2018. http://dspace.univ-setif.dz:8888/jspui/handle/123456789/1437.

King P. T. "Inflammation in Chronic Obstructive Pulmonary Disease and Its Role in Cardiovascular Disease and Lung Cancer." *Clinical and Translational Medicine* 4, no. 1 (December 2015): 68.

Koh, K. J., A. L. Pearce, G. Marshmann, et al. "Tea Tree Oil Reduces Histamine-Induced Skin Inflammation." *British Journal of Dermatology* 147, no. 6 (December 2002): 1212–17.

Liju, V. B., K. Jeena, and R. Kuttan. "An Evaluation of Antioxidant, Anti-inflammatory, and Antinociceptive Activities of Essential Oil from *Curcuma longa* L." *Indian Journal of Pharmacology* 43, no. 5 (September–October 2011): 526–31.

Mangprayool, T., S. Kupittayanant, and N. Chudapongse. "Participation of Citral in the Bronchodilatory Effect of Ginger Oil and Possible Mechanism of Action." *Fitoterapia* 89 (September 2013): 68–73.

McGeachie, M. J. "Childhood Asthma Is a Risk Factor for the Development of Chronic Obstructive Pulmonary Disease." *Current Opinion in Allergy and Clinical Immunology* 17, no. 2 (April 2017): 104–9.

Murdoch, J. R., and C. M. Lloyd. "Chronic Inflammation and Asthma." *Mutation Research* 690, nos. 1–2 (August 7, 2010): 24–39.

Narke, D., M. Kurade, K. Dholakia, et al. "Limonene Reduces Airway Hyperreactivity and Inflammation through Activation of A2A Adenosine Receptors." *FASEB Journal* 31, no. S1 (April 2017): 820.1.

Ou, M.-C., Y.-F. Lee, C.-C. Li, et al. "The Effectiveness of Essential Oils for Patients with Neck Pain: A Randomized Controlled Study." *Journal of Alternative and Complementary* 20, no. 10 (October 2014): 771–79.

Ramos Alvarenga, R. F., B. Wan, T. Inui, et al. "Airborne Antituberculosis Activity of *Eucalyptus citriodora* Essential Oil." *Journal of Natural Products* 77, no. 3 (March 28, 2014): 603–10.

Silva, G. L., C. Luft, A. Lunardelli, et al. "Antioxidant, Analgesic and Anti-inflammatory Effects of Lavender Essential Oil." *Anais da Academia Brasileira Ciencias* 87, suppl. 2 (August 2015): 1397–408.

Silva, J., W. Abebe, S. M. Sousa, et al. "Analgesic and Anti-inflammatory Effects of Essential Oils of Eucalyptus." *Journal Ethnopharmacology* 89, nos. 2–3 (December 2003): 277–83.

Silva, J. K., P. L. B. Figueiredo, K. G. Byler, et al. "Essential Oils as Antiviral Agents, Potential of Essential Oils to Treat SARS-CoV-2 Infection: An In-Silico Investigation." *International Journal of Molecular Science* 21, no. 10 (May 2020): 3426.

Sun, Z., H. Wang, J. Wang, et al. "Chemical Composition and Anti-inflammatory, Cytotoxic and Antioxidant Activities of Essential Oil from Leaves of *Mentha piperita* Grown in China." *PLoS One* 9, no. 12 (2014): e114767.

Taher, Y. A., A. M. Samud, F. E. El-Taher, et al. "Experimental Evaluation of Anti-inflammatory, Antinociceptive and Antipyretic Activities of Clove Oil in Mice." *Libyan Journal of Medicine* 10, no. 1 (2015): 28685.

Thuy, B. T. P., T. T. A. My, N. T. T. Hai, et al. "Investigation into SARS-CoV-2 Resistance of Compounds in Garlic Essential Oil." *ACS Omega*, 5, no. 14 (March 31, 2020): 8312–20.

Tisserand Institute. "Are Eucalyptus and Peppermint Oils Safe for Young Children?" Accessed December 16, 2020. https://tisserandinstitute.org/learn-more/kids-inhalation-safety.

Ueno-Iio, T., M. Shibakura, K. Yokota, et al. "Lavender Essential Oil Inhalation Suppresses Allergic Airway Inflammation and Mucous Cell Hyperplasia in a Murine Model of Asthma." *Life Sciences* 108, no. 2 (June 2014): 109–15.

University of Maryland Medical Center. "Roman Chamomile." https://umm.edu/health/medical/altmed/herb/roman-chamomile.

Wang, H., L. Song, W. Ju, et al. "The Acute Airway Inflammation Induced by PM2.5 Exposure and the Treatment of Essential Oils in Balb/c Mice." *Scientific Reports* 7 (March 9, 2017): 44256.

World Health Organization. "The Top 10 Causes of Death." December 9, 2020. https://www.who.int/news-room/fact-sheets/detail/the-top-10-causes-of-death.

Worth, H., C. Schacher, and U. Dethlefsen. "Concomitant Therapy with Cineole (Eucalyptole) Reduces Exacerbations in COPD: A Placebo-Controlled Double-Blind Trial." *Respiratory Research* 10, no. 1 (July 22, 2009): 69.

Wu, S., K. B. Patel, L. J. Booth, et al. "Protective Essential Oil Attenuates Influenza Virus Infection: An In Vitro Study in MDCK Cells." *BMC Complementary and Alternative Medicine* 10, no. 1 (November 15, 2010): 69.

Zhou, X. M. "Preventive Effects of *Citrus reticulata* Essential Oil on Bleomycin-Induced Pulmonary Fibrosis in Rats and the Mechanism." *Journal of Chinese Integrative Medicine* 10, no. 2 (February 2012): 200–9.

Chapter 14: DIABETES AND OBESITY

Alexandrovich, I., O. Ralovitskaya, E. Kolmo, et al. "The Effect of Fennel (*Foeniculum vulgare*) Seed Oil Emulsion in Infantile Colic: A Randomized, Placebo-Controlled Study." *Alternative Therapies in Health and Medicine* 9, no. 4 (July–August 2003): 58–61.

Asnaashari, S., A. Delazar, B. Habibi, et al. "Essential Oil from *Citrus aurantifolia* Prevents Ketotifen-Induced Weight-Gain in Mice." *Phytotherapy* 24, no. 12 (December 2020): 1893–97.

Cardoso, S., and P. I. Moreira. "Diabesity and Brain Disturbances: A Metabolic Perspective." *Molecular Aspects of Medicine* 66 (April 2019): 71–79.

Cardoso, S., R. Seiça, and P. I. Moreira. "Diabesity and Brain Energy Metabolism: The Case of Alzheimer's Disease." *Advanced Neurobiology* 19 (September 2017): 117–50.

Chung, M. J., S.-Y. Cho, M. J. H. Bhuiyan, et al. "Anti-diabetic Effects of Lemon Balm (*Melissa officinalis*) Essential Oil on Glucose- and Lipid-Regulating Enzymes in Type 2 Diabetic Mice." *British Journal of Nutrition* 104, no. 2 (July 2010): 180–88.

Firmin, M. W., A. L. Gillette, T. E. Hobbs, et al. "Effects of Olfactory Sense on Chocolate Craving." *Appetite* 105 (October 2016): 700–4.

Hubert, H. B., M. Feinleib, P. M. McNamara, et al. "Obesity as an Independent Risk Factor for Cardiovascular Disease: A 26-Year Follow-Up of Participants in the Framingham Heart Study." *Circulation* 67, no. 5 (May 1983): 968–77.

Kalra, S. "Diabesity." *Journal of the Pakistan Medical Association* 63, no. 4 (March 31, 2013): 532–34.

Key, T., E. A. Spencer, and G. K. Reeves. "Symposium 1: Overnutrition: Consequences and Solutions. Obesity and Cancer Risk: Conference on 'Over- and undernutrition: Challenges and Approaches.'" *Proceedings of the Nutrition Society* 69, no. 1 (December 3, 2009): 86–90.

Kim, S.-J., K.-S. Kim, Y.-M. Choi, et al. "A Clinical Study of Decrease Appetite Effects by Aromatherapy Using *Foeniculum vulgare* Mill (Fennel) to Female Obese Patients." *Journal of Korean Medicine for Obesity Research* 5, no. 1 (2005): 9–20.

Lee, S.-C., W.-X. Xu, L.-Y. Lin, et al. "Chemical Composition and Hypoglycemic and Pancreas-Protective Effect of Leaf Essential Oil from Indigenous Cinnamon (*Cinnamomum osmophloeum* Kanehira)." *Journal of Agricultural and Food Chemistry* 61, no. 20 (May 22, 2013): 4905–13.

Lin, L.-Y., C.-H. Chuang, H.-C. Chen, et al. "Lime (*Citrus aurantifolia* (Christm.) Swingle) Essential Oils: Volatile Compounds, Antioxidant Capacity, and Hypolipidemic Effect." *Foods* 8, no. 9 (September 7, 2019): 398.

Mesfin, M., K. Asres, and W. Shibeshi. "Evaluation of Anxiolytic Activity of the Essential Oil of the Aerial Part of *Foeniculum vulgare* Miller in Mice." *BMC Complementary and Alternative Medicine* 14 (August 23, 2014): 310.

Oboh, G., I. A. Akinbola, A. O. Ademosun, et al. "Essential Oil from Clove Bud (*Eugenia aromatica*

Kuntze) Inhibit Key Enzymes Relevant to the Management of Type-2 Diabetes and Some Pro-oxidant Induced Lipid Peroxidation in Rats Pancreas In Vitro." *Journal of Oleo Science* 64, no. 7 (2015): 775–82.

Ostad, S. N., M. Soodi, M. Shariffzadeh, et al. 2001. "The Effect of Fennel Essential Oil on Uterine Contraction as a Model for Dysmenorrhea, Pharmacology and Toxicology Study." *Journal of Ethnopharmacology* 76, no. 3 (August 2001): 299–304.

Powell, A. "Obesity? Diabetes? We've Been Set Up." *Harvard Gazette*, March 7, 2012. https://news.harvard.edu/gazette/story/2012/03/the-big-setup/.

Rather, M. A., B. A. Dar, S. N. Sofi, et al. "*Foeniculum vulgare*: A Comprehensive Review of Its Traditional Use, Phytochemistry, Pharmacology, and Safety." *Arabian Journal of Chemistry* 9, suppl. 2 (November 2016): S1574–S1583.

Reed, J. A., J. Almeida, B. Wershing, et al. "Effects of Peppermint Scent on Appetite Control and Caloric Intake." *Appetite* 51, no. 2 (September 2008): 393.

Saeedi, P., I. Petersohn, P. Salpea, et al. "Global and Regional Diabetes Prevalence Estimates for 2019 and Projections for 2030 and 2045: Results from the International Diabetes Federation Diabetes Atlas, 9th edition." *Diabetes Research and Clinical Practice* 157 (November 1, 2019). https://www.diabetesresearchclinicalpractice.com/article/S0168-8227(19)31230-6/fulltext.

Sebai, H., S. Selmi, K. Rtibi, et al. "Lavender (*Lavandula stoechas* L.) Essential Oils Attenuate Hyperglycemia and Protect against Oxidative Stress in Alloxan-Induced Diabetic Rats." *Lipids in Health and Disease* 12 (December 28, 2013): 189.

Selmi, S., K. Rtibi, D. Grami, et al. "Rosemary (*Rosmarinus officinalis*) Essential Oil Components Exhibit Anti-hyperglycemic, Anti-hyperlipidemic and Antioxidant Effects in Experimental Diabetes." *Pathophysiology* 24, no. 4 (December 2017): 297–303.

Shen, J., A. Niijima, A. Tanida, et al. "Olfactory Stimulation with Scent of Lavender Oil Affects Autonomic Nerves, Lipolysis and Appetite in Rats." *Neuroscience Letters* 383, nos. 1–2 (July 22–29, 2005): 188–93.

Talpur, N., B. Echard, C. Ingram, et al. "Effects of a Novel Formulation of Essential Oils on Glucose-Insulin Metabolism in Diabetic and Hypertensive Rats." *Diabetes, Obesity & Metabolism* 7, no. 2 (March 2005): 193–99.

Tremmel, M., U.-G. Gerdtham, P. M. Nilsson, et al. "Economic Burden of Obesity: A Systematic Literature Review." *International Journal of Environmental Research and Public Health* 14, no. 4 (April 19, 2017): 435.

Ward, Z. J., S. N. Bleich, A. L. Cradock, et al. "Projected U.S. State-Level Prevalence of Adult Obesity and Severe Obesity." *New England Journal of Medicine* 381 (December 2019): 2440–50.

World Health Organization. "Obesity and Overweight." April 1, 2020. https://www.who.int/news-room/fact-sheets/detail/obesity-and-overweight.

World Obesity Federation. *Atlas of Childhood Obesity*. London: World Obesity Federation, 2019. http://s3-eu-west-1.amazonaws.com/wof-files/WOF_Childhood_Obesity_Atlas_Report_Oct19_V2.pdf.

Yen, H.-F., C.-T. Hsieh, T.-J. Hsieh, et al. "In Vitro Anti-diabetic Effect and Chemical Component Analysis of 29 Essential Oils Products." *Journal of Food and Drug Analysis* 23, no. 1 (March 2015): 124–29.

Chapter 15: FATTY LIVER

Al-Okbi, S. Y., D. A. Mohamed, T. E. Hamed, et al. "Protective Effect of Clove Oil and Eugenol Microemulsions on Fatty Liver Dyslipidemia as Components of Metabolic Syndrome." *Journal of Medicinal Food* 17, no. 7 (July 2014): 764–71.

Alsanea, S., and D. Liu. "BITC and S-Carvone Restrain High-Fat Diet-Induced Obesity and Ameliorate Hepatic Steatosis and Insulin Resistance." *Pharmacological Research* 34, no. 11 (November 2017): 2241–49.

Asadollahpoor, A., M. Abdollahi, and R. Rahimi. "*Pimpinella anisum* L. Fruit: Chemical Composition and Effect on Rat Model of Nonalcoholic Fatty Liver Disease." *Journal of Research in Medical Sciences* 22 (March 15, 2017): 37.

Asghari, A., A. A. Khaki, A. Rajabzadeh, et al. "A Review on Electromagnetic Fields (EMFs) and the Reproductive System." *Electronic Physician* 8, no. 7 (July 2016): 2655–62.

British Liver Trust. "Statistics: Liver Disease Crisis." Accessed December 16, 2020. https://britishliver trust.org.uk/about-us/media-centre/statistics.

de Oliveira, J. R., S. E. A. Camargo, and L. D. de Oliveira. "*Rosmarinus officinalis* L. (Rosemary) as Therapeutic and Prophylactic Agent." *Journal of Biomedical Science* 26, no. 5 (January 2019): 1–22.

Dorin, J. "The Worst Disease You've Never Heard Of." Cedars Sinai. May 7, 2017. https://www .cedars-sinai.org/discoveries/2017/05/worst-disease-youve-never-heard.html.

Farzaei, M. H., M. Zobeiri, F. Parvizi, et al. "Curcumin in Liver Diseases: A Systematic Review of the Cellular Mechanisms of Oxidative Stress and Clinical Perspective." *Nutrients* 10, no. 7 (July 1, 2018): 855.

Huang, X., X. Liu, and Y. Yu. "Depression and Chronic Liver Diseases: Are There Shared Underlying Mechanisms?" *Frontiers in Molecular Neuroscience* 10 (May 8, 2017): 134.

Kim, E., Y. Choi, J. Jang, et al. "Carvacrol Protects against Hepatic Steatosis in Mice Fed a High-Fat Diet by Enhancing SIRT1-AMPK Signaling." *Evidence-Based Complementary and Alternative Medicine* 2013, no. 3 (February 2013): 290104.

Lai, Y.-S., W.-C. Lee, Y.-E. Lin, et al. "Ginger Essential Oil Ameliorates Hepatic Injury and Lipid Accumulation in High Fat Diet-Induced Nonalcoholic Fatty Liver Disease." *Journal of Agricultural and Food Chemistry* 64, no. 10 (March 16, 2016): 2062–71.

Lin, L.-Y., C.-H. Chuang, H.-C. Chen, et al. "Lime (*Citrus aurantifolia* (Christm.) Swingle) Essential Oils: Volatile Compounds, Antioxidant Capacity, and Hypolipidemic Effect." *Foods* 8, no. 9 (September 2019): 398.

Maurice, J., and P. Manousou. "Non-alcoholic Fatty Liver Disease." *Clinical Medicine* 18, no. 3 (June 2018): 245–50.

National Institute of Diabetes and Digestive and Kidney Diseases. "Definition & Facts of NAFLD &

NASH." November 2016. https://www.niddk.nih.gov/health-information/liver-disease/nafld
-nash/definition-facts.

Özbek. H., S. Uğraş, H. Dülger, et al. "Hepatoprotective Effect of *Foeniculum vulgare* Essential Oil."
Fitoterapia 74, no. 3 (April 2003): 317–19.

Rašković, A., I. Milanović, N. Pavlović, et al. "Antioxidant Activity of Rosemary (*Rosmarinus officinalis*
L.) Essential Oil and Its Hepatoprotective Potential." *BMC Complementary and Alternative Medicine* 14 (July 7, 2014): 225.

Tisserand, R., and R. Young. *Essential Oil Safety: A Guide for Health Care Professionals,* 2nd ed., 517.
London: Churchill Livingstone, 2013.

Yin, X., J. Yang, T. Li, et al. "The Effect of Green Tea Intake on Risk of Liver Disease: A Meta
Analysis." *International Journal of Clinical and Experimental Medicine* 8, no. 6 (June 15, 2015):
8339–46.

Chapter 16: INFLAMMATORY BOWEL DISEASES

Agah, S., A. M. Taleb, B. Moeini, et al. "Cumin Extract for Symptom Control in Patients with Irritable
Bowel Syndrome: A Case Series." *Middle East Journal of Digestive Diseases* 5, no. 4 (October 2013):
217–22.

Alammar, N., L. Wang, B. Saberi, et al. "The Impact of Peppermint Oil on the Irritable Bowel Syndrome: A Meta-analysis of the Pooled Clinical Data." *BMC Complementary and Alternative Medicine* 19, no. 1 (January 17, 2019): 21.

Bastani, M., Z. Mousavi, J. Asgarpanah, et al. "Biochemical and Histopathological Evidence for Beneficial Effects of *Pelargonium graveolens* Essential Oil on the Rat Model of Inflammatory Bowel
Disease Research." *Journal of Pharmacognosy* 6, no. 2 (March 2019): 77–84.

Béjaoui, A., H. Chaabane, M. Jemli, et al. "Essential Oil Composition and Antibacterial Activity of
Origanum vulgare Subsp. *glandulosum* Desf. at Different Phenological Stages." *Journal of Medicinal
Food* 16, no. 12 (December 2013): 1115–20.

Bukovská, A., S. Cikos, S. Juhás, et al. "Effects of a Combination of Thyme and Oregano Essential
Oils on TNBS-Induced Colitis in Mice." *Mediators of Inflammation* 2007, no. 4 (February 2007):
23296.

Centers for Disease Control and Prevention. "Data and Statistics: Inflammatory Bowel Disease Prevalence (IBD) in the United States." Last reviewed August 11, 2020. https://www.cdc.gov/ibd/
data-statistics.htm.

Cho, J. Y., H.-J. Chang, S.-K. Lee, et al. "Amelioration of Dextran Sulfate Sodium-Induced Colitis in
Mice by Oral Administration of Beta-Caryophyllene, a Sesquiterpene." *Life Sciences* 80, no. 10
(February 13, 2007): 932–39.

Dictionary.com. "Gut." Accessed December 17, 2020. https://www.dictionary.com/browse/gut?s=t.

Donatini, B., and I. Le Blaye. "Medicinal Sulphur Polypore Mushroom *Laetiporus sulphureus* (Agaricomycetes) Plus Tiny Amounts of Essential Oils Decrease the Activity of Crohn Disease." *International Journal of Medicinal Mushrooms* 21, no. 3 (2019): 267–73.

The Free Dictionary. "Bowel." Accessed December 17, 2020. https://medical-dictionary.thefreedictionary.com/bowel.

Hawrelak, J., T. Cattley, and S. P. Myers. "Essential Oils in the Treatment of Intestinal Dysbiosis: A Preliminary In Vitro Study." *Alternative Medicine Reviews* 14, no. 4 (December 2009): 380–84.

Keshavarz, A., M. Minaiyan, A. Ghannadi, et al. "Effects of *Carum carvi* L. (Caraway) Extract and Essential Oil on TNBS-Induced Colitis in Rats." *Research in Pharmaceutical Sciences* 8, no. 1 (January–March 2013): 18.

Liju, V. B., J. Jeena, and R. Kuttan. "Gastroprotective Activity of Essential Oils from Turmeric and Ginger." *Journal of Basic and Clinical Physiology and Pharmacology* 26, no. 1 (January 2015): 95–103.

Logan, A. C., and T. M. Beaulne. "The Treatment of Small Intestinal Bacterial Overgrowth with Enteric-Coated Peppermint Oil: A Case Report." *Alternative Medicine Reviews* 7, no. 5 (October 2002): 410–17.

Madisch, A., C. J. Heydenreich, V. Wieland, et al. "Treatment of Functional Dyspepsia with a Fixed Peppermint Oil and Caraway Oil Combination Preparation as Compared to Cisapride. A Multicenter, Reference-Controlled Double-Blind Equivalence Study." *Arzneimittelforschung* 49, no. 11 (November 1999): 925–32.

Rashidian, A., P. Rooho, S. Mehrzadi, et al. "Protective Effect of *Ocimum basilicum* Essential Oil Against Acetic Acid-Induced Colitis in Rats." *Journal of Evidence-Based Complementary and Alternative Medicine* 21, no. 4 (November 2015): NP36–NP42.

Sapra, B., S. Jain, and A. K. Tiwary. "Percutaneous Permeation Enhancement by Terpenes: Mechanistic View." *AAPS Journal* 10, no. 1 (2008): 120–32.

Thapa, D., P. Louis, R. Losa, et al. "Essential Oils Have Different Effects on Human Pathogenic and Commensal Bacteria in Mixed Faecal Fermentations Compared with Pure Cultures." *Microbiology* 161, pt. 2 (February 2005): 441–49.

Thompson, A., D. Meah, N. Ahmed, et al. "Comparison of the Antibacterial Activity of Essential Oils and Extracts of Medicinal and Culinary Herbs to Investigate Potential New Treatments for Irritable Bowel Syndrome." *BMC Complementary and Alternative Medicine* 13 (November 28, 2013): 338.

Toden, S., A. L. Theiss, X. Wang, et al. "Essential Turmeric Oils Enhance Anti-inflammatory Efficacy of Curcumin in Dextran Sulfate Sodium-Induced Colitis." *Scientific Reports* 7, no. 1 (December 2017): 814.

Yu, X., G. Yang, H. Jiang, et al. "Patchouli Oil Ameliorates Acute Colitis: A Targeted Metabolite Analysis of 2,4,6-Trinitrobenzenesulfonic Acid-Induced Rats." *Experimental and Therapeutic Medicine* 14, no. 2 (August 2017): 1184–92.

Chapter 17: PARKINSON'S DISEASE AND EPILEPSY

Agatonovic-Kustrin, S., E. Kustrin, and D. W. Morton. "Essential Oils and Functional Herbs for Healthy Aging." *Neural Regeneration Research* 14, no. 3 (March 2019): 441–45.

Ambrosio, L., M. C. Portillo, C. Rodríguez-Blázquez, et al. "Living with Chronic Illness Scale: International Validation of a New Self-Report Measure in Parkinson's Disease." *NPJ Parkinson's Disease* 2 (October 20, 2016): 16022.

Bahr, T. A., D. Rodriguez, C. Beaumont, et al. "The Effects of Various Essential Oils on Epilepsy and Acute Seizure: A Systematic Review." *Evidence-Based Complementary and Alternative Medicine* 2019 (May 22, 2019): 6216745.

Cho, J. Y., H.-J. Chang, S.-K. Lee, et al. "Amelioration of Dextran Sulfate Sodium-Induced Colitis in Mice by Oral Administration of Beta-Caryophyllene, a Sesquiterpene." *Life Sciences* 80, no. 10 (February 13, 2007): 932–39.

El Alaoui, C., J. Chemin, T. Fechtali, et al. "Modulation of T-type Ca2+ Channels by Lavender and Rosemary Extracts." *PloS One* 12, no. 1 (October 26, 2017): e0186864.

Hartsel, J. A., J. Eades, B. Hickory, et al. "*Cannabis sativa* and Hemp." Chapter 53 in *Nutraceuticals*, edited by R. C. Gupta, 735–54. Cambridge, MA: Academic Press, 2016.

Hussain, S. A., R. Zhou, C. Jacobson, et al. "Perceived Efficacy of Cannabidiol-Enriched Cannabis Extracts for Treatment of Pediatric Epilepsy: A Potential Role for Infantile Spasms and Lennox-Gastaut Syndrome." *Epilepsy Behavior* 47 (June 2015): 138–41.

Mathew, T., V. Kamath, R. S. Kumar, et al. "Eucalyptus Oil Inhalation–Induced Seizure: A Novel, Underrecognized, Preventable Cause of Acute Symptomatic Seizure." *Epilepsia Open* 2, no. 3 (September 2017): 350–54.

Medline Plus. "Living with a Chronic Illness—Reaching Out to Others." Last reviewed August 4, 2018. https://medlineplus.gov/ency/patientinstructions/000602.htm.

National Health Service. "Causes: Restless Legs Syndrome." Last reviewed August 6, 2018. https://www.nhs.uk/conditions/restless-legs-syndrome/causes.

Pagan, F., M. Hebron, E. H. Valadez, et al. "Nilotinib Effects in Parkinson's Disease and Dementia with Lewy Bodies." *Journal of Parkinson's Disease* 6, no. 3 (July 11, 2016): 503–17.

Parkinson's Foundation. "Statistics." Accessed December 17, 2020. https://www.parkinson.org/Understanding-Parkinsons/Statistics.

Pavithra, M. "Effect of *Cymbopogon flexuosus* (Lemongrass Oil) against Rotenone-Induced Parkinsonism in Rats." Dissertation, The Tamil Nadu Dr. M.G.R. Medical University Chennai, 2017.

Puschmann, A., R. F. Pfeiffer, A. J. Stoessl, et al. "A Family with Parkinsonism, Essential Tremor, Restless Legs Syndrome, and Depression." *Neurology* 76, no. 19 (May 10, 2011): 1623–30.

Rekha, K. R., and R. I. Sivakamasundari. "Geraniol Protects Against the Protein and Oxidative Stress Induced by Rotenone in an In Vitro Model of Parkinson's Disease." *Neurochemical Research* 43, no. 10 (October 2018): 1947–62.

Santos, N. A. G., N. M. Martins, F. M. Sisti, et al. "The Neuroprotection of Cannabidiol against MPP^+-Induced Toxicity in PC12 Cells Involves trkA Receptors, Upregulation of Axonal and Synaptic Proteins, Neuritogenesis, and Might Be Relevant to Parkinson's Disease." *Toxicology In Vitro* 25, 1 pt. B (December 25, 2015): 231–40.

Semyanov, A., M. C. Walker, D. M. Kullman, et al. "Tonically Active GABAA Receptors: Modulating Gain and Maintaining the Tone." *Trends in Neurosciences* 27, no. 5 (May 2004): 262–69.

Silvestro, S., S. Mammana, E. Cavalli, et al. "Use of Cannabidiol in the Treatment of Epilepsy: Efficacy and Security in Clinical Trials." *Molecules* 24, no. 8 (April 2019): 1459.

Tisserand, R., and R. Young. *Essential Oil Safety: A Guide for Health Care Professionals,* 2nd ed., 519, 557, 585. London: Churchill Livingstone, 2013.

UCLA Cannabis Research Initiative. Accessed December 17, 2020. https://cannabis.semel.ucla.edu.

UConn Health. "Epilepsy and Movement Disorders." Department of Surgery, Neurosurgery. Accessed December 17, 2020. https://health.uconn.edu/neurosurgery/patient-care/brain/epilepsy-and -movement-disorders.

Viveros-Paredes, J. M., R. E. González-Castañeda, J. Gertsch, et al. "Neuroprotective Effects of β-Caryophyllene against Dopaminergic Neuron Injury in a Murine Model of Parkinson's Disease Induced by MPTP." *Pharmaceuticals* 10, no. 3 (July 6, 2017): 60.

Waldman N. "Seizure Caused by Dermal Application of Over-the-Counter Eucalyptus Oil Head Lice Preparation." *Clinical Toxicology* 49, no. 8 (August 2011): 750–51.

Appendix A: DISEASE-BUSTING HEALTHY LIFESTYLE HACKS

Centers for Disease Control and Prevention. "How You Can Prevent Chronic Diseases." Last reviewed September 15, 2020. https://www.cdc.gov/chronicdisease/about/prevent/index.htm.

Recommended Resources

To help you along the journey, we have created a series of demo videos on preparing several of the essential oil remedies and recipes featured in *The Essential Oils Apothecary*. Each of the videos contains extra insights into the strategies and information covered in this book. You can access these videos free at EOApothecary.com.

These resources will help you on your journey as you follow the guidelines outlined in this book. If you have any questions or a testimonial you'd like to share, please contact us at Support@NaturalLivingFamily.com. We always love to read the healing stories that flow through our inbox, telling us how essential oils have changed people's lives!

Essential Oils Apothecary Package (Free Gift)

- Recipe demo videos
- Starter checklists, shopping guides, and more
- EOApothecary.com

Educational RESOURCES

Essential Oils for Abundant Living Masterclass

- Free viewing of our video series to help you use essential oils the right way
- EssentialOilsForAbundantLiving.com

The Healing Power of Essential Oils Book

- With more than 150 effective recipes and natural remedies
- HealingPowerOfEssentialOils.com

The Essential Oils Diet Book

- A complete healthy lifestyle plan powered by essential oils
- EssentialOilsDiet.com

Dr. Z's Essential Oils Club

- Our library of online resources
- EssentialOilsClub.info

Natural Living RESOURCES

Toxic-Free Healthy Home Makeover Tour

- Free viewing of Mama Z's video series showing you how we've detoxed our home
- MamaZHealthyHome.com

Organic Gardening Made Easy

- Free viewing of Mama Z's organic gardening class
- MamaZGardening.com

Fit40 and Beyond

- Free viewing of Mama Z's home exercise class (suitable for all fitness levels)
- MamaZExercise.com

Gluten-Free Italian Cooking Class

- Free viewing of Mama Z's popular cooking class (learn how to make your favorite Italian recipes allergy-friendly)
- MamaZItalian.com

Simple Sensational Salads

- Free viewing of Mama Z's popular cooking class (allergy-friendly salads have never tasted so good)
- MamaZSalads.com

Hope for Breast Cancer

- Free viewing of our award-winning documentary featuring one brave young mom's journey as she traveled the world, customizing her own integrative cancer treatments
- HopeForBreastCancer.com

Essential PRODUCTS

- Visit NaturalLivingFamily.com/how-to-be-healthy/—for a list of all the health products, supplements, books, and educational resources we recommend.

Aromatherapy REFERENCE BOOKS, TEXTS, AND CERTIFICATION COURSES

- Atlantic Institute of Aromatherapy: AtlanticInstitute.com
- Buckle, Jane. *Clinical Aromatherapy: Essential Oils in Healthcare*, 3rd ed. (St. Louis, MO: Churchill Livingstone, 2014).
- Price, Len, and Shirley Price. *Understanding Hydrolats: The Specific Hydrosols for Aromatherapy: A Guide for Health Professionals*. (London: Churchill Livingstone, 2004).
- Price, Shirley, and Len Price. *Aromatherapy for Health Professionals*, 4th ed. (London: Churchill Livingstone, 2011).
- Rose, Jeanne. *375 Essential Oils and Hydrosols* (Berkeley, CA: Frog, 1999).
- Sheppard-Hanger, Sylla. *The Aromatherapy Practitioner Reference Manual*, 2 vols. (Tampa, FL: Atlantic Institute of Aromatherapy, 1997).

- Tisserand, Robert, and Rodney Young. *Essential Oil Safety: A Guide for Health Care Professionals*, 2nd ed. (London: Churchill Livingstone, 2013).

Environmental WORKING GROUP HEALTH AND SAFETY GUIDES

- EWG's Skin Deep Cosmetics Database: EWG.org/skindeep
- EWG's Guide to Healthy Cleaning: EWG.org/guides/cleaners
- EWG's Food Scores: EWG.org/foodscores

Acknowledgments

Our sincere love and heartfelt gratitude to God, and to all of the behind-the scenes people He put in our path who helped make this book a reality.

To Mom and Dad Frawley, yay, we did it. Again! ;) You supported us to chase our dreams, and look what happened. Without you, our global Bible health ministry would not exist and this book would never have been written. We are also eternally grateful for everything that you have taught us about business and work ethics, and for inspiring us to never settle for anything but God's best in our lives.

To Papa Enoch, your ministry has inspired thousands to live for Christ and to seek the abundant life through many of the principles shared in this book. Through your mentorship, you helped lay the foundation for much of what is written in these pages, and we are grateful for the time that you spent teaching us these eternal truths.

To Miss Alex Chapman, Miss Natalie, and Miss Kayla, for helping with the kid-dos during those long hours and for being Mama Z's right-hand gals for all things natural living. We all love you!

To Whit, Elizabeth, Angela, Erica, Christa, Kyle, Dee, Sev, Bev, April, Carrie, Derek, Shant, Chris, and the entire NaturalLivingFamily.com team, your hard work and determination have been priceless! Thank you so much for all that you do to make NaturalLivingFamily.com the number one most-visited website devoted to biblical health on the planet!

To Maggie Greenwood-Robinson, for your brilliant insight and savvy word-smithing. And to Gina Badalaty, for your research support and help with sifting through the medical literature. Your help putting together this manuscript was absolutely priceless. You are a gem, and it has been an honor to work with you on this project.

To our literary agents, John Maas and Celeste Fine Folch, for your advocacy, your hard work, and your role as our trusted guides. You are the best! To the wonderful team at Harmony Books: Marnie Cochran, Katherine Leak, Christina Foxley, Danielle Curtis, Tammy Blake, Connie Capone, and the unsung heroes in the fact-checking and copyediting departments—all we can say is "Wow!" You are the dream team, and we couldn't have asked for a better group of professionals to make all of this happen.

Index

drug interactions, 312, 313, 314
for energy/alertness, 61
for Parkinson's and epilepsy, 294, 296
for stress and anxiety, 92–93
lemon myrtle, 61, 159, 312, 313, 314
lemon tea tree, 61, 312, 313, 314
lethargy. *See* fatigue
libido, 140–52
  basics, 140–41
  gentle vaginal lubricant, 142
  oils and blends for, 143–52
lifestyle uses. *See* healthy lifestyle practices and uses
lime, 29, 108
  for appetite, 173
  for liver health, 267
  for mental clarity/alertness, 61, 63
  for obesity/weight loss, 219, 249
limonene, 101, 107–8, 201, 202, 219, 220
linalool, 149, 159, 181, 201
  for Alzheimer's, 170
  for appetite, 205
  cardiovascular health and, 224
  for depression and substance abuse, 110–11, 113, 114
  oils containing, 86
  for pain relief, 135, 136–39
  Parkinson's/epilepsy and, 290, 296
linalyl acetate, 86, 87, 149
Litsea. *See* may chang
liver damage, risk of, 32
liver disease, 260–70, 271
  basics, 260–63
  oils and blends for, 107, 263–70
lubricants, 141–42, 150

mandarin, 29, 76, 108, 199, 239, 276–77
March, Lyn, 177
marjoram, 231. *See also* sweet marjoram; wild marjoram
massage and massage oils, 21, 306. *See also* body oils, creams, and roll-ons

aromatherapeutic hand massage, 91–92, 112, 168
for common ailments of the elderly, 173–75
mastic, 199
matcha:
  EO-Powered Matcha Latte, 124–25, 189
  Spearminty Iced Matcha Latte, 270
maximum daily oral dose, 32, 227–28
may chang, 61, 76, 173, 174, 312, 313, 314
MCT oil, 23–24
medications, conventional. *See* conventional medical approaches; *specific medications and therapies*
meditation, 63, 305
Melissa. *See* lemon balm
memory loss, 174. *See also* Alzheimer's and dementia; cognitive problems
mental illness, 97–99. *See also* anxiety; depression and substance abuse
menthol, 201, 230, 231, 237
metabolic syndrome, 212, 219–20, 261
microbiome, essential oils and, 274–75, 279
  Microflora-Friendly Capsule, 279, 280
migraines, 28, 82, 123, 135, 174
Mojay, Gabriel, 37
mood disorders. *See* anxiety; depression and substance abuse; mental illness
mood elevation, 97
  oils and blends for, 87, 91, 102–7, 110–15, 117, 171–72
mountain savory, 61. *See also* savory
MyGreenFills products, 43
myrrh, 63, 174
myrtle, 76, 175, 199, 230, 253–54, 312, 313

NAFLD (nonalcoholic fatty liver disease), 5, 261–63
  oils and blends for, 263–70
NASH, 261, 265, 269
nausea, 275, 283
nebulizers, 19–20
necklaces, aromatherapy, 16
neroli, 63, 86, 87, 89–90, 150, 169, 174
neurological disorders. *See* Alzheimer's and dementia; epilepsy; Parkinson's disease
niaouli, 175, 230
nicotine, 6, 80, 100, 229. *See also* smoking
  nicotine cravings, 115–16
Nigella. *See* black seed
nonalcoholic fatty liver disease (NAFLD), 5, 261–63
  oils and blends for, 263–70
nonalcoholic steatohepatitis (NASH), 261, 265, 269
NSAIDs (non-steroidal anti-inflammatory drugs), 179–80, 187
nut grass, 199
nutmeg, 173, 174
nutrition. *See* diabetes and obesity; diet and nutrition; weight loss

obesity. *See* diabetes and obesity; weight loss
oils. *See* body oils, creams, and roll-ons
ointments. *See* body oils, creams, and roll-ons
olive oil, 23
opoponax, 63
oral use. *See* internal use
orange, 55–56, 101, 108. *See also* bitter orange; blood orange; sweet orange; wild orange
  for cancer, 199
  for mental clarity/alertness, 61, 63
  for respiratory health, 240
  for sleep, 174
  for stress and anxiety, 88–89

About the Authors

The author of the national bestseller *The Healing Power of Essential Oils* and *The Essential Oils Diet* (with Sabrina Ann Zielinski), Dr. Eric Zielinski has pioneered natural living and biblical health education since 2003. Trained as an aromatherapist, public health researcher, and chiropractor, Dr. Z started DrEricZ.com (now NaturalLivingFamily.com) in 2014 with his wife, Sabrina Ann, to help people learn how to safely and effectively use natural remedies such as essential oils.

Sabrina Ann Zielinski is a certified group fitness instructor, health coach, lactation consultant, and natural health guru. The mastermind behind the allergy-friendly food recipes and do-it-yourself remedies featured on the Zielinskis' website, she's known as "Mama Z" to many mamas who are looking for natural ways to care for their families.

Now visited by more than three million natural health seekers every year, NaturalLivingFamily.com has rapidly become the number one online source for biblical health and nonbrand essential oils education.

The Zs live in Atlanta with their five children.

Also by

THE ZIELINSKIS

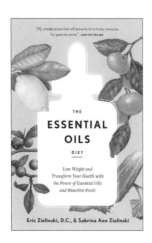

THE ESSENTIAL OILS DIET

Harness the power of essential oils
and bioactive foods to help you achieve
and maintain a healthy weight
and abundant health.

THE HEALING POWER OF ESSENTIAL OILS

Recipes and expert advice
for using essential oils in your health
routine and creating a sustainable,
non-toxic home.

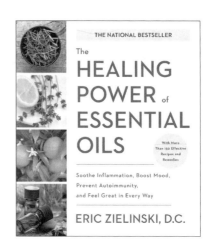

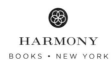

HARMONY

BOOKS • NEW YORK

Available wherever books are sold